MW01611713

Handbook of Community-Based
Participatory Research

Handbook of
Community-Based
Participatory Research

EDITED BY STEVEN S. COUGHLIN

SELINA A. SMITH

and

MARIA E. FERNANDEZ

OXFORD
UNIVERSITY PRESS

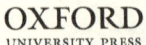

Oxford University Press is a department of the University of Oxford. It furthers
the University's objective of excellence in research, scholarship, and education
by publishing worldwide. Oxford is a registered trade mark of Oxford University
Press in the UK and certain other countries.

Published in the United States of America by Oxford University Press
198 Madison Avenue, New York, NY 10016, United States of America.

Library of Congress Cataloging-in-Publication Data
Names: Coughlin, Steven S. (Steven Scott), 1957– editor. | Smith,
Selina A., editor. | Fernandez, Maria E. (Maria Eulalia), editor.
Title: Handbook of community-based participatory research / edited by
Steven S. Coughlin, Selina A. Smith, Maria E. Fernandez.
Other titles: Community-based participatory research
Description: Oxford ; New York : Oxford University Press, [2016] | Includes
bibliographical references and index. | Description based on print version
record and CIP data provided by publisher; resource not viewed.
Identifiers: LCCN 2016031904 (print) | LCCN 2016030512 (ebook) |
ISBN 9780190652241 (e-book) | ISBN 9780█████258 (e-book) |
ISBN 9780190652234 (paperback : alk█████)
Subjects: | MESH: Community-Ba███████████████rch
Classification: LCC R850 (print███████████ NLM W 84.3 |
DDC 610.72/4—dc23
LC record available at h████████████6031904

9 8 7 6 5 4 3 2 1

Printed by Webcom Inc., Canada

Contents

Preface

As a collaborative approach to research, community-based participatory research (CBPR) equitably includes all partners in the research process and often involves partnerships between academic and community organizations with the goal of increasing the value of the research product for all partners. In the past, social scientists and researchers who focused on disease prevention tended to conduct studies of social phenomena and community problems with an "outsider's approach" which distanced the research from the participants' daily lives. This approach was questioned by theorists such as Kurt Lewin and Paulo Freire, who proposed more participatory and inclusive methods. As detailed in chapter 1 by Steven Coughlin, Selina Smith, and Maria Fernandez, and in several other chapters in this volume, current perspectives seek to address the complexity of the human experience and the differential power that sometimes exists between academic researchers and research participants.

Community-based participatory research is linked to other social justice–informed methodologies to research (e.g., action research, participatory action research, and participatory learning and action) that attempt to empower communities to address the root causes of inequality and identify their own problems and appropriate solutions. Community-based participatory research strives to acknowledge and implement the participants' needs, behaviors, and beliefs concerning their well-being. Community-based participatory research takes into account the strengths and insights that community and academic partners bring to framing health problems and developing solutions. Not all research that is conducted in communities (community-placed research) is participatory in nature. Rather, CBPR and related approaches to community-engaged research occur across a continuum, as discussed in chapter 2 by Steven Coughlin and Wonsuk Yoo. In its purest form, CBPR involves true partnerships between academic researchers and community members.

This book on CBPR is an important addition to Oxford University Press's outstanding line of books on public health and related topics because of widespread interest in CBPR; health disparities; public health research involving racial and ethnic minority communities; the health of immigrants; women's health; maternal and child health; infant mortality; cancer screening; prevention of cardiovascular disease, hypertension, obesity, and diabetes; cigarette smoking, physical activity, and diet; HIV/AIDS prevention; faith-based health interventions; gay, lesbian, bisexual, and transgender health; mental health; substance abuse; sexual assault and violence; urban health; rural health; environmental health and environmental justice; global health; research ethics; and public health ethics. This volume complements and explicates closely related developments such as community-based evaluative research, community-engaged research, and the National Institutes of Health (NIH) Clinical and Translational Science Awards.

This book is likely to be a useful resource for public health researchers, practitioners, and members of communities who are challenged by health disparities. This book will be of interest to practicing public health professionals from various public health disciplines (epidemiology, behavioral science, health communications, community engagement, nutrition, environmental health, health disparities, and global health) and to members of nonprofit organizations, community-based organizations, and members of community coalitions and health advocacy organizations. Many contributors to this book are nationally and internationally recognized for their work. The chapters were contributed by experts from a variety of backgrounds and disciplines. Notably, several of the authors who contributed to this volume are members of community-based organizations, community coalitions, and nonprofit organizations in the United States, Canada, Great Britain, and Switzerland. While editing this book with his coeditors, Steven Coughlin served as a member of both the Connect-to-Protect community coalition on HIV/AIDS among young people in Memphis, Tennessee, and the Mayor's Health Task Force Healthy Active Living Working Group in Lawrence, Massachusetts. Maria Fernandez was founder of Latinos in a Network for Cancer Control (LINCC) in Texas.

We are grateful to our families and close friends who supported us in this multiple-year effort. We would thank Chad Zimmerman, our editor with Oxford University Press, and his assistant Chloe Layman. In addition, we are grateful to our professional colleagues and students at the Rollins School of Public Health at Emory University (S.S.C.); the University of Tennessee College of Medicine Department of Preventive Medicine (S.S.C.); the University of Massachusetts Lowell Division of Public Health (S.S.C.); the University of Massachusetts Center for Clinical and Translational Sciences (S.S.C.); the Augusta University College of Health Sciences (S.S.C.); the Institute for Public and Preventive Health at the University of Augusta (S.A.S.); the Department of Family Medicine at the Medical College of Augusta (S.A.S.); and the University of Texas at Houston School of

Public Health (M.E.F.). Selina Smith was supported by a grant awarded to the Augusta University Institute of Public and Preventive Health by the National Cancer Institute (R01CA166785).

S.S.C.
Augusta, Georgia
S.A.S.
Augusta, Georgia
M.E.F.
Houston, Texas

Contributors

Leland K. Ackerson, ScD, MPH
Graduate Public Health Program
 Coordinator
Associate Professor
Department of Community Health
 and Sustainability
University of Massachusetts, Lowell
Lowell, Massachusetts

Tobia Henry Akintobi, PhD, MPH
Associate Professor and Associate
 Dean, Community Engagement
Director, Prevention Research Center
Director, Evaluation and Institutional
 Assessment
Associate Professor
Department of Community Health
 and Preventive Medicine
Morehouse School of Medicine
Atlanta, Georgia

Benjamin E. Ansa, MD, MSCR
Senior Research Associate
Institute of Public and
 Preventive Health
Augusta University
Augusta, Georgia

Peter Baltrus, PhD
Associate Professor of Community
 Health and Preventive Medicine
National Center for Primary Care
Morehouse School of Medicine
Atlanta, Georgia

Shanice Battle, MPH
Department of Psychiatry
Center for Maternal Substance Abuse
 and Child Development
Emory University School of Medicine
Atlanta, Georgia

Allyson S. Belton, MPH
Associate Project Director
Satcher Health Leadership Institute
Morehouse School of Medicine
Atlanta, Georgia

Mara Bird, PhD
Director
Center for Latino Community
 Health, Evaluation and Leadership
 Training
California State University,
 Long Beach
Long Beach, California

Daniel Blumenthal, MD, MPH
President, American College of
    Preventive Medicine
Professor Emeritus
Department of Community Health
    and Preventive Medicine
Morehouse School of Medicine
Atlanta, Georgia

Deborah Bowen, PhD
Professor
Department of Bioethics and
    Humanities
School of Medicine
University of Washington
Seattle, Washington

Ulrike Brizay, PhD
University of Applied Science, FH
Erfurt, Germany

Steven S. Coughlin, PhD
Associate Professor
Department of Clinical and Digital
    Health Sciences
College of Allied Health Sciences
Augusta University
Augusta, Georgia
Adjunct Professor
    of Epidemiology
Rollins School of Public Health
Emory University
Atlanta, Georgia

Pamela Daniels, MBA, MPH, PhD
Epidemiologist
Morehouse School of Medicine
Atlanta, Georgia

Maria E. Fernandez, PhD
Director, Center for Health Promotion
    and Prevention Research
University of Texas at Houston, School
    of Public Health
Professor, Health Promotion and
    Behavioral Sciences
Houston, Texas

**Maria Eugenia
Fernandez-Esquer, PhD**
Associate Professor of Health
    Promotion and Behavioral
    Sciences
University of Texas Health Science
    Center at Houston, School of
    Public Health
Houston, Texas

Jennifer Glick, PhD, MPH
Department of Global Community
    Health and Behavioral Sciences
School of Public Health and Tropical
    Medicine
Tulane University
New Orleans, Louisiana

Jason Globerman, MSc
Ontario HIV Treatment Network
Toronto, Canada

David Gogolishvili, MPH
Ontario HIV Treatment Network
Toronto, Canada

Lina Golob, MSc
International AIDS Society
Geneva, Switzerland

Erin N. Haynes, DrPH, MS
Associate Professor
Director, Clinical and Translational
    Research Training Program
Director, Community Outreach and
    Engagement Core, Center for
    Environmental Genetics
Division of Epidemiology
Department of Environmental Health
University of Cincinnati, College of
    Medicine
Cincinnati, Ohio

Shirin Heidari, PhD
Director
Reproductive Health Matters
London, United Kingdom

Harry J. Heiman, MD, MPH
Director, Division of Health Policy
Satcher Health Leadership Institute
Morehouse School of Medicine
Atlanta, Georgia

Natalia I. Heredia, MPH
Predoctoral fellow, PhD candidate
University of Texas Health Science
  Center at Houston, School of
  Public Health
Houston, Texas

LaShawn M. Hoffman
Chair, Community Coalition Board
Prevention Research Center
Morehouse School of Medicine
Atlanta, Georgia

Kisha B. Holden, PhD, MSCR
Associate Professor, Department of
  Psychiatry and Behavioral Sciences
Department of Community Health
  and Preventive Medicine
Interim Director, Satcher Health
  Leadership Institute
Morehouse School of Medicine
Atlanta, Georgia

Cheryl L. Holt, PhD
Associate Professor, Behavioral and
  Community Health
Director, CHAMP (Community
  Health Awareness, Messages, and
  Prevention) Lab
Codirector, Center for Health Behavior
  Research
Coleader for Population Science Program
  in the Greenebaum Cancer Center
University of Maryland
College Park, Maryland

Farrah Jacquez, PhD
Associate Professor
Department of Psychology
University of Cincinnati
Cincinnati, Ohio

Carolyn M. Jenkins, DrPH, MSN, RN, RD, LD, FAAN
Professor and Ann Darlington
  Edwards Endowed Chair in
  Nursing
Director for Center for Community
  Health Partnerships
Codirector, SCTR Community
  Engagement
Medical University of South Carolina
Charleston, South Carolina

Carl Kendall, PhD
Director, Center for Global
  Health Equity
Professor, Department of Global
  Community Health and Behavioral
  Sciences
School of Public Health and Tropical
  Medicine
Tulane University
New Orleans, Louisiana

Stephani S. Kim, MPH
Doctoral Student
Division of Epidemiology
Department of Environmental
  Health
University of Cincinnati, College of
  Medicine
Cincinnati, Ohio

Heather Kitzman-Ulrich, PhD
Director, Research and Development
Diabetes Health & Wellness Institute
Baylor Scott and White Health
Dallas, Texas
Adjunct Assistant Professor
Department of Behavioral and
  Community Health
School of Public Health
University of North Texas Health
  Science Center
Fort Worth, Texas

Yen-Chi L. Le, PhD
Project Manager II, Adjunct Faculty
Healthcare Transformation Initiatives
    Department
University of Texas Health Science
    Center at Houston, McGovern
    Medical School
Houston, Texas

Rodney Lyn, PhD, MS
Associate Professor and Associate
    Dean for Academic Affairs
School of Public Health
Georgia State University
Atlanta, Georgia

Kelly G. McGauhey
Center for Health Promotion and
    Prevention Research
University of Texas Health Science
    Center at Houston, School of
    Public Health
Houston, Texas

Annie L. Nguyen, PhD, MPH
Assistant Professor
Department of Family Medicine
Keck School of Medicine
University of Southern California
Los Angeles, California

Tonny J. Oyana, PhD
Director of Spatial Analytics and
    Informatics Core,
Research Center for Health
    Disparities, Equity, and the
    Exposome
Professor, Department of Preventive
    Medicine
University of Tennessee Health
    Science Center
Memphis, Tennessee

Britt Riot-Ellis, PhD
Founding Dean
College of Health Science and Human
    Services
California State University,
    Monterey Bay
Seaside, California

Latrice Rollins, PhD, MSW
Assistant Director of Evaluation and
    Institutional Assessment
Prevention Research Center
Department of Community Health
    and Preventive Medicine
Morehouse College of Medicine
Atlanta, Georgia

Sean B. Rourke, PhD, FCAHS
Scientific and Executive Director
Ontario HIV Treatment Network
Professor of Psychiatry
University of Toronto
Scientist, Li Ka Shing Knowledge
    Institute of St. Michael's Hospital
Toronto, Canada

David Seal, PhD
Professor and Vice-Chair
Doctoral Programs Director
Department of Global Community
    Health and Behavioral Sciences
School of Public Health and Tropical
    Medicine
Tulane University
New Orleans, Louisiana

Selina A. Smith, PhD, MDiv
Director, Institute of Public and
    Preventive Health
Professor and Curtis G. Hames, MD,
    Distinguished Chair
Department of Family Medicine,
    Medical College of Georgia
Augusta, Georgia

Lisa M. Vaughn, PhD
Professor, Pediatrics
Cincinnati Children's Hospital
    Medical Center
University of Cincinnati College of
    Medicine
Cincinnati, Ohio

Alice Welbourn, PhD
Founding Director
Salamander Trust
London, United Kingdom

Glenda Wrenn, MD, MSHP
Assistant Professor
Department of Psychiatry and
    Behavioral Sciences
Morehouse School of Medicine
Atlanta, Georgia

Wonsuk Yoo, PhD
Associate Director, Data
    Coordinating Center
Institute of Public and
    Preventive Health
Associate Professor
College of Dental Medicine
Augusta University
Augusta, Georgia

Emily Youngblom, MPH
Institute of Public Health
    Genetics
University of Washington
Seattle, Washington

1

Overview of Community-Based Participatory Research

STEVEN S. COUGHLIN, PHD, SELINA A. SMITH, PHD, MDIV,

AND MARIA E. FERNANDEZ, PHD

This chapter provides an introduction to community-based participatory research (CBPR), a collaborative approach to research that equitably involves all partners, including community members affected by the health topic being addressed, organizational representatives, and academic researchers, in the research process. This approach includes partnerships between academic and community organizations with the goal of increasing the value of the research product for all partners and sustaining its impact on population health. Community-based participatory research addresses health disparities and inequities in diverse communities including groups that are socially disadvantaged, marginalized, stigmatized, or that have suffered historical injustices. It takes into account the strengths and insights that community and academic partners bring to framing health problems and developing solutions. As illustrated throughout this volume, CBPR approaches have been used to address a wide variety of health topics, including environmental hazards, HIV/AIDS, maternal and child health, cancer, cardiovascular disease, diabetes, obesity, cigarette smoking, substance abuse, and mental health. The combination of experiences of community members with public health science provides a deeper understanding of complex social phenomena, thereby providing more relevant interventions and increasing the likelihood that the interventions will be effective and that they will be adopted, implemented, and sustained in real-world settings. The CBPR research paradigm represents a fundamental shift in academic researchers' views of community residents, from patients and research subjects who may benefit from medical advances to essential partners who can energize their communities to develop and implement effective, sustainable interventions to improve health and eliminate health disparities.

What Is Community-Based Participatory Research?

Community-based participatory research is a collaborative approach to research in which the research process is driven by an equitable partnership that is formed between relevant community members, organizational representatives, and academic researchers; the CBPR framework uses this partnership with the aim of increasing the value of the research product for all partners. Community-based participatory research takes advantage of the unique strengths and insights that community and academic partners each bring to framing health problems and developing solutions. Community members, organizational representatives, and academic researchers participate in and share control over all phases of the research process from assessment—discovering the community's health needs— to dissemination—developing strategies to increase the adoption, implementation, and maintenance of evidence-based interventions (EBIs) in communities and healthcare settings. Community-based participatory research approaches facilitate and accelerate research translation so that research produces pragmatic results capable of leading to positive and sustainable community change.

In the past, social scientists and researchers who focused on disease prevention tended to engage in studies of social phenomena and community problems with an "outsider's approach," which distanced the research from the participants' daily lives. Lewin[1] and Freire[2] questioned the "outsider's approach" and proposed more participatory and inclusive approaches to research. Current perspectives seek to address the complexity of the human experience and the differential power that sometimes exists between academic researchers, representatives of community groups, and research participants.

"The CBPR research paradigm represents a fundamental shift in academic researcher's views of community residents, from patients and research subjects who may benefit from medical advances to essential partners who can energize their communities to develop effective, sustainable interventions to improve health and eliminate health disparities."[3]

Rather than focusing solely on health problems or other concerns, the CBPR framework highlights community resilience, resources, and opportunities for positive growth.[4] It places emphasis on shared decision-making, co-learning, reciprocal transfer of expertise between partners, and mutual ownership of research products.[5] Partners also strive to acknowledge and act on participants' needs, behaviors, and beliefs concerning their own well-being. Community-based participatory research is linked to other social-justice-informed approaches to research, such as action research and participatory action research, that empower communities to address the root causes of inequity and identify their own problems and appropriate solutions; thus CBPR efforts typically do not focus on the individual only. Instead, CBPR fits within an ecological perspective about the determinants of adverse health outcomes and includes consideration of individual-level risk factors, multiple social determinants of health, and structural problems such as poverty, unemployment, homophobia/transphobia, racism, and lack of access to primary healthcare.

PROCESS

The starting point for a CBPR project typically includes a health needs assessment, a focused literature review, and a review of published and unpublished data to identify priority health concerns. Epidemiologic data about the geographic and social distribution and determinants of health concerns in a community are also useful for planning purposes. For example, such data may include age-adjusted morbidity and mortality rates at the zip code or county level broken down by race, ethnicity, or other factors, or geospatial information about educational attainment, household income, or the availability of primary healthcare and public transportation. The needs assessment process should be carried out using the same principles of CBPR as all other phases of the research effort. Gathering community member feedback can be done through a variety of methods, such as obtaining information through in-depth interviews of key informants or soliciting feedback during community advisory board meetings. Including community representatives as integral members of the planning group, however, helps ensure participation throughout the planning process. Planning groups including community partners should explore existing sources of data and the need for new data collection and should participate collaboratively in the interpretation of findings.[6] The CBPR approach requires academic researchers to listen to the voices of community residents before a shared decision is made about which health topics to address first. Thus, although seat belt use may be an important public health concern in a community, and an academic researcher may wish to compete for funding for a study of the effectiveness of an intervention to increase seat belt use, community residents and representatives of community organizations may give priority to projects that address breast cancer screening and survival among African American women or disparities in infant mortality by race, ethnicity, or socioeconomic status.

The importance of addressing community priorities is emphasized in a definition of CBPR provided by the Kellogg Foundation Community Health Scholars Program. According to this definition, CBPR "equitably involves all partners with a research topic of importance to the community with the aim of contributing knowledge and action for social change to improve community health and eliminate health disparities."

Several principles of CBPR have been identified: the need to ensure openness, trust, and power sharing among partners; the need for a genuine partnership approach; capacity-building of community partners; and the importance of shared decision-making, colearning, shared ownership of research products, applying findings to benefit all partners, and including community partners in all phases of the research from the identification of health priorities to evidence translation and the dissemination of research findings.[7] Another principle of CBPR is having an ecological perspective about the determinants of adverse health outcomes and considering individual-level risk factors; multiple social determinants of illness; and structural problems such as poverty, unemployment, homophobia/transphobia, racism, and lack of access to primary healthcare.

Previous authors have noted that CBPR should move toward action through the translation of findings and their application in the community.[5,8-10] This may include changes in practice or policies through policy advocacy, additional research, or evaluation to understand how to intervene effectively.

USE OF COMMUNITY-BASED PARTICIPATORY RESEARCH

The CBPR approach to public health research and evaluation has grown in popularity in recent years. This is evidenced by an increase in peer-reviewed journal articles on CBPR and major funding initiatives from leading and private foundations.[3,7,11,12] Contributing to the popularity of CBPR is that it addresses health disparities and inequities in diverse communities including groups that are socially disadvantaged, marginalized, stigmatized, or have suffered historical injustices.[5]

In the United States and other countries, CBPR approaches have been used to address a wide variety of health topics. Many CBPR projects have been conducted in mid- and low-income countries where public health concerns include infant mortality, infectious diseases such as malaria, and food insecurity. The development and implementation of effective interventions for complex health problems, such as HIV/AIDS in socially disadvantaged or marginalized communities, are strengthened from the perspectives of community members and academic researchers.[10] The combination of experiences from community members and public health scientists provides a deeper understanding of complex social phenomena, thereby providing more relevant interventions and increasing the likelihood that the interventions will be successful.[10]

The discussions that follow cover several CBPR principles and provide an account of how innovation and creativity are hallmarks of CBPR research and evaluation. The first is an account of the importance of CBPR to addressing health disparities in diverse communities.

Addressing Health Disparities

As an orientation to research, CBPR is useful for addressing health disparities and inequities in diverse communities, including groups that are disadvantaged, marginalized, or stigmatized. In many countries, including the United States, pronounced health disparities exist across population groups defined by a variety of demographic factors.[13] Efforts to reduce and eliminate disparities among racial and ethnic minorities in the United States include a seminal report by the Institute of Medicine and the landmark 1985 US Department of Health and Human Services Heckler Report on variations in health status among non-White populations.[14-15] Over the past three decades, health professionals have made increasing efforts to define the causes of health disparities and to identify effective ways to promote greater equity in healthcare access and outcomes.[13] Recently, national goals to reduce and eliminate health disparities and achieve health equity were set through the Healthy People initiative.[16] Racial minorities in the United States are more likely than Whites to die from many common diseases including breast cancer, cardiovascular disease, and HIV/AIDS, and have higher rates of infant mortality.[13] While overall health status continues to improve for all populations in the United States, there is little improvement in racial disparities.

The CBPR approach to health research offers advantages to addressing health disparities in diverse populations. For example, many health disparities and inequities are best addressed at multiple—individual, group, neighborhood, community, society, and policy—levels.[10] Structural problems and social determinants of disease, such as poverty, unemployment, inadequate or substandard housing, the stigmatization of persons living with HIV/AIDS, and lack of primary healthcare, can be addressed through CBPR approaches.[17] Community-based participatory research offers promise for addressing health disparities because this process combines insights of community members with scientific knowledge to provide a deeper understanding of complex phenomena, thereby providing more relevant health interventions and increasing the likelihood that the interventions will be effective and sustainable.[10]

Shared Decision-Making

The strength the CBPR approach has in addressing health disparities comes from its principle of shared decision-making between partners so that community members, organizational representatives, and academic researchers participate in and share control over all phases of the research process: assessment, definition of the problem, selection of research methods, data collection, data analysis, and the interpretation and dissemination of findings.[5] Power sharing helps to ensure that all those with a stake in the research or evaluation effort can have their voices heard.[10] For example, when Native American communities are fully involved in developing and implementing health promotion programs, a common result is culturally relevant and potentially sustainable approaches for improving community health.[4] As in-group members, Native American residents are in a position to know whether the research methods are culturally appropriate and how to best recruit participants.[18] Because of shared decision-making and its partnership approach to research, the CBPR process is able to use the strengths and insights that community and academic partners bring to framing health problems and developing solutions.

Building and sustaining trust is essential in all aspects of CBPR. Community members may distrust researchers from outside organizations because of a history of prejudice, discrimination, or marginalization of minority communities by healthcare systems, or earlier experiences of helicopter research, when researchers enter a community, collect data, and leave without providing any information or direct benefits to the community.[18] Community participation and shared decision-making help to ensure that the study objectives are relevant to the community, that the methods of accomplishing the objectives are practical and acceptable to residents, and that the study findings are shared and provide direct benefits to the community.

Community Advisory Boards

In order for CBPR projects to successfully use shared decision-making, a community advisory board composed of CBPR partners should be established if one does not exist. Many community advisory boards include community members, patients, representatives from local nonprofit organizations and faith-based institutions, teachers, business owners, primary care providers, and representatives from local hospitals or clinics. In projects undertaken in collaboration with Native American tribes, tribal elders generally serve as valued members of the community advisory board.[19] Community advisory board members and academic researchers work together to plan and monitor CBPR studies. For a given project, some members of the community advisory board may be more involved than others depending on their interests and time commitments. In addition, the community residents and organizational representatives who are part of the community advisory board may change over time.

Academic researchers who engage a community advisory board in order to plan and conduct CBPR projects must foster communication and seek to develop trust within the partnership. The focus should be on encouraging equitable participation and establishing norms for working together.[19] To build a partnership, academic researchers can confer with people in their institution who have existing community partnerships for guidance on approaching community gatekeepers. Local public health departments, agencies, nonprofit organizations, and coalitions may also be helpful in establishing partnerships.[6]

Potential partners may differ in priorities, such as the extent to which they focus on research versus delivery of health services, acquiring new scientific knowledge versus building infrastructure, or publishing versus informing policy change. Communication styles and approaches to decision-making are also likely to vary across partnership organizations, which is why establishing norms for working order is important.[18-19] Building and sustaining a CBPR partnership requires a long-term commitment of time and effort by the partners.[10]

Reciprocal Transfer of Expertise

One of the benefits of CBPR partnerships is that they create space for colearning, the reciprocal transfer of expertise, and mutual ownership of research products between community and academic partners.[5] The process of colearning brings academic researchers and community members together and helps community participants to increase control and self-ownership of their health lives.[4] For this to be successful, academic researchers must respect nonacademic knowledge and expertise and support an egalitarian relationship with community members.

Community partners can help develop new hypotheses, provide new ideas for intervention and delivery, and contribute to research and evaluation activities by advising and participating in recruitment and retention of study participants.[18] The expertise provided by community partners takes into account the social, cultural, and economic realities of community residents who are potential participants. Academic partners provide knowledge about the extent of the health or social problems in the community from an epidemiologic perspective, potential study designs and implementation approaches, and how to test hypotheses about evidence-based health interventions with scientific rigor.[18]

Sustainability, Evidence Translation, and Dissemination of Research Findings

A core principle of CBPR is increasing community capacity,[7] yet challenges in increasing capacity to implement and maintain effective interventions in communities persist. Rhodes et al.[10] noted, "By working in partnership, individual and community-level capacities are developed. These capacities may include an increased understanding of how to affect change among individuals and within communities, and the development of community mobilization, problem-solving, and even public speaking skills." Community-based participatory research can help ensure that programs are developed with dissemination and sustainability in mind and can improve community capacity and increase the potential that the interventions will be adopted, implemented, and sustained. For example, community engagement can facilitate integration of programs into existing health systems [20] by employing CBPR processes during the development of interventions, or adaptation of existing evidence-based interventions. Collaboration between partners in data analysis and dissemination of research findings can also contribute to the use and usefulness of data for improving community programs and health systems.

The translation of CBPR findings to address public health concerns helps to ensure that the research has pragmatic results that lead to the greatest possible benefit. The CBPR approach increases the potential of the translational sciences to develop, implement, and disseminate effective public health interventions in diverse communities. Implementation and dissemination are defined as strategies to adopt evidence-based health interventions in order to effect change within specific community settings.[20] Relative to nonparticipatory research studies that do not involve partnerships with community residents or organizations, findings from CBPR studies are more likely to be disseminated to diverse audiences and to be translated into useful outcomes, such as improvements in policy. For example, CBPR partners may wish to adapt an EBI for increasing physical activity and healthy eating, previously shown to be effective in a randomized trial conducted in an urban population, to a rural population that includes more seniors, persons with chronic illnesses such as obesity and diabetes, and persons with low health literacy. The CBPR approach is helpful for translating specific findings from controlled trials to real-world settings in diverse communities.[20] The input received from community partners who understand the community's culture, language, and other contextual factors helps to maximize the external validity of the health intervention. In attempting to translate evidence from one setting to another, researchers and their community partners must consider variability in culture, resources, and community acceptance of research.

Innovations in Health Promotion and Community-Based Participatory Research

Community-based participatory research is not a specific qualitative or quantitative research method but rather an orientation to research; there is no single approach to CBPR. Rather, this orientation to research encompasses an array of diverse approaches to community-based research that have been refined and improved over time. Innovation in community-based research and the development of creative approaches for engaging and empowering community members are hallmarks of CBPR, as they have been over the past decade or two.[4]

The incorporation of photovoice, a method of telling personal community stories through photographs, into CBPR studies highlights the creativity of the CBPR approach.[4,21-23] Photovoice is especially useful as a method of health needs assessment and fits well with CBPR principle of equitable partnership. When Casteden et al.[24] used photovoice in a CBPR project conducted with an indigenous community in Canada, the researchers found that the process was culturally relevant, fostered trust between researchers and community members, and created a sense of ownership regarding the information that was collected.[24] Other researchers have incorporated community arts events into CBPR projects. Chung et al.[25] collected survey data at art events in an African American community in Los Angeles as part of a CBPR project on depression care. The researchers used photography exhibits, group discussions, and story readings as catalysts for responses that were obtained through the survey.[25]

Summary

The CBPR research paradigm discussed in this chapter and throughout this book represents a fundamental shift in academic researcher's views of community residents from subjects who may benefit from medical advances to essential partners who can add value and efficacy to research processes and products.[18] Academic researchers and community members who are engaged in CBPR seek to democratize the production of knowledge in ways that transform research from a top-down process driven by scientific experts into one of colearning and coproduction.[26] The benefits of CBPR for community partners include learning new skills and becoming members of engaged communities that are taking charge of their own health.[26] A key principle of CBPR is increasing the capacity of community members in research and program implementation.[7,10] By increasing community and researcher capacities, all partners gain an enhanced understanding of effective community mobilization and how to incite change among individuals within their unique community setting.

References

1. Neill, S.J. "Developing Children's Nursing Through Action Research." *Journal of Child Health Care* 2 (1998): 11–15.
2. Freire, P. "Creating Alternative Research Methods: Learning to Do It by Doing It." In *Creating Knowledge: A Monopoly*, ed. B. Hall, A. Gillette and R. Tandon. New Delhi: Society for Participatory Research in Asia, 1982; pp. 29–37.
3. Wallerstein, N. and Duran, B. "The Conceptual, Historical, and Practice Roots of Community-Based Participatory Research and Related Participatory Traditions." In *Community-Based Participatory Research for Health*, ed. M. Minkler and N. Wallerstein. San Francisco, CA: Jossey-Bass, 2003; pp. 27–52.
4. Gray, N., Ore de Boehm, C., Farnsworth, A. and Wolf, D. "Integration of Creative Expression into Community Based Participatory Research and Health Promotion with Native Americans." *Family and Community Health* 33 (2010): 186–92.
5. Viswanathan, M., Eng, E., Ammerman, A., et al. *Community-Based Participatory Research: Assessing the Evidence* (Evidence Report/Technology Assessment no. 99). Rockville, MD: Agency for Healthcare Research and Quality, 2004.
6. Bartholomew Eldredge, L.K., Markham, C.M., Ruiter, R.A.C., Fernández, M.E., Kok, G., Parcel, G.S., eds. *Planning Health Promotion Programs: An Intervention Mapping Approach* (4th ed.). San Francisco, CA: Jossey-Bass, 2016.
7. Israel, B.A., Schulz, A.J., Parker E.A., et al. "Review of Community-Based Research: Assessing Partnership Approaches to Improve Public Health." *Annual Review of Public Health* (1998): 173–202.

8. Cornwall, A. and Jewkes, R. "What Is Participatory Research?" *Social Science and Medicine* 41 (1995): 1667–76.

9. Minkler, M. "Community-Based Research Partnerships: Challenges and Opportunities. *Journal of Urban Health* 82 (2005): ii3–ii12.

10. Rhodes, S.D, Malow, R.M. and Jolly, C. "Community-Based Participatory Research (CBPR): A New and Not-so-New Approach to HIV/AIDS Prevention, Care, and Treatment." *AIDS Education and Prevention* 22 (2010): 173–83.

11. Centers for Disease Control and Prevention, and Agency for Toxic Substances and Disease Registry Committee on Community Engagement. *Principles of Community Engagement.* Atlanta, GA: US Department of Health and Human Services, 1997.

12. Institute of Medicine. *Promoting Health: Intervention Strategies from Social and Behavioral Research.* Washington, DC: National Academy Press, 2000.

13. Adler, N.E. and Rehkopf, D.H. "U.S. Disparities in Health: Descriptions, Causes, and Mechanisms." *Annual Review of Public Health* 29 (2009): 235–52.

14. Heckler, M. *Report of the Secretary's Task Force on Black and Minority Health.* Washington, DC: US Department of Health and Human Services, 1985.

15. Institute of Medicine. *Unequal Treatment: Confronting Racial and Ethnic Disparities in Health Care.* Washington, DC: National Academy Press, 2002.

16. Braveman, P.A., Kumanyika, S., Fielding, J., et al. "Health Disparities and Health Equity: The Issue Is Justice." *American Journal of Public Health* 101 (2011): S149–55.

17. Eriksen, M. and Rothenberg, R. "Editorial." *Health Education Research* 27 (2012): 553–4.

18. Horowitz, C.R., Robinson, M. and Seifer, S. "Community-Based Participatory Research from the Margin to the Mainstream: Are Researchers Prepared?" *Circulation* 19 (2009): 2633–42.

19. Baldwin, J.A., Johnson, J.L. and Benally, C.C. "Building Partnerships Between Indigenous Communities and Universities: Lessons Learned in HIV/AIDS and Substance Abuse Prevention Research." *American Journal of Public Health* 99 Suppl 1 (2009): S77–82.

20. Wallerstein, N. and Duran, B. "Community-Based Participatory Research Contributions to Intervention Research: The Intersection of Science and Practice to Improve Health Equity." *American Journal of Public Health* 100 Suppl 1 (2010): S40–6.

21. Wang, C., Yuan, Y.L. and Feng, M.L. "Photovoice as a Tool for Participatory Evaluation: The Community's View of Process and Impact." *Journal of Contemporary Health* 4 (1996): 47–9.

22. Wang, C. and Pies, C. "Family, Maternal, and Child Health Through Photovoice." *Maternal and Child Health Journal* 8 (2004): 95–102.

23. Moffitt, P. and Vollman, A. "Photovoice: Picturing the Health of Aboriginal Women in a Remote Northern Community." *Canadian Journal of Nursing Research* 36 (2004): 189–201.

24. Castleden, H., Garvin, T. and Huu-ay-aht First Nation. "Modifying Photovoice for Community-Based Participatory Indigenous Research." *Social Sciences and Medicine* 66 (2008): 1393–405.

25. Chung, B., Jones, L., Jones, A., et al. "Using Community Arts Events to Enhance Collective Efficacy and Community Engagement to Address Depression in an African American Community." *American Journal of Public Health* 99 (2009): 237–44.

26. Balazs, C.L. and Morello-Frosch, R. "The Three R's: How Community Based Participatory Research Strengthens the Rigor, Relevance and Reach of Science." *Environmental Justice* 6 2013. doi: 10.1089/env.2012.0017.

2

Community-Based Participatory Research Study Approaches Along a Continuum of Community-Engaged Research

STEVEN S. COUGHLIN, PHD AND WONSUK YOO, PHD

This chapter provides an overview of research methods that have commonly been used in community-based participatory research (CBPR), including qualitative research methods such as focus groups and intervention research with a quasi-experimental or randomized controlled design. Mixed-methods approaches and dissemination and translation research are also discussed. To illustrate specific research approaches, examples of CBPR are presented.

Community-based participatory research occurs across a continuum of community-engaged research, from true collaborative studies in which community members, representatives of community-based organizations, and other stakeholders are equal partners with academic researchers and are involved in study planning, conduct, and dissemination of research findings, to studies conducted by academic researchers that are community-*placed* but in which community members are not true partners and academic researchers retain full control over the research.[1] In some community studies, which are not truly *participatory*, community leaders are asked for their endorsement of the projects and for guidance in identifying community residents for focus groups and to serve as interviewers and lay health advisors, but they do not contribute to the design of the research or have a role in interpreting the findings.[2]

Focus Groups and Other Qualitative Research Methods

Focus groups are used to obtain, from a group of people, qualitative information about their feelings, opinions, knowledge, attitudes, and beliefs related to a health problem or intervention such as breast cancer in women or barriers to screening mammography.[3] Usually focus group participants are invited to attend a few weeks before the session. At the time of the invitation, they are provided with general information about the purpose of the focus group discussion but not with detailed information, so that their responses are spontaneous.[4] The group sessions are led by a skilled moderator, who strives to elicit candid responses to a list of questions. To maximize the value of the information obtained from the participants, the questions must be carefully prepared in advance.[4] The sessions are generally documented through written notes and audio recordings, so that the transcripts can be reviewed and analyzed by the researchers. Several commercially available computer software programs, including Atlas.ti (www.atlasti.com) and NVIVO (http://www.qsrinternational.com/product) are available for content analysis and thematic analysis of focus group transcripts.

Focus group participants are ordinarily selected because they have certain characteristics. For example, in a study of colorectal cancer screening among Haitian Americans, focus group participants were recruited who were Haitian American adults between the ages of 50 and 69, and the group sessions were stratified by sex (male, female) and age categories (50 to 64, 65 to 69 years). The participants were also selected so that they were diverse with respect to the amount of time they had lived in the United States. Because focus group participants are generally not selected randomly, the results are interpreted as suggestive but not definitive.[5] Even though the results may not be representative, focus groups provide a convenient and flexible approach for obtaining qualitative data and preliminary insights at relatively low cost.[4]

In addition to providing qualitative information about the feelings, opinions, beliefs, and attitudes of a group of people about a health topic, such as cancer or cancer screening, focus groups can also be useful for pretesting intervention materials used in CBPR studies. For example, mass media intervention materials such as billboards or public service announcements can be pretested by presenting draft materials to focus group participants and asking them for their opinions or reactions to the materials.[4] Group discussions can provide feedback and stimulate ideas for improving prototype materials or storyboards with public health messages, to ensure that they are acceptable to the target population, persuasive, and likely to be effective in changing behaviors.[6]

Types of Intervention Strategies

Several different types of intervention strategies are commonly used in CBPR. They include intervention strategies such as one-on-one education (i.e., one individual providing information or motivation to another, in person or by telephone), small group education (i.e., delivering information in a classroom or other group setting), and small media such as informational pamphlets, brochures, letters, or videos.[7] Other intervention strategies include mass media (i.e., informational messages delivered to large audiences through newspapers, billboards, radio, or television) and client reminders such as letters, postcards, or telephone messages.[7] Interventions can also be aimed at providers or healthcare systems (e.g., the use of provider reminders and incentives) and at structural or environmental changes such as increasing the availability of bicycle paths or hiking trails; providing healthy, low-cost food through farmers markets; or increasing the availability of screening mammography by use of mobile mammography vans. Community-based participatory research studies can also involve health policy interventions such as the promotion of legislative smoking bans in public places or laws requiring the use of bicycle helmets. Most CBPR interventions are multicomponent in that they involve the use of two or more intervention strategies (e.g., small group education combined with mass media).

INTERVENTION RESEARCH METHODS

Community health interventions, including those involving CBPR, are undertaken when adequate time, financial resources, and scientific expertise are available for study design, data collection, and statistical analysis of quantitative data. The individuals who deliver the health intervention and collect information for process evaluation, impact evaluation, and outcome evaluation are members of the study team. In designing and accomplishing intervention studies, attention must be given to minimizing potential sources of statistical bias (for example, selection bias, information bias, and bias due to uncontrolled confounding by extraneous variables) and to the internal and external validity of the information obtained in the study. To determine whether a health intervention is effective, one or more control groups are needed so that there is a basis for comparison. The group(s) that is randomly assigned to receive the health intervention is known as the experimental group. In situations where it is feasible to allocate research participants randomly to experimental and comparison groups, study designs involving randomized controlled trials offer considerable scientific rigor.

Since the late 1940s, the randomized controlled trial has become the gold standard in biomedical research.[8] In such studies, the research participants are randomly assigned to treatment conditions after informed consent is obtained and inclusion and exclusion criteria are applied. In community health research, randomized designs are often used in CBPR studies of interventions for disease prevention or early detection. These include studies in which the intervention is at the level of individual research participants and those in which groups of people (e.g., elementary schools, neighborhoods, or military combat units) or whole communities are randomized to receive or not receive the health intervention.

In intervention studies, measurements can be obtained before the health intervention begins (i.e., pre-test), after the intervention ends (i.e., post-test), and at one or more times while the intervention is underway.[4] Measurement data are commonly obtained by use of surveys that can be administered by telephone interview, in person, or via postal survey questionnaires. In some studies, additional data are obtained from clinical or hospital records (e.g., recorded information about receipt of mammograms or Papanicolaou tests).

Examples of experimental (randomized) study designs include pre-test/post-test designs with an experimental group(s) and control group(s), post-test-only designs with an experimental group(s) and control group(s), and time-series designs.[4] In time-series studies, measurements are obtained both before and after a health intervention is implemented. Potential threats to the internal validity of randomized controlled studies include lack of concealment of allocation, secular changes in comparison groups, contamination of the comparison group, and inadequate sample sizes.[9] Problems with external validity, for example, when results from randomized controlled trials involving carefully selected and highly motivated volunteers cannot be translated to routine practice, can also occur.

Over the last two decades, cluster randomized controlled trials (CRTs) have been increasingly used in CBPR. Cluster randomized controlled trials are also known as group randomized trials or community randomized trials. The key element of these trials is that individual observations are nested within groups or clusters, such as communities, and the intervention is applied to the cluster. The clusters of individuals are randomized to receive different interventions or to serve as comparison groups. The units of randomization are diverse, for example, clinics, communities, practice groups, schools, or worksites. The intervention is delivered to and affects groups of people rather than individuals. The individuals within the same communities or clusters are often correlated with each other, since they live in similar conditions. Due to similarities among individuals within clusters, the variance of the study is inflated, which leads to reduction in statistical efficiency.[10] The degree of reduction in efficiency depends on the size of the average cluster and on intraclass correlation coefficients (ICC). An ICC can be interpreted as the standard Pearson correlation between any two responses in the same cluster or as the proportion of overall variation that can be responsible for the between-cluster variation. The variance inflation also affects the sample size requirement. The statistical power of a CRT may be substantially less than that of a similar-sized, individually randomized trial, since participants within any cluster are more likely to have similar outcomes.

As an example of a CRT that was conducted using a CBPR approach, the Faith, Activity, and Nutrition Program targeted both physical activity and healthy eating in 74 African Methodist Episcopal churches in South Carolina.[11] A total of 1,257 members of the churches participated. Data were collected from 2007 to 2011. The churches were randomized to either an immediate 15-month intervention or a delayed intervention (control churches). A CBPR approach guided the development and implementation of the intervention, which consisted of full-day training and a full-day cook training. Participants also received a stipend and 15 months of mailings and technical assistance calls to support implementation of the intervention. The primary outcomes of interest were self-reported moderate-to-vigorous-intensity physical activity, self-reported fruit and vegetable consumption, and measured blood pressure. Measurements were obtained at baseline and at 15 months. An intention-to-treat analysis was performed using repeated measures analysis of variance (ANOVA), with testing of group × time interactions, controlling for church clustering and size and participant age, gender, and education.[11] In addition, post hoc covariance analysis (ANCOVAs) was performed for participants with complete measurements. There was a significant intervention effect in self-reported leisure time physical activity ($p = .02$) but no effect for other outcomes. The ANCOVA analyses showed an intervention effect for self-reported leisure time physical activity ($p = .03$) and self-reported fruit and vegetable consumption ($p = .03$). The researchers concluded that the program showed small but significant increases in self-reported leisure time moderate-to-vigorous-intensity physical activity and that the program had potential for broad dissemination and reach.[11]

QUASI-EXPERIMENTAL AND NONRANDOMIZED STUDY DESIGNS

Despite the utility of randomized study designs in minimizing bias due to extraneous confounding factors, they are not always feasible or ethical. For example, randomized studies of group interventions aimed at changing laws and policies and improving healthcare systems may not be feasible.[9] Nonrandomized study designs and quasi-experimental studies have also been used in CBPR and program evaluation. Although attention is required to control potential confounding factors and to minimize statistical bias, carefully designed, nonrandomized studies offer useful alternatives to studies that involve random assignment of research participants or groups of people. If the generalizability of results obtained in randomized controlled trials is of concern, results obtained in nonrandomized studies of less highly selected populations may be of particular interest. Alternatives to randomized controlled trials include use of multiple baseline measurements across settings or interrupted time-series designs in which the intervention is introduced sequentially at experimentally determined times in different settings.[12] There are also examples of successful quasi-experimental studies involving a pre-test/post-test design with a comparison group. Similar pre-test measurement results between the intervention and comparison groups suggest that the groups were comparable before the beginning of the health intervention.[4] One advantage of quasi-experimental and nonexperimental studies is that they may have greater external validity, that is, the results may be more likely to apply to other populations or contexts.[9]

As an example of a quasi-experimental study that was conducted using a CBPR approach, Ralston et al.[13] undertook a church-based longitudinal intervention study aimed at reducing cardiovascular disease risk in mid-life and older African Americans. The study incorporated a longitudinal pre-test/post-test design with a comparison group. The intervention was guided by the transtheoretical model of behavior change.[14] Community-based participatory research was used to discover research ideas, identify community advisors, and recruit churches (three intervention and three comparison) in two counties in North Florida. A community advisory committee that included pastors, government officials, and representatives of health agencies was established. Measurement data were collected at baseline through self-report questionnaires and clinical assessments. This study is currently underway.

Multilevel Health Intervention Studies

Health disparities and inequities are best addressed at multiple levels including individual, neighborhood, group, community, social, and policy levels.[15] Several CBPR studies have used the socioecological model to plan multilevel health interventions.[16] According to this model, health interventions can be aimed at the individual, the social, or interpersonal level (e.g., friends, family, coworkers), the organizational level (e.g., healthcare providers and employers), and the structural or environmental level (e.g., the built environment). Health interventions can also be aimed at the level of the community or public policy. In practice, health intervention research (e.g., community context, organizational setting, policy environment) is often multilevel and crosses socioecological levels, even when it is not conducted or reported as such.[17]

Dissemination and Implementation Research

Dissemination refers to the active promotion or support of a health program to encourage its widespread adoption.[18] This includes the adaptation, evaluation, implementation, and maintenance of an intervention that has been shown to be effective. In contrast, diffusion is the passive process by which a health program becomes routine practice. Even when research findings are published, successful evidence-based programs only rarely diffuse passively to become routine practice. Instead, active efforts are needed to disseminate research-tested health interventions to other communities.[18] Dissemination requires foresight, long-term planning, and support. The potential for dissemination should be a consideration throughout the planning, implementation, evaluation, and reporting stages of health intervention research.[18] The dissemination and translation of CBPR findings to address public health concerns helps ensure that the research has pragmatic results that lead to the greatest possible benefit.

There can be barriers to the dissemination of effective health interventions, including intensive time requirements, high cost, a requirement for a high level of staff expertise, and a failure to consider future user needs when developing the intervention. Programs that are well packaged, modular, readily customized, and self-sustaining are more likely to be disseminated.[18] In conducting dissemination and implementation studies, researchers should evaluate program maintenance, sustainability, and costs and select representative populations.[19]

The CBPR approach increases the potential of the translational sciences to develop, implement, and disseminate effective public health interventions in diverse communities.[20] Relative to nonparticipatory research studies that do not involve partnerships with community residents or organizations, findings from CBPR are more likely to be disseminated to diverse audiences and to be translated into useful outcomes, such as improvements in policy.[21]

There are several definitions of implementation and dissemination research. Here, we are concerned with strategies to adapt evidence-based health interventions in order to effect change within specific community settings. In attempting to translate evidence from one setting to another, researchers and their community partners must consider variability in culture, resources, and community acceptance of research. For example, evidence-based interventions for increasing colorectal cancer screening that were developed for African Americans and found to be effective can be adapted for use in promoting colorectal cancer screening among other groups (e.g., Haitian Americans) and tested for effectiveness in randomized controlled trials or quasi-experimental studies. To maintain fidelity and minimize loss of impact of the intervention, evidence-based strategies and theoretical models and frameworks should be used to guide the adaptation of interventions.[22,23]

Several theories and frameworks have been proposed for use in dissemination and implementation research.[24] Diffusion of innovations theory and the reach, efficacy, adoption, implementation, maintenance (RE-AIM) framework have been used to adapt evidence-based interventions in studies involving dissemination and implementation research.[18,23] The diffusion of innovations theory addresses the process by which new ideas (e.g., innovative health interventions) are adopted by a target group or community.[25] People who are "innovators" or "change agents" are respected leaders who will implement the intervention and influence public opinion. "Early adopters" are persons or organizations who will adopt an intervention before others in the community and who readily see the value or utility of the intervention.[25] The RE-AIM dimensions for dissemination of an evidence-based health intervention include its reach (the percentage of the target population that comes into contact with it), effectiveness (whether the intervention achieves its targeted outcomes), adoption (the percentage of target settings and organizations that use it), implementation (how many staff within a setting or organization try it), and maintenance (whether the intervention produces lasting effects at the individual and setting level).[18,26] Other considerations are whether the intervention reaches those who are most in need and whether it is adopted by organizations serving underserved or high-risk populations.[18]

Summary

The diverse array of research methods discussed in this chapter is applicable to CBPR studies and other types of community-based research. Community-based participatory research occurs across a continuum of community-engaged research, from true collaborative studies in which community members, members of community-based organizations, and other stakeholders are involved in study planning, conduct, and dissemination of research findings, to studies conducted by academic researchers that are community-*placed* but in which community members are not equal partners in the research. When community members and representatives of community organizations are true partners in the research, the CBPR approach increases the potential of the translational sciences to develop, implement, and disseminate effective public health interventions in diverse communities.[20]

Additional methods are needed for controlling bias in nonrandomized study designs and for increasing the external validity of randomized controlled studies.[9] Alternatives to randomized controlled trials include use of multiple baseline measurements across settings or interrupted time-series designs in which the intervention is introduced sequentially at experimentally determined times in different settings.[12]

The focus of this chapter is on types of study designs used in CBPR studies and evaluation projects. Other methodologic issues relate to the identification and measurement of independent variables, mediating variables, and outcome variables. For example, in CBPR studies aimed at increasing routine cancer screening, methodologic considerations require that the increase in screening should be the main outcome variable rather than indirect factors such as client knowledge, attitudes, or intention to be screened.[9] Although the ultimate goal of such studies is to reduce cancer mortality, measuring cancer incidence and mortality is generally impractical because of the large sample sizes and duration of follow-up that are required. When the measurement of outcome variables (e.g., uptake of cancer screening) is based on self-reported information, there is a need for assessment of the reliability and validity of the information so that the potential for measurement bias can be assessed.[9]

References

1. Blumenthal, D.S., Hopkins, E., III, and Yancey, E. "Community-Based Participatory Research: An Introduction." In *Community-Based Participatory Research: Issues, Methods, and Translation to Practice*, ed. D.S. Blumenthal, R.J. DiClemente, R.L. Braithwaite and S.A. Smith. New York: Springer, 2013; pp. 1–17.
2. Hatch, J., Moss, N., Saran, A., et al. "Community Research: Partnership in Black Communities." *American Journal of Preventive Medicine* 9 Suppl 6 (1993): 27–31.

3. Gilmore, G.D. *Needs and Capacity Assessment Strategies for Health Education and Health Promotion*, 4th ed. Burlington, MA: Jones & Bartlett Learning, 2012.

4. McKenzie, J.F., Beiger, B.L. and Thackeray, R. *Planning, Implementing, and Evaluating Health Promotion Programs*, 6th ed. New York: Pearson, 2013.

5. Schechter, C., Vanchieri, C. and Crofton, C. "Evaluating Women's Attitudes and Perceptions in Developing Mammography Promotion Messages." *Public Health Reports* 105 (1990): 253–7.

6. NCI. *Making Health Communication Programs Work: A Planner's Guide, Pink Book.* Bethesda, MD: National Cancer Institute, August 2004.

7. Breslow, R.A., Rimer, B.K., Baron, R.C., et al. "Introducing the Community Guide's Reviews of Evidence on Interventions to Increase Screening for Breast, Cervical, and Colorectal Cancer." *American Journal of Preventive Medicine* 35 Suppl 1 (2008): S14–20.

8. Coughlin, S.S., ed. *Ethics in Epidemiology and Clinical Research: Annotated Readings.* Newton, MA: Epidemiology Resources, 1995.

9. Vernon, S.W., Briss, P.A., Tiro, J.A. and Warnecke, R.B. "Some Methodologic Lessons Learned from Cancer Screening Research. *Cancer* 101 Suppl 5 (2004): 1131–45.

10. Yoo, W., Mayberry, R., Bae, S., He, Q. and Singh, K. "A Study of Effects of Multicollinearity in the Multivariable Analysis." *International Journal of Applied Science and Technology* 4 (2014): 9–19.

11. Wilcox, S., Parrot, A., Baruth, M., et al. "The Faith, Activity, and Nutrition Program: A Randomized Controlled Trial in African-American Churches." *American Journal of Preventive Medicine* 44 (2013): 122–31.

12. Shadish, W.R., Cook, T.D. and Campbell, D.T. *Experimental and Quasi-Experimental Design for Generalized Causal Inference.* Boston: Houghton Mifflin, 2002.

13. Ralston, P.A., Lemacks, J.L., Wickrama, K., et al. "Reducing Cardiovascular Disease Risk in Mid-Life and Older African Americans: A Church-Based Longitudinal Intervention Project at Baseline." *Controlled Clinical Trials* 38 (2014): 69–81.

14. Prochaska, J.O., Redding, C.A. and Evers, K.E. "The Transtheoretical Model and Stages of Change." In *Health Behavior and Health Education: Theory, Research and Practice*, ed. K. Glanz, B.K. Rimer and F.M. Lewis. San Francisco, CA: Jossey-Bass, 2002; pp. 97–121.

15. Rhodes, S.D., Malow, R.M. and Jolly, C. "Community-Based Participatory Research (CBPR): A New and Not-So-New Approach to HIV/AIDS Prevention, Care, and Treatment." *AIDS Education and Prevention* 22 (2010): 173–83.

16. Breslow, L. "Social Ecological Strategies for Promoting Healthy Lifestyles." *American Journal of Health Promotion* 10 (1996): 253–7.

17. Neta, G, Glasgow, R.E., Carpenter, C.R., et al. "A Framework for Enhancing the Value of Research for Dissemination and Implementation." *American Journal of Public Health* 105 (2015): 49–57.

18. Glasgow, R.E., Marcus, A.C., Bull, S.S. and Wilson, K.M. "Disseminating Effective Cancer Screening Interventions." *Cancer* 101 Suppl 5 (2004): 1239–50.

19. Orlandi, M.A., Landers, C., Weston, R. and Haley, N. "Diffusion of Health Promotion Innovations." In *Health Behavior and Health Education: Theory, Research, and Practice*, ed. K. Glanz, F.M. Lewis and B.K. Rimer. San Francisco: Jossey-Bass, 1990; pp. 270–86.

20. Wallerstein, N. and Duran, B. "Community-Based Participatory Research Contributions to Intervention Research: The Intersection of Science and Practice to Improve Health Equity." *American Journal of Public Health* 100 Suppl 1 (2010): S40–6.

21. Balazs, C.L. and Morello-Frosch, R. "The Three R's: How Community Based Participatory Research Strengthens the Rigor, Relevance and Reach of Science." *Environmental Justice* 6 (2013). doi: 10.1089/env.2012.0017

22. Allen, J.D., Linnan, L.A. and Emmons, K.M. "Fidelity and Its Relationship to Implementation Effectiveness, Adaptation, and Dissemination." In *Dissemination and Implementation Research in Health: Translating Science to Practice*, ed. R.C. Brownson, G. Colditz and E. Proctor. New York: Oxford University Press, 2012; pp. 281–304.

23. Tu, S.P., Chun, A, Yasui, Y., et al. "Adaptation of an Evidence-Based Intervention to Promote Colorectal Cancer Screening: A Quasi-Experimental Study." *Implementation Science* 9 (2014). Web. <http://www-implementationscience.com/content/9/1/85>

24. Tabak, R.G., Khoong, E.C., Chambers, D.A. and Brownson, R.C. "Bridging Research and Practice: Models for Dissemination and Implementation Research." *American Journal of Preventive Medicine* 43 (2012): 337–50.

25. Rogers, E.M. *Diffusion of Innovations*, 4th ed. New York: Free Press, 1995.

26. *RE-AIM 2004*. Web. <http://www.re-aim.org>

3

Research Methods and Community-Based Participatory Research

Challenges and Opportunities

CARL KENDALL, PHD, ANNIE L. NGUYEN, PHD, MPH,

JENNIFER GLICK, PHD, MPH, AND DAVID SEAL, PHD

A chapter describing research methods used in community-based participatory research (CBPR) has the difficult task of describing not only the wide range of research methods used in CBPR but also activities not normally thought of as research methods—approaching communities, building and maintaining trust, forming and supporting partnerships, identifying topics for research, participating in community activities, and staying connected beyond the scope of the research. Our conception of this task, then, is not that there are unique methods to be used in CBPR, but that CBPR is a process of using research methods and methodology with communities. Acknowledging the large literature that exists, we examine these processes through three less-discussed topics: challenges in the ethical review process; challenges for faculty promotion and tenure; and lessons learned through critical analyses of community research within a CBPR framework. At the root of many of these challenges is the misconception that CBPR does not provide a rigorous approach to scientific research. To overcome this perception, CBPR publications need to provide sufficient information about the process and context of implementation to build an empirical base for discussing methodology and advancing the science of CBPR. Publishing reporting guidelines for CBPR would advance the implementation and evaluation of CBPR.

Community-based participatory research has won a large following and substantial support in public health for explicitly recognizing the advantages of community participation in community-based research and amplifying that to include the engagement of community members in activities meant to prevent or ameliorate illness or injury. Direct involvement not only encourages community support and buy-in but also provides access and insight into community processes in ways that are difficult to achieve through conventional research. The success of CBPR is reflected in the large and growing number of CBPR projects and publications, and the number of courses taught on CBPR.

Describing research methods used in CBPR should focus on how methods can be introduced to make them accessible to community members, and how decisions that relate to defining the problem, developing research questions, identifying and implementing discrete data collection methods, and analyzing results can be taught to and used by lay participants. While the methodology of social science can be compiled in compendia and taught, the community collaborative approach is much less amendable to definitive and generalizable methods. In contrast, social science research relies on processes that are uniform, codified, and shared. This creates challenges for explaining how CBPR works and accounting for the full range of potential outcomes (e.g., the benefits and positive experiences that community partners may obtain by playing an important role in CBPR studies). These challenges and dynamics are sometimes expressed in terms of measures of the quality of the research and methodological rigor. Descriptions of how CBPR works have led to a large literature on CBPR concepts and methods, often focused on implementing CBPR through university-community partnerships.

This literature is daunting. Using Google Scholar, we identified 23,700 publications using the search term "community-based participatory research" as of March 21, 2016, and 751 articles using the search term "community-based participatory research methods." In addition to the current volume, a number of comprehensive books exist such as the one edited by Israel, Eng, Schulz, and Parker.[1] As Israel et al. note in their preface:

> As opportunities for conducting and learning about CBPR expand, so does the demand for knowledge and skills in the area. Practitioners and scholars ask for information about specific participation structures and procedures.... They ask how specific data collection methods, such as survey questionnaires, in-depth interviews, focus groups, ethnography, and mapping can be designed and implemented to follow participatory principles.[2, p.7]

What, then, does this chapter add? First we clarify the discussion of methods used in CBPR. Our conception is not that there are unique methods to be used in CBPR, but that CBPR is a process of using research methods and methodology in community research. We examine these processes through three less-discussed topics: challenges in the ethical review process; challenges for faculty promotion and tenure; and lessons learned through critical analyses of community research within a CBPR framework.

The chapter is organized into five sections: (1) A brief introduction to CBPR methods and how they are framed; (2) issues related to institutional review board (IRB) procedures; (3) how the organization of review and promotion in academia makes CBPR difficult, especially for junior researchers; (4) lessons learned from CBPR, focusing on processes and methods in the field; (5) conclusions and recommendations.

Introduction

At times, CBPR, which might be called a strategy or approach, is termed a method without differentiating it from specific methods or techniques such as sampling, observations, or interviews. In fact, the list of methods applicable to CBPR is very long, for example, interviews, focus groups, narratives, cognitive mapping, social mapping, and conversation analysis. Community-based participatory research also involves activities not normally thought of as research methods, for example, approaching communities and building trust, forming and supporting partnerships, maintaining trust, identifying topics for research, participating in community activities, and staying connected beyond the scope of the research.

The confusion around what is meant by "method" is not unique to CBPR but extends to other forms of social immersive research, such as ethnography. From an academic point of view, Crotty[3] argues that the confusion lies with not differentiating the terms "methods" and "methodology," and not recognizing that both terms are embedded in layers of both an epistemology and a theoretical perspective. Methodology, in this construction, is the strategy, plan of action, process, or design lying behind the choice and use of particular methods that link the choice and use of methods to the desired outcomes. Methods are defined as the techniques or procedures used to gather and analyze data related to a research question, hypothesis, or proposition. Therefore, CBPR is a methodology rather than a set of methods. Israel et al.[2] recognize this distinction when they discuss adopting methods to CBPR. On the other hand, CBPR is among that class of research that physically colocates the researcher in a community setting over time, with the inevitable and requisite erosion of boundaries between researcher and subject, and the establishment of social relationships and friendships. These two constructions of "methods" are quite different, and certainly extend beyond the research activities commonly described in the methods sections of scientific articles.

Community-based participatory research encompasses community collaboration and goal setting, as well as a wide range of qualitative and quantitative data collection techniques. While these data collection methods are appropriate for researcher driven studies, an additional set of techniques is required for the process of implementing CBPR. These techniques and components are much broader constructions than the data collection techniques described as methods. Israel et al.[2, p.12] characterize them as core components or phases in conducting CBPR:

1. Forming partnerships
2. Assessing community strengths and dynamics

3. Identifying priority health concerns and research questions
4. Designing and conducting etiologic intervention and/or policy research
5. Feeding back and interpreting research findings
6. Disseminating and translating research findings

With the exception of number 4, which relates to conventional research, the literature often discusses techniques for developing these components of CBPR. Of course, a number of techniques can be used to accomplish these phases, but no definitive set of activities is associated with each component.

Further complicating this discussion is the overlap between "methodology" and "method" as used by different authors, and the paucity of studies carefully detailing the techniques used in implementing CBPR. For example, partnerships are formed in CBPR, but the myriad details of how rapport was established and maintained, how crises were overcome, and how existing academic structures that do not support community partnerships are circumnavigated are not published. Using narrow criteria for defining and evaluating methods, two systematic reviews of CBPR have been published. Salimi et al.[4] completed a systematic review exploring the usefulness of CBPR. In their introduction, the authors noted the obvious and growing advantages of CPPR, especially community involvement to leverage program effects and reduce inequalities. The dilemmas of discussing CBPR methods are apparent in the systematic review flow chart in the article. Over the time period 2000–2009, the authors identified over 14,000 articles with the words "community-based participatory research" and "participatory action research" in the title, but the authors identified only 70 articles with sufficient detail about design and only 8 designed so that the effects of CBPR could be quantitatively evaluated. While not a direct assessment of the methods used in CBPR, it does create the impression that much of CBPR is in the preparation and intent, rather than in generating measureable outcomes.

A second review of clinical trials associated with CBPR has been published.[5] This paper reviewed 369 trials in racial and ethnic minority populations identified in PubMed and the Cumulative Index of Nursing and Allied Health Literature (CINAHL) conducted in North America during the period 2003–2010. The review identified 19 trials with sufficient detail and rigor to be included in the study. The review demonstrated positive outcomes for CBPR to recruit and retain minority populations in trials, and positive outcomes for intervention effects. Since minorities suffer health disparities and are underrepresented in trials, such effects are promising for addressing health disparities in these populations. The two reviews, while generally positive for CBPR outcomes, manifest the tension between academic expectations and utility and use of CBPR, as well as the difficulties of systematically reviewing CBPR methods. These challenges include incomplete descriptions of methods and incomplete documentation in published studies.

Issues Related to Institutional Review Boards

One commonly encountered challenge when conducting high quality CBPR work within an academic institution is the ethical review process. An IRB, also known as an independent ethics committee, ethical review board, or research ethics board, is a committee established to ensure that human research is conducted in accordance with all federal, institutional, and ethical guidelines. As discussed by Coughlin and Ackerson in chapter 5, the purpose of the IRB is to assure that appropriate steps are taken to protect the rights and welfare of humans participating as subjects in a research study.

Formal review procedures for institutional human subject studies were originally developed in direct response to research abuses in the 20th century. Tangible results include the National Research Act of 1974 and the development of the Belmont Report, which outlined the primary ethical principles in human subjects review; these include "respect for persons," "beneficence," and "justice."[6] These ethical principles are operationalized in terms of forms and procedures that require constant updating as new research models are developed, as our understanding of the risks, potential harms, and benefits of research are improved, and as new ethical issues emerge. While the ethical issues of testing a drug in a double-blinded randomized control trial may be well understood, IRBs have been slow to adapt their policies and procedures to accommodate different methodologies and methods. This is especially true for the review of CBPR protocols.

Institutional review boards have been criticized for relying on conceptions of research that privilege biomedical, clinical, and experimental designs, therefore penalizing research that deviates from this model.[7,8] Institutional review boards are often less familiar with social science and especially CBPR procedures. Descriptions of such research may not provide definitive sample sizes or sample selection procedures. They may not provide a specific guide or instrument to be used uniformly, or be able to consent each participant. When community members conduct research, they may not be ethically certified, or the IRBs may be uncomfortable with their level of training. Many social scientists, CBPR focused and otherwise, have argued that their research is not understood by IRBs and that IRBs impose unnecessary and time-consuming bureaucratic processes that do nothing to ensure the ethical well-being of research subjects. This is reflected in the institutional structures of ethical review boards. Flicker et al.[7] reviewed forms and guidelines commonly used by public health IRBs in the United States and Canada to assess if and how the forms reflected common CBPR experiences. The authors found that ethical review forms and guidelines overwhelmingly operate within a biomedical framework that rarely takes into account common CBPR experiences. They are primarily focused on assessing risks to individuals and not to communities and continue to perpetuate the notion that the domain of knowledge production is the sole right of academic researchers. Researchers concluded that IRBs might be unintentionally placing communities at risk by continuing to use procedures inappropriate or unsuitable for CBPR.[7]

Another concern is that IRB members often have only biomedical expertise and lack a working knowledge of CBPR; proposals are often misunderstood or held to inappropriate stipulations. While every institution may not have the capacity and internal expertise to have all research types represented on an IRB, it is important to seek that expertise. A possible solution offered by Guta et al.[8] is that IRBs can solicit external expertise from researchers at other institutions in the form of a one-time consultation, similar to journals and funding agencies.

A commonly discussed challenge regarding IRB approval for CBPR research relates to the time it takes to complete IRB procedures. Institutional review boards have been accused of having a clunky, bureaucratic default mode that is excessively and unnecessarily time-consuming.[9,10] As Gunsalus noted, "In too many cases, the focus is on form over ethical substance: counting what can be counted, rather than focusing instead on what counts."[10] Community-based participatory research does not necessarily follow the IRB-prescribed expectations of the provision of all materials and plans at the initiation of the project. Community-based participatory research uses iterative and emergent processes in the field to develop many of these materials, which have been met with confusion and resistance by IRBs. Institutional review boards are often more familiar with hypotheticodeductive approaches to research.[11] Flexibility is needed with respect to research designs that evolve in the field. Delays due to the need for IRB approval of a new iteration of study materials are a source of frustration. Delays are compounded when projects require multiple reviews by different IRBs, as each IRB may have a different application and requirements. In some CBPR partnerships, community representatives act as an informal IRB with ethical standards that arguably may be higher and more relevant than the university IRB's standards.[12] Time delays can pose problems for community partners who may operate under rapid timelines and not be accustomed to the lengthy administrative timelines of many academic institutions. Lengthy delays also present challenges to community partners such as low-income collaborators relying on stipends/incentives for their project-related expenses or students who need to complete assignments by the end of their academic term.

Some common CBPR data collection and dissemination methods, such as photovoice, pose novel ethical challenges to IRBs. As discussed by Coughlin and Yoo in chapter 2, photovoice is a participatory health-promotion strategy in which people use cameras to document their health and work realities, and may use these powerful images to communicate with policy makers when advocating for change in their communities.[13] Similar to other data collection approaches whereby community members gather sensitive data, unique ethical implications arise. For example, when capturing images there is the potential for invasion of privacy. Further issues arise regarding representation, participation, ownership of images, and so forth While ethical protocols exist for photovoice methods, communication of these protocols to IRBs is often unprecedented and can raise concerns.

Recommendations to improve the IRB process for CBPR research include (1) recruit reviewers with CBPR and related experience, as well as community advocates, to join ethical review boards;[8,12,14] (2) provide mutual education between IRB staff, researchers, and community review boards to maximize CBPR understandings and each stakeholder's requirements to ensure ethical research;[7,812,14] (3) encourage improved communication, relationship building, and mutual education between IRB staff and researchers;[8,12,14] and (4) encourage IRBs to remain flexible where variances from the protocol do not constitute a material change in risk to participants and their communities.[8]

Advancement and Promotion for Researchers

For new investigators, the structure of and expectations for promotion and tenure (P&T) at academic institutions present multiple barriers toward engaging in CBPR-driven projects, particularly those using qualitative methods of inquiry. Traditional, discipline-driven academia can create an environment that is challenging, and sometimes even hostile, toward CBPR.[15] A study published by Marrero et al.[16] demonstrated that among the tenure and tenure-track faculty surveyed at three research universities, only 35% of faculty agreed or strongly agreed that community-engaged research was recognized and rewarded during the P&T process. Only 28% of surveyed faculty agreed or strongly agreed that the P&T process encourages publication in sources that disseminate community-engaged research, and 16% of faculty agreed or strongly agreed that members of the P&T committees have a broad understanding of community-engaged scholarship. Given this collective sentiment, junior faculty may be encouraged by senior mentors to hold off on engaging in CBPR until the stages of mid or late career. These challenges related to perceptions of CBPR importance and potential for recognition and reward are compounded by the challenges of engaging in qualitative research.

Qualitative research can be more time-consuming than quantitative research. in addition, the process of CBPR is time-consuming and often includes a "preresearch" period of community engagement where time is spent developing rapport before the official research process begins.[17] For tenure-track faculty who are well aware of the ticking of the so-called tenure clock, time plays a significant factor when considering research approaches and designs. Completing research projects, obtaining extramural funding, and publishing a threshold number of manuscripts are all expected to occur within a certain time frame. Thus, opportunities for quicker turnaround are enticing. For example, consider the steps required to complete secondary data analyses of existing datasets compared to a qualitative study using individual interviews. In instances where the dataset is de-identified, secondary data analyses may be exempt from IRB review and analyses can begin as soon as the data are acquired. A study using qualitative interviews would be subject to IRB review and approval, including review of participant recruitment, primary data collection, and analysis. As researchers, especially junior researchers, develop their field relationships and interviewing skills, all these procedures, materials, and respondents may change dramatically. Research institutions typically offer support for investigators who need assistance with quantitative analyses through biostatistical cores that can offer assistance on a pay-per-project or hourly basis. There are few comparable institutional support structures for qualitative research.

Building a publication list is an important part of the P&T process. Publication of research findings can play a role in building community partner trust or can destroy trust. There may be community objections to publishing accounts that offend certain members or recount a less-than-perfect path to success. Publication, which rarely benefits the community directly and often highlights the university partner, can lead to the suspicion of academic intentions.

When publications are forthcoming, there are various challenges to publishing CBPR and qualitative findings in general, particularly in high-impact journals. Journal reviewers and editors may lack sufficient knowledge or experience with CBPR to assess methods, study rigor, or implications. Authors are often forced to translate the methods and findings in a way that fits more traditional, scientific manuscript frameworks, and devote less space in the article highlighting unique features of the collaboration that may be most exciting to community partners.[18] Community-based participatory research products such as presentations, brochures, webcasts, and information sheets may be more important for community partners and for dissemination of findings, but have little value in academia compared to peer-reviewed publications.

Building a program of research in a focused area is an essential component of succeeding in academia as well as in competing for funding. Investigators, particularly junior investigators, need to be articulate and develop an expertise in a specific area of research. While this is possible to do within the paradigm of community-based research, participatory research allows the room and freedom for priority areas to emerge from the coupling of academic with community needs. Thus, researchers who engage in true CBPR must be open to the possibility of shifting their priority topics to sufficiently address the top needs of the community with which they are working. The flexibility that is required in this approach does not fit well with the fairly strict, discipline-focused structure of academia. It does not conform to many of the requirements of tenure and promotion. All investigators, not only junior investigators, are faced with the pressures of obtaining external federal funding in a challenging funding climate. The NIH success rate hovered below 20% (18.1% across all institutions) in fiscal year 2014 compared with 31.5% in fiscal year 2000.[19] Given the limited funds available, funders have to issue priority funding areas. This may not favor investigators who engage in CBPR and particularly those who use qualitative methods. The systematic review of published qualitative studies by Gagliardi and Dobrow[20] showed that less than half of the studies reported a funding source and only 26% of articles reported a federal or state funding source.

These challenges should not dissuade researchers from engaging in CBPR, particularly if the science of the project is enhanced or made more rigorous by CBPR approaches. Rather, investigators must maintain awareness of the challenges to CBPR and anticipate these challenges in much the same way investigators are trained to anticipate challenges to aspects of any research protocol or project such as recruitment setbacks or delays and issues with participant retention. The unique nature of CBPR simply presents a different set of challenges for investigators to consider and to tackle. Certainly, this may require investigators to examine and gather information about the culture and policies of their own institution regarding P&T, to perform a sort of environmental scan, in order to determine how to divide their time and resources. Community-based participatory research is but one approach to community-engaged work, and researchers need to find their own personal balance between the pros and cons of engaging in such work at different points in their careers.

Lessons Learned

Earlier in this chapter, we discussed Israel et al.'s[2] core components of CBPR. In this concluding section, we examine these components and phases and offer insight into potential challenges of their implementation. We also offer suggestions for overcoming these challenges, drawing on multiple CBPR projects that we have been involved with.

FORMING PARTNERSHIPS

There are many levels of partnership, ranging from networking, cooperating, coordinating, to collaborating.[21] Networking involves low levels of time and trust. Cooperating requires moderate levels of time and trust, as well as some sharing of turf. Coordinating requires high levels of time and trust and moderate sharing of turf. Collaborating requires maximum levels of time, trust, and turf sharing. Transcendent partnership involves partners working together on endeavors of mutual interest irrespective of a person's community and/or academic background. Transcendent partnership involves working **WITH** each other, not doing **TO** or doing **FOR** one another.

Community-academic partnerships are most likely to succeed when partners have (1) a clear understanding of the strengths and limitations each organization brings to the partnership; (2) a strong belief in and commitment to compromise and equality as essential components of partnership; and (3) clearly established guidelines or a memorandum of understanding to guide the partnership process. For example, one author of this chapter has had a collaborative community partnership with the lesbian, gay, bisexual, and transgendered (LGBT) community in a Midwestern city for almost two decades. The partnership includes both programmatic and scientific health promotion projects, as well as shared service on advisory groups, in support of improving the health and wellness of LGBT persons. This collaboration builds on their respective scientific and programmatic strengths. Well-defined and time-tested guidelines for decision-making and communication developed and refined over time in their lengthy history enables their investigative team to quickly initiate project activities if funded. Such strategies include (1) a written agreement outlining individual and shared responsibilities, decision-making processes, and budget allocations and (2) regular team meetings, phone conversations, and e-mail correspondence. Budgets are equally distributed, and often the majority of funds are allocated to the community partners.

Although each partner has specific tasks related to their areas of expertise within any given project, our partnership plan ensures that project decisions are made through consensus agreement between community and academic leadership in close consultation with our auxiliary partners. The executive director of the lead community partner and the lead investigator of the academic team frequently serve as co-principal investigators on their collaborative project. For multisite projects, both individuals have an equal role in the representation of the investigative team at national meetings, and they jointly share project oversight. All project decisions are made through consensus, and both individuals have complete veto power on any decision. When rare differences do arise, they are resolved through discussion and compromise. Their collaboration, which synthesizes unique scientific and programmatic expertise, increases the likelihood of developing programs and interventions that are (1) scientifically efficacious, (2) programmatically appropriate, and (3) responsive to community needs, values, and priorities.

ASSESSING COMMUNITY STRENGTHS AND DYNAMICS

Community-academic research projects typically have an advisory or leadership board. Ideally, these boards are composed of those individuals with a documented history of community accomplishment related to project implementation. Boards that are filled by community and/or academic representatives due to their name reputation or title, without front-line accomplishment or experience with community-academic partnership, often have diminished success and influence. The most successful boards we have worked with are composed of leaders who work closely with the community regardless of their title or status, and would continue to do so even if no current project existed. These boards operate most successfully when there is shared leadership and power within the operating structure. Ways to promote these goals are (1) having a cofacilitator structure where a community leader and an academic/public health representative coplan and cofacilitate meetings, (2) having more community representatives than non-community representatives on the board, and (3) creating an environment where experiential knowledge is valued equally to academic knowledge.

IDENTIFYING PRIORITY HEALTH CONCERNS AND RESEARCH QUESTIONS

Too often, researchers have tried to impose participatory research on communities based on funding opportunities, high profile issues in the media, current sociopolitical agendas, or emerging epidemiological trends. This approach does not take into account community priorities, which may not align with research or public health agendas. Nor does this approach take into consideration the context in which the chosen research issue is embedded. Further, many research concerns are embedded in social inequalities, historical injustices, and involve challenges related to race, gender, power, and turf. Identifying a research area of mutual interest often takes considerable discussion of priorities, potential approaches, feasibility issues, organizational structure, and operating processes. This must be accomplished through dialogue, compromise, and consensus among partners. Unless the research team has a strong relationship with the community and had a history of successfully navigating these issues, the partnership and project are unlikely to succeed.

Rigorous community needs assessments can be important tools for understanding community priorities, the community's understanding of the underlying determinants of identified research questions, and sources of insight into potential solutions. They also can be a vehicle for developing community rapport and creating community relationships. For example, in a CBPR violence reduction project, one of the authors of this chapter was the lead investigator on an initial 18-month multicomponent community needs assessment.[22] The first step was a pair of community forums designed to introduce the initiative to the larger community and elicit community views on the definition of violence, its causes, and its prevention. At the forums, attended by over 125 people, a call for applications to serve on the project steering committee was issued. Subsequently, a steering committee was convened and began meeting regularly over an 18-month period to (1) establish specific, long-term goals of the project; (2) develop a detailed implementation plan to reduce violence and increase community capacity to conduct violence prevention projects; and (3) provide leadership and oversight of project activities.

In addition to the steering committee, a community asset team conducted a series of community forums, workgroups, and assessments to elicit community perspectives on the definition of violence, its underlying causes, priority populations to target for prevention, and recommendations for intervention. Staff first conducted 62 individual interviews with key informants from a broad spectrum of community sectors including grass-roots and community leaders, community-based agencies, social-service agencies, school systems (public, private, charter), faith-based institutions, business, public, law enforcement, judicial/legal agencies, neighborhood associations, medical and mental health providers, funders, academia, media, and the arts. Staff also conducted analyses of 10 high-risk zip codes in the target city to identify and map community assets and needs. A summary report of these two assessments was prepared and discussed in three focus groups with 16 stakeholders who had participated in the interviews. Participant feedback was elicited about the face validity of the report and the implications of the findings for violence prevention efforts. Key recommendations of these community assessment activities were that the violence prevention efforts should focus on youth, take a comprehensive approach to prevention, and involve diverse community partnerships.

Subsequently, two additional community forums attended by 169 participants to present findings from the stakeholder interviews, stakeholder focus groups, and community mapping analyses elicited additional feedback about (1) how to build alliances and navigate community politics in local prevention efforts, (2) best strategies to listen to and give voice to youth, (3) novel ideas to address youth violence in the target city, (4) how best to deliver technical assistance resources to existing initiatives that were currently addressing youth violence prevention, and (5) training and education needed to advance policy addressing youth violence.

All of the activities listed above were designed to elicit information to inform the steering committee and the community about stakeholder definitions of violence, its causes, and its prevention. Next, four community action workgroups (involving 64 stakeholders who participated in one or more workgroups) were convened to translate the community assessment findings into concrete action recommendations for consideration by the steering committee. These community action workgroups made recommendations around four broad content areas: (1) community coalition building and collaboration, (2) community-academic capacity, (3) policy and advocacy development, and (4) youth asset development. Workgroup participants were recruited through open invitations at the 2009 community forums and through an e-distribution list. The workgroups were facilitated by steering committee members and community leaders. Both large- and small-group discussion formats were used to generate action recommendations.

The final phase of the community assessment was designed to elicit youth perspectives on violence, its causes, and its prevention. We conducted 18 individual interviews with high-risk youth recruited in street settings through key informant contacts. We also conducted six focus groups with youth ($n = 64$) recruited through agencies that serve high-risk youth. Finally, we held two youth summits ($n = 140$ participants) to present findings from the youth interviews and focus groups, elicit feedback about what we learned, and hear youth testimonials about their own experiences with violence. Summary reports of all these activities were then combined into a comprehensive summary report that was widely distributed to stakeholders throughout the city.

DESIGNING AND CONDUCTING ETIOLOGIC, INTERVENTION, AND/OR POLICY RESEARCH

At the conclusion of the needs assessment phase described in the previous section, a new community-academic board was formed to translate the needs assessment into a call for proposals from community coalitions interested in violence-prevention implementation grants targeting youth. Some of the board members had also served during the needs assessment phase, while others were new to the process. The board was purposively composed of a 2:1 community to academic member representation. The translation was done using a rigorous and systematic process. All community action recommendations identified in the community needs assessment were extracted and pasted into the appropriate level of the socioecological model (SEM) (i.e., individual, interpersonal, neighborhoods-schools, societal). Within the SEM model, the community action recommendations were conceptually organized and redundancies merged. This framework and associated community action recommendations were then embedded within the a priority programmatic framework established by the prior steering committee, including (1) prevent and intervene early with youth 0–11 years of age; (2) motivate and influence youth 12–17 years of age; and (3) educate, develop, catalyze, and convene across all youth to build capacity for violence prevention with neighborhoods, schools, and the broader community. Finally, through multiple meetings and considerable discussion, the board reached consensus about the parameters of the call for proposals.

The call for proposals required multiagency community coalitions, which may or may not involve academic partners, to develop a plan for a multifaceted youth violence prevention intervention, in accordance with the broad programmatic goals, that was culturally appropriate, feasible, and acceptable to the communit(ies) that the coalition planned to involve. The proposals had to include information about how the coalition was derived, how they planned to work together, and how they would involve youth leadership and community advisory groups. Thus, within the broad parameters of the call for proposals, each coalition had considerable autonomy to develop a locally tailored proposal. The coalitions who were selected to receive funding then were partnered with an academic leadership team who worked collaboratively with the coalition to translate their proposal into a logic model, develop measureable outcomes for their proposed activities, and provide collaborative coordination of the multiple coalitions that were selected. A separate academic team was contracted for the project to provide rigorous and independent evaluation of the agreed on outcomes.

FEEDING BACK AND INTERPRETING
RESEARCH FINDINGS

Successful community–academic partnerships do not cease when the data have been collected. They also continue through the analyses, interpretation, and dissemination phases. There are many methods to involve community in this phase of the project. Sometimes community members have conducted the analyses in partnership with the academic members. They also can provide member feedback about the validity of the interpretation of the findings or help provide understanding of counterintuitive or contradictory findings. In other cases, they provide thoughtful discussion about the findings, their interpretation, and their implications. Involving community in thoughtful review and discussion of the data and their interpretation can enhance the validity and meaningfulness of final reports and manuscripts.

Related, many community–academic partnerships fail because institutions are reluctant to acknowledge their shortcomings and accept outside criticism. The authors have been involved in CBPR efforts in which the academic institution sponsoring the project was resistant to including anything in their study reports that reflected poorly on the institution. For example, in one community needs assessment, the lead academic institution received many critiques from community members such as researchers never really relinquished power or promoted equity, the institution used the community but rarely gave back, the institution promoted more image than substance, and institutional researchers became nonexistent in community as soon as they got their data. Within community-academic partnerships, it is essential to be transparent and to let the data speak. All too often, researchers pick and choose the key points of needs assessments or outcome data that support their underlying agenda or desired outcome. This type of censorship of data to protect the institution results in a lack of transparency that damages community relationships. Rather than reject these critiques, researchers could acknowledge them and use them as an opportunity to begin a dialogue of the ways that this project could be done differently.

TRANSLATING AND DISSEMINATING
RESEARCH FINDINGS

Researchers should avoid jargon and fancy conceptual models meant to impress academics. Elegant conceptual models and terminology are fine for academic presentations, but the best community presentations are when academics present concepts in straightforward lay language. Similarly, community presentations of data are best when focused on a summary of key findings without lots of statistics. Successful community dissemination is best focused on interpreting the findings and on how best to use the information to improve programs and services. Another successful strategy is to include of key community partners as copresenters who can present the findings in their own words and lead discussion.

Other Lessons Learned

TRUST IN THE TEAM

It is also important that academic leadership be actively involved with the community partners and the day-to-day research activities. This can be accomplished through attendance at regular team meetings, regular site visits to understand the context of the staff's daily work environment, and regular meetings with community partner leadership to ensure everyone remains aligned in their goals and operating procedures. Creating field teams in which community staff work side-by-side with research staff toward shared outcomes can enhance this process.

Front-line staff are the pulse of a CBPR project. They are in the community on a daily basis and are usually in the best position to understand what is going on. Give staff considerable autonomy to do their jobs without micromanagement. The academic's job is to make sure the project operates within the scientific parameters outlined in the community- and IRB-approved protocol and to ensure scientific fidelity. Further, front-line staff should be deeply involved in the development of specific project implementation protocols. When community staff are involved in the implementation of the research project, it is essential that academics trust their expertise and experience. Recognize that community-based staff may work in different ways than academic staff. Regardless of formal educational training, community staff can contribute considerable experiential expertise. Respecting and learning from this expertise is important in community partnerships.

In many CBPR projects, academics may seek different skills and backgrounds in their staff hires versus community leadership. It is important that each side respect their respective hires. It can be beneficial to form a personnel review team that gives equal voice to both the community and academic leadership in a joint review process for both community and academic hires. This helps to ensure that the hires will be received by the community while having the capacity to conduct research. Related, all staff should be evaluated by their ability to achieve project goals within the parameters of the research design, not by whether they rigidly adhere to institutional operating norms. Recognition of the unique skills and expertise brought by research staff who come from community versus academic backgrounds is important in building strong teams. Good leadership will recognize these respective strengths and utilize their staff accordingly.

EMBRACE CRITICS

One author has had experiences in which organizers of community boards and forums have purposively rejected key informants and experts (both academic and community members) because they are openly critical of the organizing body. Rather, they should accept the critiques and work to overcome them. It is preferable to have our critics at the table having their voice heard rather than offering vocal outside criticism. Including them at the table allows the ability to have open dialogue to find points of compromise. It can be helpful to ask the most vocal critics to meet for coffee or lunch to learn more about their views and their work, or visit their agency and learn more about the setting in which they work.

Related, team settings that encourage dissent and critical reflection as a way of improving the final design and operating procedures result in higher quality design and implementation, as well as happier, more cohesive teams. We recommend considering any staff critique as long as it is thoughtful and respectful and offers an alternative for the team to consider.

BUILDING AND SUSTAINING PARTNERSHIPS

Building partnerships takes time and investment. One good way to show commitment to, and gain the trust of, community organizations and residents is to be visible at community meetings, events, forums, and so forth. This lets people know that you care about their community beyond the research. It allows people the opportunity to get to know you as a person, not just a researcher. Be available and willing to provide technical assistance, training, and guidance to community agencies who seek your assistance. Do this willingly and without strings attached or requests. The development of social capital within the community can be an important enabler of developing partnerships. Community members are much more willing to listen to researcher ideas when they know that an individual is committed to the community and actively participates in it.

Conclusions and Recommendations

The experience of implementing CBPR is often presented in case studies that can capture the rich multidimensional nature of collaborations. While specific data collection activities can be described and presented, few published CBPR studies provide the detail required for an evaluation of methods. In addition, few publications provide sufficient information about the process and context of CBPR implementation to build an empirical base for discussing methodology. In lacking this platform from which to discuss methodology in a way that is unique to CBPR, we also lack an appropriate way to evaluate CBPR. Instead, CBPR is evaluated and assessed against the standards of traditional forms of scientific inquiry, which fails to capture and appreciate the unique aspects of CBPR that make it successful. This is reflected in the challenges that CBPR academic researchers face with policies and practices in regard to IRB and promotion and tenure. This is also reflected in the tension that exists when researchers perform their work within the broader institutional culture, which may not support the nontraditional academic practices of sharing power and decision-making with communities. What is needed is appropriate guidelines for describing CBPR methodology. Israel et al.'s core components begin to map out such a guide. Publishing guidelines such as consolidated criteria for reporting qualitative research (COREQ)[23] and Strengthening the Reporting of Observational Studies in Epidemiology (STROBE)[24] for CBPR would include both a description of method and of methodology, as discussed in this chapter. Details that make articles overlong, and documentation of specific steps in the research can be appended electronically to the article. Such steps will advance our collective understanding of how best to implement and evaluate CBPR.

References

1. Caldwell, W. B., et al. "Community Partner Perspectives on Benefits, Challenges, Facilitating Factors, and Lessons Learned from Community-Based Participatory Research Partnerships in Detroit." *Prog Community Health Partnersh* 9.2 (2015): 299–311.
2. *Methods for Community-Based Participatory Research for Health* (2nd ed.). Wiley, 2012.
3. Crotty, M. *The Foundations of Social Research*. London: Sage, 1998.
4. Salimi, Y., et al. "Is Community-Based Participatory Research (CBPR) Useful? A Systematic Review on Papers in a Decade." *Int J Prev Med* 3.6 (2012): 386–93.
5. De las Nueces, D., et al. "A Systematic Review of Community-Based Participatory Research to Enhance Clinical Trials in Racial and Ethnic Minority Groups." *Health Serv Res* 47.3 Pt 2 (2012): 1363–86.
6. Department of Health and Education, et al. "The Belmont Report: Ethical Principles and Guidelines for the Protection of Human Subjects of Research." *J Am Coll Dent* 81.3 (2014): 4–13.
7. Flicker, S., et al. "Ethical Dilemmas in Community-Based Participatory Research: Recommendations for Institutional Review Boards." *Journal of Urban Health* 84.4 (2007): 478–93.
8. Guta, A., et al. "'Walking Along Beside the Researcher': How Canadian REBs/IRBs Are Responding to the Needs of Community-Based Participatory Research." *J Empir Res Hum Res Ethics* 7.1 (2012): 15–25.
9. De Vries, R., DeBruin, D. A. and Goodgame, A. "Ethics Review of Social, Behavioral, and Economic Research: Where Should We Go from Here?" *Ethics and Behavior* 14.4 (2004): 351–68.
10. Gunsalus, C.K. "The Nanny State Meets the Inner Lawyer: Overregulating While Underprotecting Human Participants in Research." *Ethics and Behavior* 14.4 (2004): 369–82.
11. Bledsoe, C. H., et al. "Regulating Creativity: Research and Survival in the IRB Iron Cage." *Northwestern University Law Review* 101.2 (2007): 593–641.
12. Shore, N. "Community-Based Participatory Research and the Ethics Review Process." *Journal of Empirical Research on Human Research Ethics* 2.1 (2007): 31–41.
13. Wang, C.C. and Redwood-Jones, Y.A. "Photovoice Ethics: Perspectives from Flint Photovoice." *Health Education and Behavior* 28.5 (2001): 560–72.

14. Wolf, Leslie E. "The Research Ethics Committee Is Not the Enemy: Oversight of Community-Based Participatory Research." *Journal of Empirical Research on Human Research Ethics* 5.4 (2010): 77–86.

15. Nyden, P. "Academic Incentives for Faculty Participation in Community-Based Participatory Research." *J Gen Intern Med* 18.7 (2003): 576–85.

16. Marrero, D.G., et al. "Promotion and Tenure for Community-Engaged Research: An Examination of Promotion and Tenure Support for Community-Engaged Research at Three Universities Collaborating Through a Clinical and Translational Science Award." *Clin Transl Sci* 6.3 (2013): 204–8.

17. D'Alonzo, K. T. "Getting Started in CBPR: Lessons in Building Community Partnerships for New Researchers." *Nurs Inq* 17.4 (2010): 282–8.

18. Bordeaux, B. C., et al. "Guidelines for Writing Manuscripts About Community-Based Participatory Research for Peer-Reviewed Journals." *Prog Community Health Partnersh* 1.3 (2007): 281–8.

19. NIH Report. "Research Project Success Rates by NIH Institites for 2014." Web. March 28, 2016.

20. Gagliardi, A.R., and Dobrow, M.J. "Paucity of Qualitative Research in General Medical and Health Services and Policy Research Journals: Analysis of Publication Rates." *BMC Health Serv Res* 11 (2011): 268.

21. Himmelman, A.T. *Collaboration for a Change: Definitions, Decision-Making Models, Roles, and Collaboration Process Guide.* Minneapolis, MN: Himmelman Consulting, 2002.

22. Seal, D. W., et al. *Medical College of Wisconsin Youth Violence Prevention Initiative: Summary Report—Development Phase, 2008–2010.* Milwaukee: Institute for Health and Society, Medical College of Wisconsin, 2010.

23. Tong, A., Sainsbury, P. and Craig, J. "Consolidated Criteria for Reporting Qualitative Research (COREQ): A 32-Item Checklist for Interviews and Focus Groups." *Int J Qual Health Care* 19.6 (2007): 349–57.

24. von Elm, E., et al. "The Strengthening the Reporting of Observational Studies in Epidemiology (Strobe) Statement: Guidelines for Reporting Observational Studies." *Prev Med* 45.4 (2007): 247–51.

4

The Use of GIS/GPS and Spatial Analyses in Community-Based Participatory Research

TONNY J. OYANA, PHD

To understand the relevance and context of geographic information systems (GIS)/global positioning system (GPS) applications for CBPR, the starting point is to recognize the significance of place, location, and distance and how they matter in every aspect of our lives. The prominence of these concepts has been further emphasized by several studies, which have suggested that most of today's health problems, especially chronic diseases, can be attributed to how and where people live. The GIS/GPS technologies have a central role in catalyzing evidence-based public health interventions, partly because current health challenges require a transdisciplinary perspective. These technologies can be used in many different ways. In this chapter, GIS/GPS technologies are highlighted that can be used to collect and analyze environmental (geospatial) datasets, which offer new scientific knowledge and insights into health problems. Robust and unbiased geospatial data and knowledge about communities can be used to deepen our understanding of public health problems, target interventions to reduce health disparities, and achieve health equity. Furthermore, personalized knowledge of individuals' or neighborhood patterns may yield specific health information that can be used to create healthier communities. The knowledge gained can enable people to lead healthier and longer lives.

Recent opportunities, as described in this chapter, demonstrate how GIS/GPS technologies can be used to facilitate the conduct of bottom-up, high-impact health disparities research. Community participants use GIS/GPS in experiential learning and colearning. The technology offers a unique opportunity for participants to engage in and contribute to the research.[1-3] This chapter also provides an up-to-date review of participatory GIS methods and analytical techniques. The chapter considers volunteered geographic health information (e.g., information provided by citizen scientists); 10 ways GIS and spatial analytics can be used for community-engaged health research; and challenges, alternative approaches, and ideas for future directions.

Mapping applications and e-health technologies have proliferated in many aspects of our daily activities. This is augmented by the wide availability of easy-to-use, user-friendly GIS/GPS-enabled tracking/sensor devices/data services on the Internet and mobile devices such as smartphones. The abundance of these emerging technologies reinforces the critical need to better integrate and use current state-of-the-art GIS/GPS tools and applications to support CBPR. They are now commonplace and are frequently used to guide our thinking and decisions.

Mapping sensor technologies have revolutionized data collection and can essentially be used to help communities in identifying, assessing, and mapping community health resources or assets. Specifically, GIS/GPS technologies can be used to collect activity-level data on where people live, play, work, worship, shop, eat, or learn. Data points representing the location of participants, service providers, food stores, farmers markets, and restaurants are automatically assigned geographic coordinates and merged, integrated, or analyzed to inform health decisions. Contextual environmental measures, including physical activity environment, recreational facilities, land use mix, and walkability score, can be compiled using GIS. Near/proximity and geospatial measures can be derived to support targeted interventions.

Review of Participatory GIS Methods

Previous authors have explored the concept of participatory GIS and community-integrated GIS.[1,4-10] The common theme from these publications suggests that participatory GIS, also referred to as community-integrated GIS, community mapping, or collaborative mapping, is largely informed by the context, and is issue-driven rather than technology-led.[1,4-8] The concept is inspired by the pressing need to emphasize the effective representation, inclusion, and active involvement of a community in the production and use of geographic information.[1,4-8]

The central tenet of participatory GIS, which is intended to empower at-risk and hard-to-reach communities, is social inclusiveness. Scientific methods and tools that empower and effectively engage a community, such as participatory GIS, have moved to the forefront. Participatory GIS has key capabilities and advantages: It can help with community health assessment through data collection and analysis, provide a learning opportunity for community stakeholders and researchers, and facilitate the determination of the most appropriate solution. Despite participatory GIS's capability, it is essential to have a true and meaningful dialogue among participants. This helps with trust building and also facilitates the successful use of scientific measurement tools, strategies, and research methods. Reaching out through encouragement and offering training support, especially to socioeconomically disadvantaged communities with low health literacy and numeracy, enables them to fully engage in the CBPR process from initial planning to implementation phase. Broadening public participation requires that community partners be given the opportunity to be involved and contribute to the community-based initiatives.[11]

The National Institute of Environmental Health Sciences (NIEHS) has endorsed six principles of effective CBPR: (1) promotes active collaboration and participation at every stage of research, (2) fosters colearning, (3) ensures projects are community-driven, (4) disseminates results in useful terms, (5) ensures research and intervention strategies are culturally appropriate, and (6) defines community as a unit of identity.[1] Other authors, including Dennis Jr. et al.,[3] Dulin et al.,[12] and Tapp and White,[10] have described the principles of the CBPR process in similar terms. Based on the six identified CBPR principles, we can infer that numerous research opportunities exist at every stage of research for the use of participatory GIS methods.

A number of interesting commentaries and groundbreaking studies in participatory GIS methods have been published in journals, newspapers, textbooks, and other reports.[1,4-10,13-15] Participatory GIS and community-integrated GIS have been applied in a wide range of contexts. These include community health needs assessment;[12,16-19] neighborhood mapping;[13,20-22] community asset mapping, tracking, and monitoring;[10,15,17] environmental risk, vulnerability, and disaster assessment;[23] spatiotemporal measures and changes;[12,18] identification of contextual factors and decision-making;[12,17,18,24-26] development of place-based health measures and interventions;[12,18,27,28] and data integration, visualization, and management needs.[2,3,12,18,29-31] Table 4.1 presents a sample of these GIS participatory applications.

Rationale for Community-Based GIS and Spatial Analytic Methods

As noted earlier, with the rapid proliferation of mobile devices and sensor technology, science has become a way of life.[32-35] Citizen scientists have empowered themselves and are using mobile devices or sensors (e.g., citizen sensors) to record their locations, daily activities, healthcare facilities, building heights, farmers markets, food stores and restaurants, blood pressure, duration of sleep, or body weight. The data are recorded using a specific metric that may consist of non-numeric or numeric attributes with a unit. Several options for data collection and infographics are available. An engaged community can define measures by attaching descriptors, blogging, goal setting, and self-monitoring or by tracking their summary health reports using infographics and other visual tools and analytics. Integrated wearable sensor technologies are available with GIS/GPS trackers and spatial analytic methods for collecting, mapping, visualizing, and analyzing data anytime, anywhere. These technologies empower citizens with

Table 4.1 **Community-Based GIS Applications in the Health Sector**

Study	Approach	Use of GIS and Spatial Analytics	Comments
Dulin et al.[12]	Outcomes measured using CBPR and Geospatial Modeling	Community health needs assessment Analysis of the patterns of healthcare access Evaluation of intervention impact over time	GIS was used in supportive role by the research team to collect data and create geospatial models
Dulin et al.[18]	Geospatial models used to target interventions in neighborhoods	Data management Implementation of interventions Data validation using qualitative methods and surveys	GIS was used in supportive role by the research team to collect data and create geospatial models GIS used to facilitate focus group discussions and decision-making Ranking variables and assigning weights using the analytic hierarchy process for input into the geospatial models Attribute assessment and evaluation
Jung[31]	Qualitative geovisualization	Children's meaning of community Social network analysis Identifying racial groups Analysis of social proximity	Community photo mapping Visualization of community resources Community mapping

Table 4.1 **Continued**

Study	Approach	Use of GIS and Spatial Analytics	Comments
Driedger et al.[29]	Health decision support system using GIS	Map production and a collaborative Web-based GIS tool EYEMAP development Mapping functionality	Web-based mapping tool Cartographic design Data sharing
Dennis et al.[3]	Participatory photo mapping	Integration of digital tools, narrative interviewing, and participatory protocols	GIS and photo mapping used to support focus group discussions
Castleden et al.[30]	Participatory photovoice	Mapping food environment Mapping open space and safety Culturally appropriate method	Community photo mapping Visualization of community resources Photovoice used to address environment and health questions
Brown et al.[2]	Physical activity and urban park benefits measured using GIS	Tested user usability of PPGIS website Use of Google maps interface Identification of park benefits Supporting urban park studies	Park classification and mapping GIS used to study physical activities and benefits
Chirowodza et al.[17]	Geospatial methods used to target HIV interventions	Community health needs assessment Identifying study sites and location Identifying contextual factors Implementation of interventions	Community mapping Visualization of community resources

(*continued*)

Table 4.1 **Continued**

Study	Approach	Use of GIS and Spatial Analytics	Comments
Hill et al.[29]	Physical activity and food environment measured using CBPR and GIS	Analysis of patterns of physical activity and food environment	GIS used to facilitate focus group discussions and decision-making
		Development of walkability index	GIS used to facilitate the discussion of causal model of geographic influences
		Implementation of interventions	
			Spatial analysis conducted to determine spatial autocorrelation
Aronson et al.,[20] Wood,[13] Deeds et al.,[21] and Topmiller et al.[22]	Neighborhood mapping	Community health needs assessment	Creation of geospatial measures
	Multilayered GIS approach	Study of urban infant mortality prevention program	Identification of neighborhood characteristics and social determinants of health
		Integration of GIS, environmental audits, group narratives, and sketch mapping	Integration of multiple levels of data into maps and perspectives into policy action
			Community mapping

timely information and actionable intelligence to engage in leisure activities and enhance healthy living.

A curiosity to learn and gain knowledge about their community's health status motivates citizens to partner with scientists. Together, they systematically ask specific research questions, formulate hypotheses, design experiments, ensure proper collection of primary data, and verify or reject the hypothesis using collected observations. Throughout the scientific process, citizen scientists are encouraged and given equal opportunity to actively engage by challenging and contributing useful ideas that promote the community's health. The ultimate goal of academic, scientific, or community partnership is to obtain credible and actionable scientific results that produce positive benefits.

O'Fallon and Dearry[1] have outlined eight key CBPR benefits to scientists and communities if there is active participation, engagement, and honest communication among all partners in the scientific process: (1) increased relevance of research question; (2) increased quantity and quality of data collection; (3) increased use and relevance of data; (4) increased dissemination; (5) research translated into policy; (6) emergence of new research questions; (7) research and intervention extended beyond specific project; (8) builds infrastructure and sustainability.

The framework presented in Figure 4.1 can be used to (1) inform the comprehensive community needs assessment process, (2) guide the action plan, (3) facilitate the design of multilevel intervention plans (from individual/micro-level to institution and community/macro-level); and (4) increase the transferability of lessons learned. The framework integrates new tools, social network analysis methods and measures, and strategies, and is fused with the knowledge and expertise of a transdisciplinary team to work on multiple datasets at the individual or population level to influence health. The framework is inspired by the CBPR approach, multilevel intervention perspectives, public health perspectives, health literacy, behavioral psychology, statistical modeling, GIS approaches, and health disparities research.[1,3,10,27,36]

Volunteered Geographic Health Information: Using Citizen Science to Collect and Visualize GIS Data

The concept of volunteered geographic information (VGI) was first inspired by Michael Goodchild in 2007 in a seminal article, "Citizens as Sensors: The World of Volunteered Geography."[32] The concept refers to user-generated content on the Internet captured either through the use of mobile sensing devices or through dissemination of maps and infographics generated using crowdsourced or open access data. Crowdsourcing simply refers to obtaining data, information, or input into a particular task or project by soliciting paid or unpaid services of a large online community.[37] For example, Twitter data can be used to disseminate health information, identify influencers and competitors, identify what is trending, measure impact and reach, map tweets and retweets, and to acquire statistics on mentions, followers, retweets, and much more. Figure 4.2 shows the intensity and location of user-generated content based on the hashtags "Memphis" and "Health" from Twitter data.

The VGI and citizen science literature has grown over the past decade, and perspectives on it are now available in a number of scientific reports.[32-35,38-40] The context, drivers, typology, standards, methods, and characteristics of VGI and citizen science have been developed and explained. The reports have detailed the role of volunteers and crowdsourcing; levels of motivation, participation, and engagement; measures and quality of data/knowledge derived from participants; sensor technologies and their benefits/limitations; and uncertainty and remaining challenges.

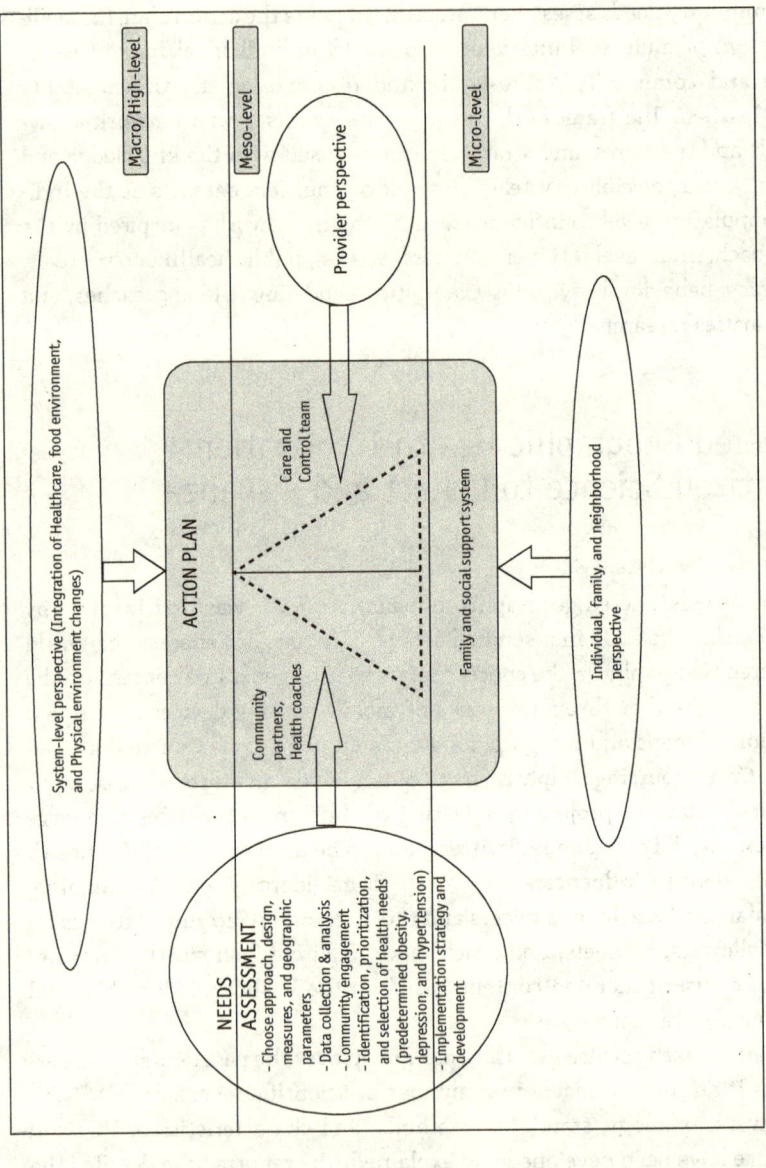

Figure 4.1 A theoretical conceptual framework that integrates a socioecological model and geographic parameters. This model can be applied to community health needs assessments, for example in the reduction of risk factors for obesity, depression, or hypertension. The needs assessment component integrates geospatial measures in the CBPR process.

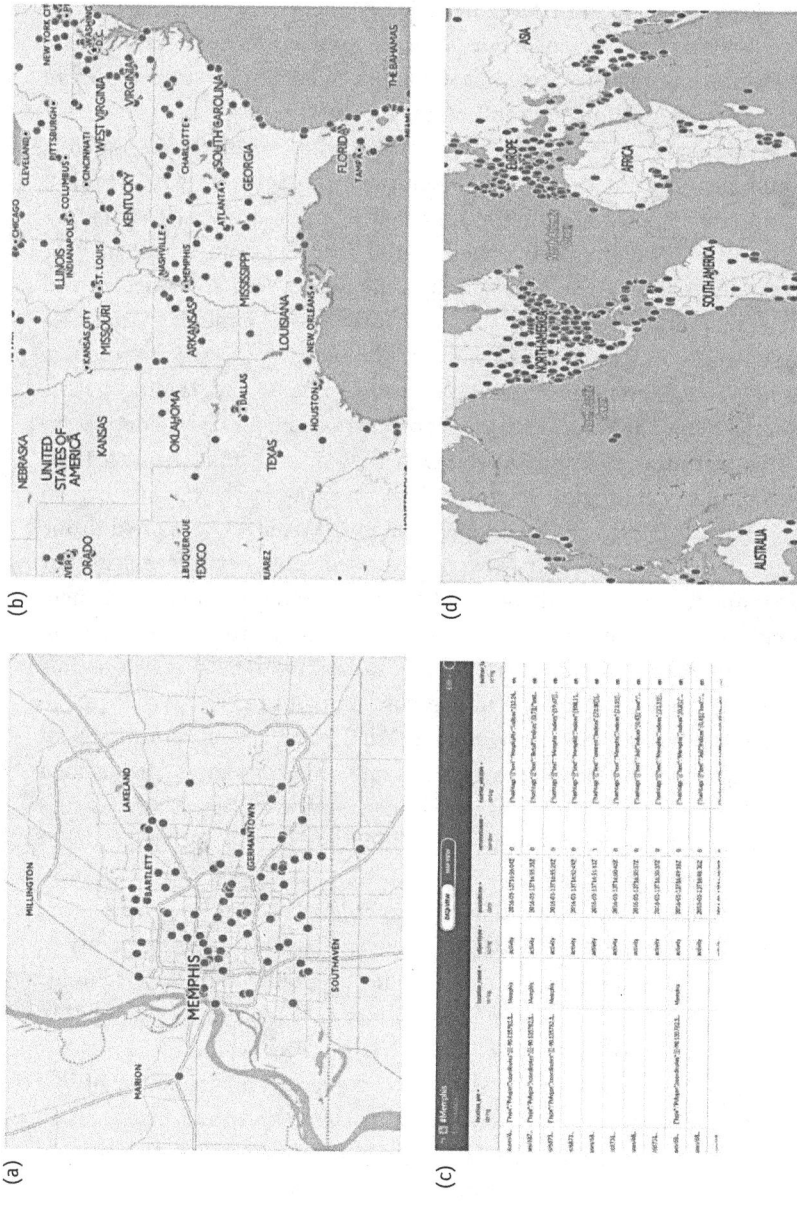

Figure 4.2 Analyzing Twitter Data with Hashtags Memphis and Health using tags for Geodata and CartoDB Dashboard as of January 14, 2016. (a) Contributions from Memphis, (b) Contributions from Southern USA, (c) Attribute table showing geotags, and (d) Contributions from the World.

Four levels of levels of participation and engagement in VGI and citizen science have been conceptualized.[34] Crowdsourcing is the lowest level, where citizens act as sensors and participate in volunteered computing. The next level is distributed intelligence, with citizens serving the role of basic interpreters and engaging in volunteered thinking. In the third level, participatory science, citizens participate in problem definition and data collection. The uppermost level is extreme citizen science. This is where citizens engage in conducting collaborative science and are involved in problem definition, data collection, and analysis.

Recent breakthroughs in GIS/GPS, location-aware technologies, mobile objects databases, embedded technology solutions (computer systems with a dedication function/task) and applications, spatiotemporal models, data science, and citizen science offer new opportunities for the advancement of VGI. For example, standards and methods through the use of Web 2.0 concepts and leading online mapping services that support content development, spatial data sharing, and decision-making have been rapidly evolving.[33,39,40] For example, through Ubuntu, a community-driven operating system, and leading online mapping services such as Google Maps, MapQuest, and OpenStreetMap, communities have significantly contributed text, photos, and images using their knowledge, skills, and strategies. OpenRelief was inspired by the disaster events in Japan in March 2011 (http://www.openrelief.org/). A newly designed drone with an open airframe monitoring capacity was used to gather information for disaster assessment to understand pre- and postdisaster periods in order to help with emergency management and relief efforts. Recent crowdsourcing projects (OpenRelief) have given drones a humanitarian and health purpose. This crowdsourcing technology was used in the post-tsunami recovery of Japan to remap the existing disaster zones (Figure 4.3). AirCasting is another example of a crowdsourcing platform for mapping health and environmental data using a smartphone (http://aircasting.org/map). It consists of wearable citizen sensors that detect changes in the environment and individuals' physiology and provides personalized and aggregated data and information.

Both theoretical and empirical claims have been made about knowledge from VGI and citizen science, and how it enables the visual anchoring of spatiality of spatial processes, critical thinking, and theory building that is accurately grounded in qualitative and quantitative data.[33,41] Flanagin et al.[42] articulated strategies to help discern the credibility of VGI and citizen science. Peer review measures and standards have been implemented to enhance the quality and credibility of VGI and citizen science. A growing number of tools, algorithms, and methods are being used to increase the credibility of VGI and citizen science data. Some common examples include the use of truth and trust metrics (e.g., coloring, accuracy, timeliness, and other metadata features), author trust and credibility, message tagging and indexing, viewing of statistics, use of key words and searches, fact and statistical checking, and data and information gathering through multiple sources, collective intelligence, and social filtering.[42,43]

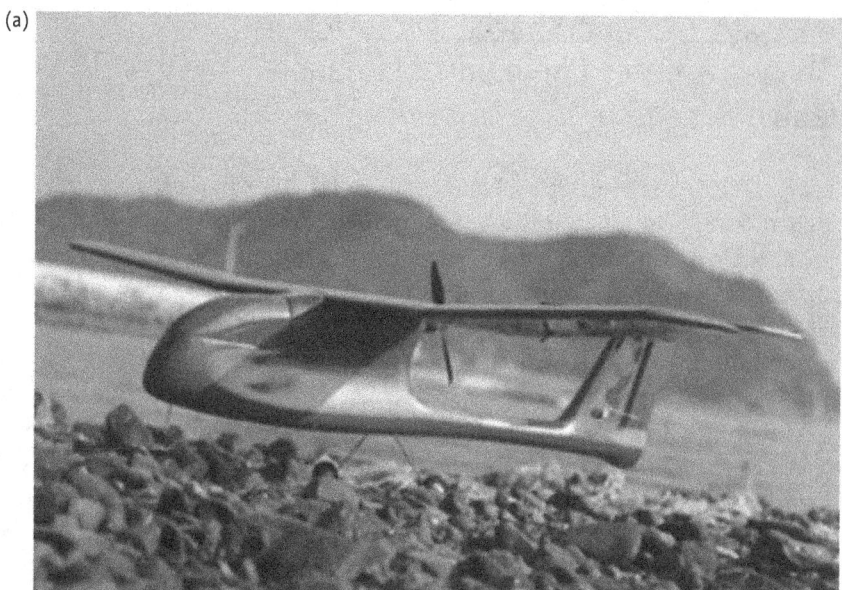

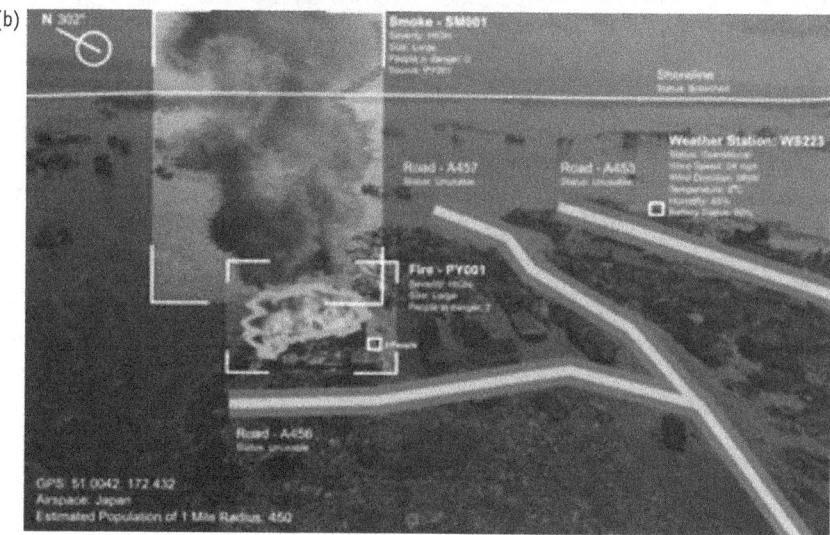

Figure 4.3 The new drone has a monitoring capacity with an open source airframe, which is designed to engage end users and application developers, doctors, and disaster workers and is equipped with sensors, video camera, real-time data-transfer capabilities, and much more. (a) OpenRelief disaster drone and (b) mapping capabilities that reveal road, danger levels, events, and weather conditions. (Courtesy of OpenRelief 2012, http://www.openrelief.org/)

Ten Ways GIS and Spatial Analytics Can Be Used for Community Engaged Health Research

Clearly, GIS/GPS is a major tool and resource for the mapping, targeting, and elimination of health disparities at the community level. There are at least ten specific ways participatory GIS and spatial analytics can be used to support and enhance community-based participatory health disparities research:

1. **Data collection, integration, and management**. Geographic information systems can be used to develop a robust data management and analytical framework. The framework facilitates the creative use of large-scale datasets for health monitoring and tracking and has a strong potential to yield effective multilevel interventions (Figure 4.4). Integration of place, time, and person-level health measures into the design of multilevel interventions through the use of smart and connected mobile health monitoring devices and sensors yields robust geospatial measures. Robust data services and study and analytical protocols must always take data collection, processing and manipulation, quality assurance and quality controls, analysis, sharing, protection, interpretation, storage, and best practices of metadata documentation into consideration.

2. **Activity-level monitoring**. Researchers and communities can use personal air quality or physical activity monitors (wearable motion- or chemical-sensing technologies) equipped with high precision GPS sensors with submeter accuracy to collect robust and unbiased geospatial measures.

3. **Understanding spatial trajectories of life course exposure**. Spatial trajectories of individuals collected with GIS/GPS tools can provide more accurate assessment of exposures to environmental or social factors when integrated with detailed GIS data, especially the data and knowledge of spatial and temporal variations of disease risk factors. Further, GIS/GPS can help researchers and communities establish reliable activity patterns and life course profiles of cohorts with a wide spectrum of environmental exposure at different spatial scales. This requires proper alignments, matching, and harmonization of primary and secondary sources of spatial and temporal datasets.

4. **Quantification of robust and unbiased geospatial measures**. Examples of common geospatial measures include:
   a. Neighborhood safety measure (crime and street lights data)
   b. Food access measure (spatial access such as proximity of restaurants, groceries, and farmers markets; temporal access measures; and spatiotemporal access measures)
   c. Physical activity measure (built environment/street connectivity, land use mix, recreational facilities, walkability score, monitors and trackers)

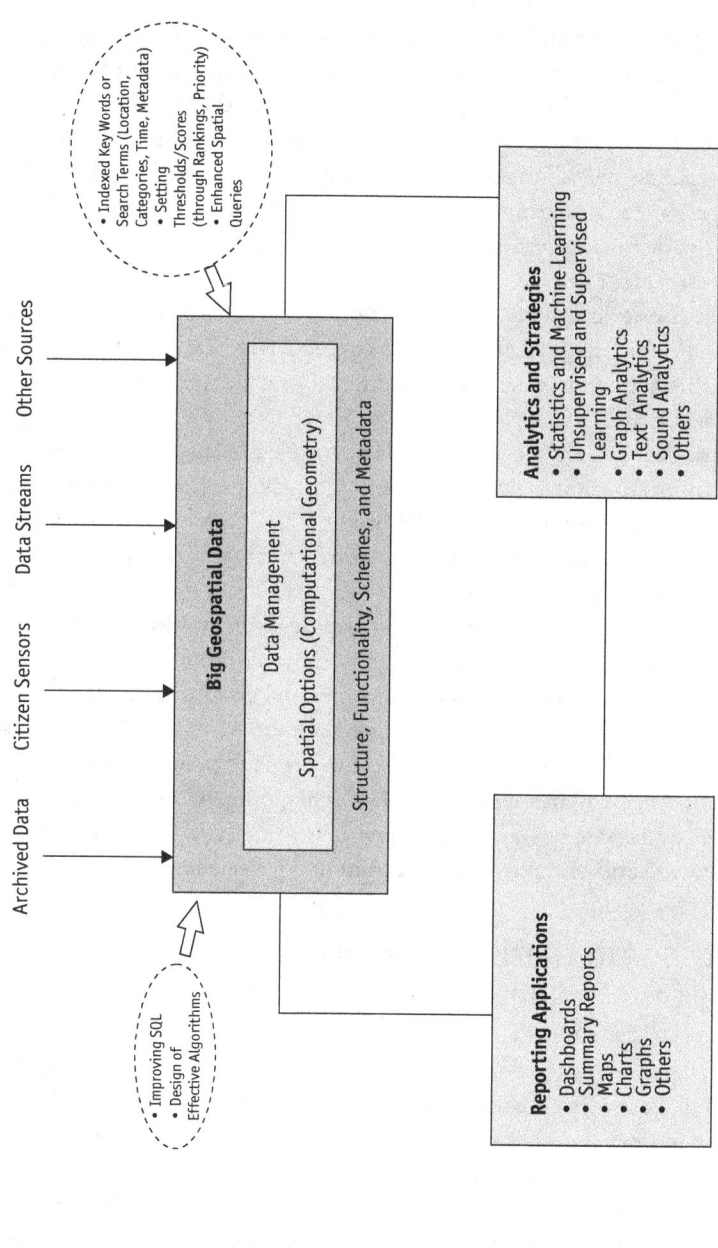

Figure 4.4 A data science approach that integrates big geospatial data, including citizen sensors, data streams, and archived data.[44]

    d. Derive near/proximity and other geospatial measures to support interventions (nearest restaurants, nearest healthcare provider, etc.)

5. **Asset mapping and tracking**. Identifying key community resources (assets) and tracking them in a timely manner can facilitate the understanding of disease dynamics and community burden.

6. **Community mapping and health needs assessment**. For example, participants can create images containing GPS data and map community resources and develop a virtual map showing a transect walk through the community enhanced by photos of specific locations for use in a needs assessment dialogue. Walking and talking to experience place has been promoted as a strong methodology for gathering rich and diverse qualitative data. Figure 4.1 shows a framework that incorporates geospatial measures for community health needs assessment.

7. **Risk assessment and risk management**. Studies have applied risk assessment and risk management concepts to develop effective guidelines and policies to mitigate and manage environmental and occupational hazards and improve human health outcomes.

8. **Mapping disease risk**. GIS/GPS tools can be used to map settings and study locations, participants, activity pattern/routines, health outcomes, healthcare providers, and risk factors. The use of GIS/GPS has been proven to be effective in many scientific reports, primarily in maximizing geographic targeting and intervention options.

9. **GIS-based multicriteria evaluation and decision-making**. Critical community dialogue can lead to valuable input for ranking and assigning weights to important health measures and outcomes and risk factors. The identification of community health priorities using a multicriteria approach helps to target intervention efforts and resources in the right places and direction.

10. **Visualization and map analytics**. Photo mapping, photovoice, data visual analytics and strategies, and other geovisualization tools can aid the effective presentation and communication of community health information.

Challenges, Alternative Approaches, and Ideas for Future Direction

Many challenges exist in the use of GIS and spatial analytic methods in CBPR work, ranging from conceptualization to implementation. For example, in working with theoretical concepts for multilevel interventions, challenges can arise in operationalizing/implementing methods for defining communities, deriving models that are congruent with community culture, and integrating these into multilevel interventions. However, evidence-based and best practices can be drawn on in order to tap into the knowledge and experience of existing transdisciplinary research. Nonetheless, there are many challenges in turning geospatial data and knowledge into meaningful community action plans. Other challenges relate to moderating factors that impact effectiveness and the quality of scientific products generated through community engagement, but reports suggest there are higher returns and benefits in engaging the community than liabilities.

Novel multiscale computational or combinatorial data approaches that link community-engaged research to crowdsourced data need to be expanded. The knowledge generated through data science can play a critical role in informing data management, analytics and strategies, and communication, especially data fusion and harmonization across a wide spectrum of studies and perspectives (Figure 4.4). Some of the key considerations for harmonizing data across cohorts must be considered, including adapting data science approaches, guidelines, and best practices that promote data exchange and sharing. Data managers running data centers for health applications need to think carefully about a number of data and information standardization protocols, such as (1) the use of common primary keys such as patient identifiers, admission identifiers, social security, and driver's license for linking data; (2) identification of secondary identifiers such as birth dates; (3) assignment of unique data identifiers that can easily be matched back to original data or other datasets and across institutions; (4) procedures for updating records and quality checks; (5) validation techniques, quality assurance, and quality control measures; (6) metadata documentation; (7) strong rationale for data standardization and missing records; (8) procedures for data aggregation that enhance protected health information (PHI) and are compliant with the Health Insurance Portability and Accountability Act (HIPAA); and (9) protection of privacy and confidentiality.

Conclusion

Researchers and communities need guidance on data integration, especially with regard to how to use GIS archived and real-time quantitative data to develop actionable health knowledge. Participatory GIS can be used to expand our understanding of disparities in health outcomes within a neighborhood, for data collection and management of health data, for visualization and analysis of health data, and to better understand activity patterns and environmental exposures of individuals over a life course. It can also be used to better understand spatial patterns of infectious diseases so that we may gain fundamental clues, knowledge, and insights as to their causes and controls, especially the relationships between pathogenic factors (causative agents, patients, vectors and hosts) and their geographic environments. Participatory GIS can be used to explore spatiotemporal trends, patterns, and relationships in socioeconomic and environmental factors that may explain disparities in health outcomes. Health disparities can be identified using mapping at different spatial scales. Spatial analysis tools and methods can be employed to obtain insights into the health outcomes of different sociodemographic and economic subgroups, and to ensure that controls and intervention groups are comparable and focused on particular areas or communities affected by health disparities.

References

1. O'Fallon, L. and Dearry, A. "Community-Based Participatory Research as a Tool to Advance Environmental Health Sciences." *Environmental Health Perspectives* 110 Suppl 2 (2002): 155–9.
2. Brown, G., Schebella, M.F. and Weber, D. "Using Participatory GIS to Measure Physical Activity and Urban Park Benefits." *Landscape and Urban Planning* 121 (2014): 34–44.
3. Dennis, S.F., Jr., Gaulocher, S., Carpiano, R.M. and Brown, D. "Participatory Photo Mapping (PPM): Exploring an Integrated Method for Health and Place Research with Young People." *Health and Place* 15.2 (2009): 466–73.
4. Abbott, J., Chambers, R., Dunn, C., et al. "Participatory GIS: Opportunity or Oxymoron?" *Notes on Participatory Learning and Action (PLA Notes)* 33 (1998): 27–34.
5. McCall, M.K. "Seeking Good Governance in Participatory-GIS: A Review of Processes and Governance Dimensions in Applying GIS to Participatory Spatial Planning." *Habitat International* 27 (2013): 549–73.
6. Elwood, S. A. "Negotiating Knowledge Production: The Everyday Inclusions, Exclusions, and Contradictions of Participatory GIS Research." *Professional Geographer* 58.2 (2006): 197–208.
7. Elwood, S. A. "Beyond Cooptation or Resistance: Urban Spatial Politics, Community Organizations, and GIS-Based Spatial Narratives." *Annals of the Association of American Geographers* 96 (2006): 323–41.
8. Dunn, C. "Participatory GIS: A people's GIS?" *Progress in Human Geography* 31 (2007): 617–38.
9. Rouse, L.J., Bergeron, S.J. and Harris, T.M. "Participating in the Geospatial Web: Collaborative Mapping, Social Networks and Participatory GIS." In *The Geospatial Web: How Geobrowsers, Social Software and the Web 2.0 are Shaping the Network Society*, ed. A. Scharl and K. Tochtermann. New York: Springer, 2007; pp. 153–8.
10. Tapp, H., White, L., Steuerwald, M. and Dulin, M. "Use of Community-Based Participatory Research in Primary Care to Improve Healthcare Outcomes and Disparities in Care." *Future Medicine* 2 (2013): 405–19.
11. Oyana, T.J., Garcia, S., Hawthorne, T., Haegele, J.A., Morgan, J. and Young, N. "Nurturing Diversity in STEM Fields Through Geography: The Past, the Present, and the Future." *Journal of STEM Education: Innovations and Research* 16.2 (2015): 20–29.
12. Dulin, M.F., Tapp, H., Smith, H.A., de Hernandez, B.U. and Furuseth, O.J. "A Community Based Participatory Approach to Improving Health in Hispanic Population." *Implementation Science* 6 (2011): 38.
13. Wood, J. "How Green Is My Valley? Desktop Geographic Information Systems as a Community Based Participatory Mapping Tool." *Area* 37.2 (2005): 159–70.
14. Wang, X., Yu, Z., Cinderby, S. and Forrester, J. "Enhancing Participation: Experiences of Participatory Geographic Information Systems in Shanxi Province, China." *Applied Geography* 28.2 (2008): 96–109.
15. Gilmore, M.P. and Young, J.C. "The Use of Participatory Mapping in Ethnobiological Research, Biocultural Conservation, and Community Empowerment: A Case Study from the Peruvian Amazon." *Journal of Ethnobiology* 32.1 (2012): 6–29.
16. Phillips, R.L., Jr., Kinman, E.L. and Schnitzer, P.G. "Using Geographic Information Systems to Understand Health Care Access." *Archives of Family Medicine* 9.10 (2000): 971–8.
17. Chirowodza, A., van Rooyen, H., Joseph, P., Sikotoyi, S., Richter, L. and Coates, T. "Using Participatory Methods and Geographic Information Systems (GIS) to Prepare for an HIV Community-Based Trial in Vulindlela, South Africa." *Journal of Community Psychology* 37.1 (2009): 41–57.

18. Dulin, M.F., Tapp, H., Smith, H.A., et al. "A Trans-Disciplinary Approach to the Evaluation of Social Determinants of Health in a Hispanic Population." *BMC Public Health* 12 (2012): 769.

19. Tanner, A.E., Reboussin, B.A., Mann, L., et al. "Factors Influencing Health Care Access Perceptions and Care-Seeking Behaviors of Immigrant Latino Sexual Minority Men and Transgender Individuals: Baseline Findings from the HOLA Intervention Study." *Journal of Health Care for the Poor and Underserved* 25.4 (2014): 1679–97.

20. Aronson, R.E., Wallis, A.B., O'Campo, P.J. and Schafer, P. "Neighborhood Mapping and Evaluation: A Methodology for Participatory Community Health Initiatives." *Maternal and Child Journal* 11.4 (2007): 373–83.

21. Deeds, B.G., Peralta, L., Willard, N., Ellen, J., Straub, D.M. and Castor, J. "Adolescent Medicine Trials Network for HIV/AIDS Interventions: The Role of Community Resource Assessments in the Development of 15 Adolescent Health Community-Researcher Partnerships. *Progress in Community Health Partnerships: Research, Education, and Action* 2.1 (2008): 31–9.

22. Topmiller, M., Jacquez, F., Vissman, A.T., Raleigh, K. and Miller-Francis, J. "Partnering with Youth to Map Their Neighborhood Environments: A Multilayered GIS Approach." *Family and Community Health* 38.1 (2015): 66–76.

23. McCall, M.K. "Participatory Mapping and Participatory GIS (PGIS) for CRA, Community DRR and Hazard Assessment." *ProVention Consortium, CRA Toolkit, Participation Resources.* Geneva: Switzerland, 2008. <http://www.ppgis.net/wp-content/uploads/2015/06/McCall-2008-ProVention-PGIS-and-CBDRR-Sept08.pdf> (accessed on April 6, 2016).

24. Jankowski, P. "Towards Participatory Geographic Information Systems for Community-Based Environmental Decision Making." *Journal of Environmental Management* 90.6 (2008): 1966–71.

25. Meng, Y. and Malczewski, J. "Web-PPGIS Usability and Public Engagement: A Case Study in Canmore, Alberta, Canada." *Journal of the Urban and Regional Information Systems Association* 22.1 (2010): 55–64.

26. Boroushaki, S. and Malczewski, J. "Participatory GIS: A Web-Based Collaborative GIS and Multicriteria Decision Analysis." *Journal of the Urban and Regional Information Systems Association* 22.1 (2010): 23–32.

27. Margolis, P.A., Stevens, R., Bordley, W., et al. "From Concept to Application: The Impact of a Community-Wide Intervention to Improve the Delivery of Preventive Services to Children." *Pediatrics* 108.3 (2001): e42.

28. Kruger, D.J., Lewis, Y. and Schlemmer, E. "Mapping a Message for Faith Leaders: Encouraging Community Health Promotion with Local Health Data." *Health Promotion Practice* 11.6 (2010): 837–44.

29. Driedger, S.M., Kothari, A., Morrison, J., Sawada, M., Crighton, E.J. and Graham, I.D. "Correction: Using Participatory Design to Develop (Public) Health Decision Support Systems Through GIS." *International Journal of Health Geographics* 6 (2007): 53.

30. Castleden. H., Garvin, T. and Huu-ay-aht First Nation. "Modifying Photovoice for Community-Based Participatory Indigenous Research." *Social Science and Medicine* 66.6 (2008): 1393–1405.

31. Jung, J. "Community Through the Eyes of Children: Blending Child-Centered Research and Qualitative Geovisualization." *Children's Geographies* 13.6 (2015): 722–40.

32. Goodchild, M.F. "Citizens as Censors: The World of Volunteered Geography." *Geojournal* 69.4 (2007): 211–21.

33. Hein, J.R., Evans, J. and Jones, P. "Mobile Methodologies: Theory, Technology and Practice." *Geography Compass* 2.5 (2008): 1266–85.

34. Haklay, M. 2012. "Citizen Science and Volunteered Geographic Information: Overview and Typology of Participation." In *Crowdsourcing Geographic Knowledge: Volunteered Geographic Information (VGI) in Theory and Practice*, ed. D. Siu, S. Elwood and M. Goodchild. Dordrecht, Netherlands: Springer, 2012; pp. 105–22.

35. Elwood, S., Goodchild, M.F. and Sui, D.Z. "Researching Volunteered Geographic Information: Spatial Data, Geographic Research, and New Social Practice." *Annals of Association of American Geographers* 102.3 (2012): 571–90.

36. Dankwa-Mullan, I. and Maddox, Y.T. "Embarking on a Science Vision for Health Disparities Research." *American Journal of Public Health* 105.S3 (2015): S369–71. doi: 10.2105/AJPH.2015.302756

37. Matthias, H., Hoßfeld, T., and Phuoc T. "Anatomy of a Crowdsourcing Platform: Using the Example of Microworkers.com." 5th IEEE *International Conference on Innovative Mobile and Internet Services in Ubiquitous Computing* (IMIS 2011), June 2011. doi: 10.1109/IMIS.2011.89

38. Tulloch, D.L. "Is VGI participation? From Vernal Pools to Video Games." *GeoJournal* 72.3 (2008): 161–71.

39. Rinner, C., Keßler, C. and Andrulis, S. "The Use of Web 2.0 Concepts to Support Deliberation in Spatial Decision-Making." *Computers, Environment and Urban Systems* 32.5 (2008): 386–95.

40. Coleman, D., Georgiadou, Y. and Labonte, J. "Volunteered Geographic Information: The Nature and Motivation of Produsers." *International Journal of Spatial Data Infrastructures Research* 4 (2009): 332–58.

41. Kwan, M. and Knigge, L. "Doing Qualitative Research Using GIS: An Oxymoronic Endeavor?" *Environment and Planning A* 38.11 (2006): 1999–2002.

42. Flanagin, A.J. and Metzger, M.J. "The Credibility of Volunteered Geographic Information." *GeoJournal* 72.3 (2008): 137–48.

43. West, A.G., Chang, J., Venkatasubramanian, K.K. and Lee, I. "Trust in Collaborative Web Applications." *Future Generation Computer Systems* 28.8 (2012): 1238–51. <http://dx.doi.org/10.1016/j.future.2011.02.007>

44. Oyana T.J. and Margai, M.F. "Data Science: Understanding Computing Systems and Analytics for Big Data." In *Spatial Analysis: Statistics, Visualization, and Computational Methods*. Boca Raton, Florida: CRC Press, Taylor and Francis, 2016; pp. 267–94.

5

Ethical Issues in Community-Based Participatory Research Studies

STEVEN S. COUGHLIN, PHD AND LELAND K. ACKERSON, SCD

Respect for communities and individuals, distributional justice, and the provision of benefits are core values and principles of community-based participatory research (CBPR). Additional values and ethical principles also underlie this approach to research in diverse communities (for example, social justice, power sharing, transparency, and trust). The ethical issues in CBPR include those that arise in all human subjects research (for example, the need for institutional review board [IRB] review and the obligation to minimize risks and potential harms while providing benefits to research participants) and additional issues that arise because of the focus on community concerns and benefits. Other ethical challenges arise because of the collaborative approach to research that involves working closely with community partners in all aspects of the research process. As highlighted throughout this book, community members, organizational representatives, and academic researchers participate in and share control over all phases of the CBPR research process including assessment and definition of the problem; selection of research methods; data collection, analysis, and interpretation; and dissemination of findings. While this collaborative approach to research can raise novel ethical challenges, it also helps to minimize potential problems such as the stigmatization of communities due to the release of sensitive data by researchers without prior consultation, communities feeling further marginalized by research, or researchers advancing their academic careers at the expense of community members, who may be left feeling overresearched or misled.[1] The CBPR approach minimizes the likelihood of research that is irrelevant or insensitive to community concerns. The inclusion of community members in the research team as equal partners helps to protect the community from harm and exploitation and supports self-determination.[2]

Community collaboration and involvement is both an ethical feature of CBPR and part of the definition of this justice-oriented approach to research. Collaboration requires sharing of experience and leadership (reciprocity), transparency, and the development of trust between academic researchers and community partners, all of which have ethical implications.[2-4] Through the hiring and training of community members, CBPR can help build community capacity to address health concerns, help to develop resources, and redress prior research that may not have offered direct benefits for participating communities.[5]

Minimizing Risks and Providing Benefits

The ethical conduct of CBPR research requires that risks and potential harms to individual research participants and the community as a whole be considered. Community members may be harmed by research findings, either because they internalize negative research results about their community or because data collected for one purpose are later used for another purpose without consent.[6] Potential adverse effects of community-based research include labeling of individuals and community, stigmatization, discrimination, increased insurance rates, and loss of community income.[7] The development of a community advisory board can help ensure that CBPR projects are sensitive to community concerns and that risks are minimized.

Healthy community advisory boards can serve several purposes, in addition to protecting the interests of potentially vulnerable populations who are involved in research projects. The Latino Family Advisory Board in Baltimore was developed in order to improve the experience of Spanish-speaking Latino families within the healthcare system at an urban health clinic with a high number of Latino patients.[8] The Board participants were specifically recruited from the clinic population to represent people from different groups within the Spanish-speaking population. This included those with disabled children, those who had difficulty using the healthcare system, those who had a long relationship with the clinic, and those who were new patients. Given proper support and training, this board provided important recommendations regarding the design of a new emergency department, a community health assessment, and a research project designed to reduce childhood overweight.

Providing benefits is also important. In order for CBPR projects to be ethical, community needs and priorities must be seriously considered and there should be tangible community benefits.[2] Both the process of doing the collaborative research and study outcomes can provide benefits, although not every CBPR project will have positive findings. The aim of CBPR research and evaluation projects is to contribute knowledge that leads to positive social change and the enhancement of community well-being.[9] The latter includes the improvement of community health and reduction or elimination of health disparities. Community-based participatory research can empower communities to address the root causes of inequality and identify their own problems and appropriate solutions. Community-based participatory research has been shown to be helpful for addressing health disparities and inequities in communities that are socially disadvantaged, marginalized, stigmatized, or that have suffered historical injustices.[10] However, it can be challenging to produce benefits for participating communities when project funds are insufficient for direct compensation or service provision.[11]

RECRUITMENT STRATEGIES

Studies of hard-to-reach populations (for example, homeless persons, undocumented workers who are not authorized to work in the country, and injection drug users) often use persons who are members of the local community or group to recruit study participants. Such recruitment strategies (for example, peer-driven recruitment or network sampling) are useful for accessing human subjects, but they also raise several ethical issues and influence the balance of risks and potential benefits of the research.[12] For the recruiters, their role may provide opportunities for employment and developing useful skills. For researchers, the use of recruiters from the local community can enhance access to potential research participants who reflect local health needs and cultural norms. The ethical challenges potentially raised by peer-driven recruitment and network-sampling strategies include the potential for recruiters to exploit their peers in the community or group in an effort to meet recruitment quotas, and for the privacy and confidentiality of research participants to be more readily violated.[12] Peer-driven recruitment is often used in small and intimate communities where breaches of privacy and confidentiality may be particularly apt to occur without appropriate precautions. There may also be a potential for some research participants or whole subgroups of people to be excluded from the research due to biases on the part of the recruiters. To minimize such problems, education and training of research staff is essential. Molyneux et al.[13] pointed to the need for participatory training for staff from the beginning of a study employing peer-driven recruitment, including training on what health research is and how participants' rights should be protected. It is also important for peer-driven recruitment to be part of a comprehensive community engagement process that takes into account scientific constraints and local needs and interests.[12]

The role of community-based organizations in the recruitment of research participants, which is common in CBPR studies, can also raise ethical concerns.[14] For example, a community-based organization may enter into a partnership with academic researchers, and use their resources in order to assist with the recruitment of participants, and the anticipated benefits may never become a reality. In addition, a community-based organization's collaboration could be viewed as a "stamp of approval" by potential research participants, even though the organization may not have the authority to formally consent to a community's participation in research.[14] Clients of the community-based organization may also feel compelled to participate in the study in order to maintain a good relationship with the organization, particularly if they are recruited by a community-based organization staff member.[14]

Researchers in a community-based chronic disease intervention study noticed this potential for coercion among participants in veterans' organizations.[15] Speculating that many veterans have a propensity to sacrifice their own needs for those of the greater good, the team implemented a two-tier consent system. At the first tier, a post leader from the veteran's organization identified potential participants for the research and asked that they take part in the study. At the second tier, group members who agreed to take part were asked to attend an individual 90-minute session in which they were fully informed of their rights as a potential research participant and were given strong assurances that their post leaders would never be told which members participated and which did not. While the majority of members still agreed to participate, a number did not indicating to the researchers that the two-tier system did its part in assuring that potential participants could maintain their autonomy during the process.

Other studies have highlighted the potential for negative effects, not only on participants in community based studies but also on the community members who do the research. One such case involved research into cervical cancer knowledge and screening practices in a community near Cape Town, South Africa.[12] The recruitment protocol was designed so that female members of the research team would locate and interview randomly selected women in the target town. Even though the interviewers were from the same community, they were often very distressed to be confronted by signs of severe poverty, malnutrition, and domestic violence among the participants that they met through their research. As a result of preliminary feedback, psychological support services were added to the research protocol in order to assist the team members. In addition, a comprehensive tailored list of support services available to all community residents was created in order to allow the interviewers to recommend help for research participants who were clearly in need.

DISSEMINATING RESULTS

The joint interpretation and dissemination of research findings are important aspects of community autonomy and can also influence the balance of risks and potential benefits. Tension can arise in CBPR studies when academic researchers seek to disseminate potentially stigmatizing research findings against the objections of community partners who are particularly concerned about the well-being of their community and its individual members. Community partners are often concerned about control of research findings that put their community in a negative light when published or reported by the media.[16] For example, some studies have focused on gang-related violence, prostitution, and environmental waste. Academic researchers may give greater weight to the need to maintain scientific objectivity and desire to publish findings in the peer-reviewed scientific literature so as to further their career. Such conflicts require careful negotiation and discussions among the research partners in order to reconcile different perspectives and to ensure that social and economic risks to communities are minimized.

Informed Consent

Informed consent provisions in health studies ensure that research participants make a free choice and also give institutions the legal authorization to proceed with the research. Investigators must disclose information that potential participants use to decide whether to consent to the study. This includes the purpose of the research, the scientific procedures, anticipated risks and benefits, any inconveniences or discomfort, and the participant's right to refuse participation or to withdraw from the research at any time (45 Code of Federal Regulations [CFR] 46). Informed consent requirements may be waived in exceptional circumstances when obtaining consent is impractical, the risks are minimal, and the risks and potential benefits of the research have been carefully considered by an independent review committee. For example, in some health studies involving the analysis of large databases of routinely collected information (for example, insurance claims data), it may not be feasible to recontact patients to ask them for their informed consent. Risks and potential harms in such studies may be very low, and risks may be further reduced by omitting personal identifiers from the computer databases. Managing informed consent can be complex in CBPR studies where community members both assist with the research and serve as research participants. Managing those dual roles can complicate the process of obtaining informed consent.[2,17]

Special considerations for obtaining informed consent may arise in public health studies of socioeconomically deprived or marginalized people. People who have limited access to health care may misunderstand an invitation to participate in a study as an opportunity to receive medical care. In addition, they may be reluctant to refuse participation when the researcher is viewed as someone in a position of authority, such as a physician or university professor. Socioeconomically deprived people may also be more motivated to participate in studies involving financial incentives for participation. A further issue is that there is often a need to translate informed consent statements into a language other than English. The important issues that arise in international research conducted by researchers from countries such as the United States and Great Britain in developing countries have also received considerable attention.

In CBPR studies, there may be a need to obtain community consent, such as when collaborative studies are proposed that focus on sovereign Native American communities or other indigenous populations. To an increasing extent, Native American tribes require studies to be approved by tribal leadership and they may also have their own IRB. For some studies, obtaining community consent may be challenging. It may not be clear who should represent or speak on behalf of a diverse community or multiple groups. In Greenland, for example, what constitutes a community varies throughout the country. Greenlanders may identify their community as a geographic location, by the language they speak, by where they grew up, by how long they have lived in Greenland, or by what kinds of activities they participate in.[18]

Distributional Justice

Community-based participatory research studies also raise issues related to distributional justice. Smith and Blumenthal[19] noted that meaningful community participation in research can help protect communities from exploitation. And CBPR can help to transfer power from academic institutions and public agencies to unempowered low-income and minority communities.[19] Academic institutions often receive large portions of government grants and cooperative agreements awarded for community-based research. The amount of funding given to community organizations that are partners in a project is often far less than that received by the university. Academic researchers can address such concerns by awarding subcontracts to community organizations based on the importance of their contribution to the study and by hiring community members to help collect the data and carry out educational interventions. In studies that use lay health advisors or "promotoras" to deliver educational interventions to community members, community advisory boards can be consulted to help determine a fair honorarium for the workers.

It is also important to consider the sustainability of health interventions that are found to be effective, after the research grant or cooperative agreement ends. Community organizations are often vital to helping to sustain effective interventions that provide benefits to community members. Their insider knowledge can often facilitate the integration of a program into existing health systems.[20] Issues surrounding the sustainability of programs can arise in developed countries such as the United States and Canada, but the frequent lack of adequate healthcare resources in low- and middle-income countries raises additional challenges. For example, in a family- and church-based HIV prevention intervention in rural Kenya, community members began to ask community advisory council members for healthcare services beyond the scope of the intervention.[21] In addition, it was not entirely clear whether the churches would be able to sustain the intervention if it were found to be effective. In general, low-cost interventions such as those that rely on volunteers are more likely to be sustainable by community organizations.

Privacy and Confidentiality Protection

Health researchers and community members who participate in CBPR studies have important obligations to reduce potential harms and risks to participants by rigorously protecting the confidentiality of their health information. Specific measures taken by researchers to protect the confidentiality of health information include keeping records under lock and key, limiting access to confidential records, discarding personal identifiers from data collection forms and computer files whenever feasible, and training staff in the importance of privacy and confidentiality protection. Other measures that have been employed to safeguard health information include encrypting computer databases, limiting geographic detail, and suppressing cells in tabulated data where the number of cases in the cell is small.

In the United States, the Health Insurance Portability and Accountability Act (HIPAA) of 1996 took effect early in 2004 after extensive discussion. The regulations provide protection for the privacy of certain individually identifiable health data, referred to as protected health information. The privacy rules permit disclosures without individual authorization to public health authorities authorized by law to collect or receive the information for the purpose of preventing or controlling disease, injury, or disability, including public health practice activities such as surveillance.

Institutional Review Board Review

The purpose of research ethics committees or IRBs is to ensure that studies involving human research participants are designed to conform to relevant ethical standards and that the rights and welfare of participants are protected. Human subjects review by such committees ensures that studies have a favorable balance of potential benefits and risks, participants are selected equitably, and procedures for obtaining informed consent are adequate. In the United States, federal regulations to protect human research subjects (45 CFR 46) have resulted in a complex IRB system. Similar safeguards exist in Canada, Great Britain, and many other countries.

Flicker et al.[1] conducted a content analysis of forms and guidelines used by IRBs in the United States and research ethics boards in Canada. They found that the ethical review forms and guidelines operate within a biomedical framework (for example, by focusing on assessing risks and benefits to individuals and not to communities) and rarely take into account CBPR principles and practices. Only 5 of the 30 forms reviewed asked about the dissemination of research findings. Flicker et al.[1] recommended that IRBs and research ethics boards engaged in reviewing CBPR protocols be provided with basic training in the principles of CBPR; that they should mandate that CBPR projects provide signed memoranda of understanding that outline the goals of the project, principles of partnership, decision-making processes, roles and responsibilities of partners, and guidelines for how the partnership will handle and disseminate data; and that they require CBPR projects to document the process by which key decisions regarding research design were made and how the affected communities were consulted. Shore[22] argued that academic institutions should establish guidelines for assessing the appropriateness of CBPR projects, which tend to be highly process oriented.

Special considerations exist for IRB review when academic researchers seek to partner with sovereign Native American tribes and nations.[23] Researchers generally have to submit research protocols and informed consent statements to multiple IRBs including the one at their own academic institution, the regional Indian Health Service IRB, and the National Indian Health Service IRB. In addition, many tribes have their own IRB or other requirements for review and approval of proposed research. Historical abuses and more recent violations of tribal information and intellectual property rights have led to more stringent requirements for data sharing and IRB review.[23,24] Sovereign tribal governments have the power to disapprove research proposals or to condition their approval. Many tribal governments have codified the terms under which research affecting their people, culture, and homeland will be conducted.[23] Researchers seeking to undertake research within the Ho-Chunk Nation's territory, for example, must apply for and secure a permit in accordance with the Ho-Chunk Nation's Tribal Research Code. The Navajo Nation has its own IRB and Human Research Code. Each Native American nation and tribe is unique, and tribal government decisions may be made with different formal and informal processes.[23]

All CBPR researchers must learn to strike a balance between research designed to improve the lives of community members and protection of potentially vulnerable communities and individuals. This struggle is exemplified by one study in a community of Alaska Natives.[25] Fearful about reports of high levels of polychlorinated biphenyls (PCBs) in blood samples, several Yupik Alaska Native communities on Saint Lawrence Island in the Bering Strait asked a statewide environmental health advocacy agency, Alaska Community Action on Toxics, to help research the concentration of contaminants in breast milk among local mothers. Communities wanted this information in order to be able to change personal behaviors to avoid harm to newborn children and to advocate for help in cleaning up sources of contaminants. The collaboration was successful in enlisting the help of researchers from several universities, who secured federal grant money to study the issue. However, the research program was repeatedly blocked over the course of a decade by the Alaska Area Institutional Review Board (AAIRB), the agency overseen by the Indian Health Service to protect the concerns of Alaska Natives taking part in research studies. This occurred despite the fact that the relevant tribal councils had provided letters of support and that the researchers had responded thoughtfully to AAIRB concerns about how the data would be collected and used, and the techniques being used to ensure the cultural appropriateness of the project.

Academic researchers must work with community partners to obtain ethical approval from their respective institutions and provide whatever ethical training is needed for community partners to seek ethical approval.[18] All research personnel should be provided with appropriate human subjects protection training.[26]

The community advisory board can help ensure that the training is culturally sensitive and provided in a way that is understandable to the community research partners. Substantial time may be needed to provide training in human subjects research ethics and to obtain ethical approval from multiple IRBs. It can be helpful for academic researchers to arrange for community partners to meet with an IRB administrator to lessen the mystique of IRB oversight, clarify the goals and process of the IRB, and further mutual trust.[16]

Discussion

The majority of CBPR research and evaluation projects lie within the domain of public health. Public health is primarily concerned with the health of the entire population, rather than the health of individuals, and emphasizes the promotion of health and the prevention of disease and disability and the collection of qualitative and quantitative health data.[27,28] Public health also recognizes the multidimensional nature of health determinants and the complex interactions of biological, behavioral, social, and environmental factors in striving to develop effective interventions.[27]

The risks and potential harms of public health interventions include ineffective, counterproductive, or harmful interventions; unanticipated consequences; and labeling or stigmatizing of individuals and communities. Undue stress on the individual's role in the cause of illness could lead to a "blame the victim" mentality. The dilemma is how to advise people that they might be at risk for potentially serious health complications without labeling them, contributing to their anxiety, or adversely affecting their well-being.

Ethical considerations for prevention trials and community interventions include an assessment of risks and benefits, the need for voluntary participation and avoidance of excessive incentives, and justice-related issues. There is a need for sensitivity to ethnic and cultural habits and norms and to avoid "top-down" planning, in which the health concerns and self-defined information needs of the target population are ignored in favor of professional preoccupations and concerns. Such concerns have been successfully addressed through CBPR. Ethical issues in health communication include the need to avoid conflicts of interest, to present facts about health hazards or health opportunities in a truthful, balanced, and timely fashion, and to avoid distorting the facts or concealing ambiguities in the scientific evidence.

The CBPR approach emphasizes colearning, the reciprocal transfer of expertise between community members and academic partners, and mutual ownership of research products.[10] The process of colearning brings academic researchers and community members together and empowers community participants to increase control and self-ownership of their health and lives.[29] Community members, organizational representatives, and academic researchers participate in and share control over all phases of the research process, including assessment, definition of the problem, selection of research methods, data collection, and analysis, interpretation, and dissemination of findings. The CBPR research paradigm represents a fundamental shift in academic researchers' views of community residents, from patients and research subjects who may benefit from medical advances to essential partners who can help explain the social determinants of illness and energize their communities to develop effective, sustainable interventions to improve health and eliminate health disparities.[30] Researchers have generally found these methods, which seek to empower communities and increase community benefits, lead to robust ethical research practices, even though important ethical challenges arise in CBPR related to community representation, distribution of resources and potential benefits, and dissemination of sensitive information.[31]

Building and sustaining trust is essential in all aspects of CBPR studies.[32] Community members may distrust researchers from outside organizations because of a history of racism, marginalization of minority communities by healthcare systems, or earlier experiences of researchers entering communities, collecting data, and leaving without providing any direct benefits or even informing residents of the results of the research.[30]

Some authors have argued that the ethical principles identified in the landmark Belmont Report, "Ethical Principles and Guidelines for the Protection of Human Subjects of Research" (respect for persons, beneficence, and justice), do not provide a comprehensive guide to research ethics in CBPR.[2,33] Respect for persons requires that an individual's decision to become a research participant must be voluntary and that special protections are afforded for those who lack the capacity to make such decisions. Beneficence requires researchers to do no harm (which is often listed separately as a principle of nonmaleficence) and to minimize risks and potential harms to human subjects while providing benefits. The principle of justice, in its various forms, requires researchers to pay attention to the fair or equitable distribution of risks and benefits. Persons who bear the risks of research should be among the first to benefit from the information gained from the research. Community-based participatory research and community-engaged research are consistent with a broader conception of justice that includes social justice.[34] Malone et al.[35] proposed expanding the number of ethical principles outlined in the Belmont Report by adding a principle of respect for communities. Whereas IRB requirements and regulations for the protection of human subjects generally focus on research participants as individuals, CBPR views research participants as both individuals and as part of a community of individuals.[33] When writing the Belmont Report and helping to craft United States federal regulations, the National Commission did not anticipate that translational research would be conducted with the active engagement of individuals and communities.[36] Although groups or communities are not human subjects under the United States federal regulations governing research, academic and community partnerships must address these issues as part of comprehensive protection for human subjects. Ross et al.[37] provided a helpful framework for considering risks in community-engaged research including risks due either to the research process or its outcomes. They also distinguished between established communities (groups that have their own organization structure and leadership outside of the research) and unstructured groups that exist because of a shared trait but do not have a defined leadership).[37] Risks to individual members of a group can occur whether or not a particular individual actually participates in the research.[38] Despite continued advances in clarifying the ethics of CBPR, there remains a need for additional conceptual work to develop a comprehensive framework for ensuring research integrity in CBPR.[2]

References

1. Flicker, S., Travers, R., Guta, A., et al. "Ethical Dilemmas in Community-Based Participatory Research: Recommendations for Institutional Review Boards." *Journal of Urban Health* 84 (2007): 478–93.
2. Mikesell, L., Bromley, E. and Khodyakov, D. "Ethical Community-Engaged Research: A Literature Review." *American Journal of Public Health* 103 (2013): e7–14.
3. Macaulay, A.C., Delormier, T., McComber, A.M., et al. "Participatory Research with Native Community of Kahnawake Creates Innovative Code of Research Ethics." *Canadian Journal of Public Health* 89 (1998): 105–8.
4. Maiter, S., Simich, L., Jacobson, N. and Wise, J. "Reciprocity: An Ethic for Community-Based Participatory Action Research." *Action Research* 6 (2008): 305–25.
5. Kennedy, C., Vogel, A., Goldberg-Freeman, C., et al. "Faculty Perspectives on Community-Based Research: I See This Still as a Journey." *Journal of Empirical Research on Human Research Ethics* 4 (2009): 3–16.
6. Glass, K.C. and Kaufert, J. "Research Ethics Review and Aboriginal Community Values: Can the Two Be Reconciled?" *Journal of Empirical Research on Human Research Ethics* 2 (2007): 25–40.
7. Williams, R.L., Willging, C.E., Quintero, G., et al. "Ethics of Health Research in Communities: Perspectives from the Southwestern United States." *Annals of Family Medicine* 8 (2010): 433–9.
8. DeCamp, L.R., Polk, S., Chrismer, M.C., Giusti, F., Thompson, D.A. and Sibinga, E. "Health Care Engagement of Limited English Proficient Latino Families: Lessons Learned from Advisory Board Development." *Progress in Community Health Partnerships* 9 (2015): 521–30.
9. Jacklin, K. and Kinoshameg, P. "Developing a Participatory Aboriginal Health Research Project: Only if It's Going to Mean Something." *Journal of Empirical Research on Human Research Ethics* 3 (2008): 53–67.
10. Viswanathan, M., Eng, E., Ammerman, A., et al. *Community-Based Participatory Research: Assessing the Evidence.* Evidence Report/Technology Assessment, no. 99. Rockville, MD: Agency for Healthcare Research and Quality, 2004.
11. Israel, B.A., Parker, E.A., Rowe, Z., et al. "Community-Based Participatory Research: Lessons Learned from the Centers for Children's Environmental Health and Disease Prevention Research." *Environmental Health Perspectives* 113 (2005): 1463–71.
12. Simon, C. and Mosavel, M. "Community Members as Recruiters of Human Subjects: Ethical Considerations." *American Journal of Bioethics* 10 (2010): 3–11.
13. Molyneux, S., Kamuya, D. and Marsh, V. "Community Members Employed on Research Projects Face Crucial, Often Under-Recognized, Ethical Dilemmas." *American Journal of Bioethics* 10 (2010): 24–6.

14. Anderson, E.E. "The Role of Community-Based Organizations in the Recruitment of Human Subjects: Ethical Considerations." *American Journal of Bioethics* 10 (2010): 20–21.

15. Whittle, J., Fletcher, K.E., Morzinski, J., et al. "Ethical Challenges in a Randomized Controlled Trial of Peer Education Among Veterans Service Organizations." *Journal of Empirical Research on Human Research Ethics* 5 (2010): 43–51.

16. Hyatt, R.R., Gute, D.M., Pirie, A., et al. "Transferring Knowledge About Human Subjects Protections and the Role of Institutional Review Boards in a Community-Based Participatory Research Project." *American Journal of Public Health* 99 Suppl 3 (2009): S526–31.

17. Khanlou, N. and Peter, E. "Participatory Action Research: Considerations for Ethical Review." *Social Science and Medicine* 60 (2005): 2333–40.

18. Rink, E., Montgomery-Andersen, R., Koch, A., et al. "Ethical Challenges and Lessons Learned from Inuuluataarneq—Having the Good Life Study: A Community-Based Participatory Research Project in Greenland." *Journal of Empirical Research on Human Research Ethics* 8 (2013): 110–8.

19. Smith, S.A. and Blumenthal, D.S. "Community Health Workers Support Community-Based Participatory Research Ethics: Lessons Learned Along the Research-to-Practice-to-Community Continuum." *Journal of Health Care for the Poor and Underserved* 23 Suppl. 4 (2012): 77–87.

20. Wallerstin, N. and Duran, B. "Community-Based Participatory Research Contributions to Intervention Research: The Intersection of Science and Practice to Improve Health Equity." *American Journal of Public Health* 100 Suppl 1 (2010): S40–6.

21. Puffer, E.S., Pian, J., Sikkema, K.J., et al. "Developing a Family-Based HIV Prevention Intervention in Rural Kenya: Challenges in Conducting Community-Based Participatory Research." *Journal of Empirical Research on Human Research Ethics* 8 (2013): 119–28.

22. Shore, N. "Re-conceptualizing the Belmont Report: A Community-Based Participatory Research Perspective." *Journal of Community Practice* 14 (2006): 5–26.

23. Harding, A., Harper, B., Stone, D., et al. "Conducting Research with Tribal Communities: Sovereignty, Ethics, and Data-Sharing Issues." *Environmental Health Perspectives* 120: (2012): 6–10.

24. Balwin, J.A., Johnson, J.L., and Bennally, C.C. "Building Partnerships Between Indigenous Communities and Universities: Lessons Learned in HIV/AIDS and Substance Abuse Prevention Research." *American Journal of Public Health* 99 Suppl 1 (2009): S77–82.

25. Saxton, D.I., Brown, P., Seguinot-Medina, S., et al. "Environmental Health and Justice and the Right to Research: Institutional Review Board Denials of Community-Based Chemical Biomonitoring of Breast Milk." *Environmental Health* 14 (2015): 90.

26. Ross, L.F., Loup, A., Nelson, R.M., et al. "Nine Key Functions for a Human Subjects Protection Program for Community-Engaged Research: Points to Consider." *Journal of Empirical Research on Human Research Ethics* 5 (2010): 33–47.

27. Childress, J.F., Faden, R.R., Gaare, R.D., et al. "Public Health Ethics: Mapping the Terrain." *Journal of Law, Medicine and Ethics* 30 (2002): 170–8.

28. Kass, N.E. "Public Health Ethics: From Foundations and Frameworks to Justice and Global Public Health." *Journal of Law, Medicine and Ethics* 32 (2004): 232–42.

29. Gray, N., Ore de Boehm, C., Farnsworth, A. and Wolf, D. "Integration of Creative Expression into Community Based Participatory Research and Health Promotion with Native Americans." *Family and Community Health* 33 (2010): 186–92.

30. Horowitz, C.R., Robinson, M. and Seifer, S. "Community-Based Participatory Research from the Margin to the Mainstream: Are Researchers Prepared?" *Circulation* 19 (2009): 2633–42.

31. Lynch, J. and Mitchell, M. "Community Engagement and the Ethics of Global, Translational Research: A Response to Sofaer and Eyal." *American Journal of Bioethics* 10 (2010): 37–8.

32. Israel, B.A., Schulz, A.J., Parker E.A., et al. "Review of Community-Based Research. "Assessing Partnership Approaches to Improve Public Health." *Annual Reviews of Public Health* (1998): 173–202.

33. Brown, P., Morello-Frosch, R., Brody, J.G., et al. "Institutional Review Board Challenges Related to Community-Based Participatory Research on Human Exposure to Environmental

Toxins: A Case Study." *Environmental Health* 9 (2010): 39. <http://www.ehjournal.net/content/9/1/39>

34. Powers, M. and Faden, R.R., eds. *Social Justice: The Moral Foundations of Public Health and Health Policy*. New York: Oxford University Press, 2006.

35. Malone, R.E., Fann, V.B., Yerger, N.D., et al. "It's Like Tuskegee in Reverse: A Case Study of Ethical Tensions in Institutional Review Board Review of Community-Based Participatory Research." *American Journal of Public Health* 96 (2006): 1914–9.

36. Dresser, R. *When Science Offers Salvation: Patient Advocacy and Research Ethics*. New York: Oxford University Press, 2001.

37. Ross, L.F., Loup, A., Nelson, R.M., et al. "Human Subjects Protection in Community-Engaged Research: A Research Ethics Framework." *Journal of Empirical Research on Human Research Ethics* 5 (2010): 5–17.

38. Hausman, D. "Group Risks, Risks to Groups, and Group Engagement in Genetics Research." *Kennedy Institute of Ethics Journal* 17 (2008): 351–69.

6

Community-Based Participatory Research Studies in Faith-Based Settings

HEATHER KITZMAN-ULRICH, PHD AND CHERYL L. HOLT, PHD

Particularly in minority communities, faith-based organizations (FBOs), such as churches, often act as portals for support and services beyond worship. This chapter discusses the role of FBOs in community engagement and specifically in health promotion. In this chapter, research using community-engaged and community-based participatory research (CBPR) processes in faith-based settings is discussed, and implications for conducting community-engaged health promotion in the FBO setting are highlighted. Recommendations for future research are also provided.

Terminology

The study of religion and its influence on health has grown in prominence as researchers and public health professionals explore ways to prevent and manage chronic diseases. To reflect spiritual and religious constructs, the terms "religion," "spirituality," and "religiosity" are often used interchangeably, although they represent distinct but, at times, overlapping concepts. Religion, defined as the practice of a specific theology, can include participation in a social organization whose members share similar theological beliefs and practices.[1] On the other hand, spirituality refers to a more personal relationship or to a connection with the divine that is larger than oneself.[2] Other terms commonly found in the scientific and popular literature, "religiosity" and "religiousness," often refer to the broad domain of religious practice, rituals, and beliefs. In this chapter, the term "religion/spirituality" is used to represent both religious practice and spirituality constructs.

Religion/Spirituality–Health Connection

Over the past few decades, there has been much research on the influence of religion and spirituality on health outcomes, including mortality. In a 2003 review by Powell and colleagues,[3] a levels-of-evidence approach was used to evaluate the relationship between religion/spirituality and health, identifying studies with minimally acceptable methodology, as some prior reviews were criticized for including studies that were methodologically weak. Powell and colleagues[3] found persuasive evidence for a protective relationship between religious service attendance and mortality. Religion/spirituality was moderately protective of cardiovascular disease. Prayer (e.g., being prayed for) was found to improve physical recovery from acute illness. However, there was insufficient evidence to support protective relationships between religious/spiritual constructs and mortality due to cancer, cancer progression, or recovery from acute illness. A longitudinal study by Oman and colleagues[4] with 6,500 individuals found that religious attendance reduced the likelihood of mortality from cardiovascular, respiratory, and digestive disorders; however many of these relationships became nonsignificant after controlling for health status, social connections, and health behaviors. In fully adjusted models, religious attendance continued to predict significantly lower mortality from all causes and for circulatory diseases.

The relationship between religion/spirituality and health is multidimensional, and findings are inconsistent, depending on study methodology and outcomes. For example, a 2009 review by Chida and colleagues,[5] which compared religion/spirituality in healthy and unhealthy individuals, found that religion/spirituality was associated with less cardiovascular disease in healthy samples, but not in unhealthy samples. Further, a longitudinal study of approximately 5,000 African American, Caucasian, Hispanic, and Asian adults failed to find a protective relationship between religious attendance or spirituality and cardiovascular disease.[6] This study, however, found high rates of obesity for individuals who attended religious services, with a dose-response relationship showing higher levels of obesity with greater religious attendance. A similar relationship was found for obesity and spirituality.

Over the years, the connection between religion/spirituality and health has garnered considerable attention, meriting two editions of the *Handbook of Religion and Health*,[7,8] which are systematic reviews of religion and health research in areas such as mental health and chronic disease, as well as reviews of the mechanistic pathways through which religion/spirituality may affect health-related outcomes. *Religion, Families, and Health: Population-Based Research in the United States* provides a review of religion and health outcomes, highlighting various population subgroups, including African Americans, Jews, and recent immigrants.[9] In sum, the relationship between religion/spirituality and health is complex; might vary by subgroups defined by disease status, ethnicity, gender, and age; and might be a broad pathway whose relationship with health is partially explained by positive mood states or other psychosocial mediators.

Explanatory Mechanisms

Several mediational or causal pathways have been hypothesized to explain the relationship between religion/spirituality and health.[10-12] Individuals who are religious or spiritual may be more likely to avoid unhealthy behaviors. For example, some religions discourage alcohol and tobacco consumption, or have specific dietary requirements, in accord with the religious view of the body as a temple. Religion or spiritual associations may offer increased access to social support networks, which have consistently been shown to provide benefits to overall health and well-being. Further, these social support networks may support positive behavioral changes that reduce risk of disease. Religion and spiritual involvement may promote positive affective states and reduce stress through mechanisms such as using religious coping strategies and prayer to buffer stress.[13] Finally, some suggest that religion and spirituality may promote health through supernatural means that are not measureable using scientific methods.[12]

Holt and colleagues, through their Religion and Health in African Americans (RHIAA) initiative, systematically tested a set of explanatory "religion-health mechanisms" derived from a review of previous literature and based on a conceptual model of the religion-health connection (see Figure 6.1). Using data from their national cohort of African American men and women, Holt and colleagues

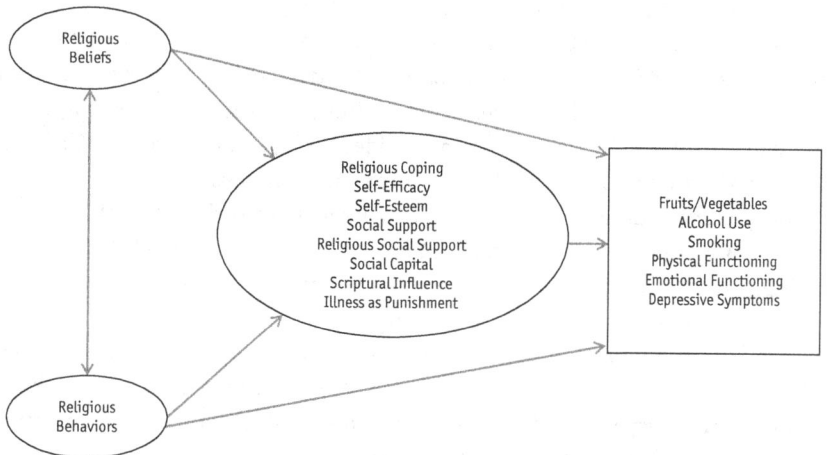

Figure 6.1 Summary model of cross-sectional mediation evidence from the RHIAA initiative.

evaluated, individually, religion–health mechanisms including positive and negative religious coping, self-efficacy, self-esteem, social support, religious social support, social capital, healthy lifestyle in accord with religious beliefs ("scriptural influence"), and illness as punishment for sin or wrongdoing.[10,14-18] Figure 6.1 provides a summary model of these mechanisms for a variety of health-related outcomes such as health behaviors, physical/emotional functioning, and depressive symptoms. The team found some support for each of the mediational models, in which the relationship between religious beliefs and behaviors was accounted for at least in part by the mediator, across a variety of health-related outcomes, including fruit/vegetable consumption, heavy drinking, emotional functioning, and depressive symptoms. This initiative provided evidence that the religion–health association often observed in African American men and women is at least partly accounted for by these mediating factors.

Church-Based Health Promotion

In view of the religion-health connection and the role of the church as a source of support and community services, the church is a favorable place for health promotion activities, both through health ministries and through partnerships with academic and other outside institutions. The term FBO is generally defined as a place of religious worship, whether that be a church, temple, mosque, or other house of worship. The term can also have a wider organizational meaning as an entity where people come together to participate in worship and religious services/activities. Faith-based organizations have distinct characteristics: Their mission is primarily of a religious nature, key roles are often held by volunteers or part-time personnel, they are nonprofit, and they often have additional service and outreach ministries. The average church size in the United States is about 75 people.[19] Faith-based organizations typically have few paid staff, and, in many cases, particularly in smaller organizations, the leader (e.g., pastor, minister, rabbi, imam) might also maintain outside employment.[19] Many FBOs have a hierarchical structure in which the leader maintains centralized decision-making authority,[19] and some are also members of a broader network such as the National Baptist Convention.[20] Financial support for FBOs is provided largely by the membership through offerings or tithes, by which members provide a proportion of monthly or yearly earnings to the church.[19]

Faith-based organizations allow workers to reach community members and deliver health promotion programming. This is particularly true in areas with documented health disparities affecting lower income and ethnic minority communities, which are often medically underserved. In order to engage FBOs in health promotion research, participatory approaches such as CBPR are often used.[21] The tenets of CBPR include equal representation from community members and researchers, community input and motivation to address a health concern, culturally relevant programs, and empowerment and education of community members. Often these CBPR partnerships are long-standing and efficiently implement initiatives based on the community's needs. In general, leadership from FBOs is essential for developing effective community–academic partnerships and for conducting CBPR and program delivery. Since FBOs are frequently a central resource for community members and have the space necessary for programming, built-in social support mechanisms, and the potential for program sustainability, they are essential components of CBPR research and community health promotion.[22] Further, in hard-to-reach populations, such as marginalized, lower income, and ethnic minority communities, integrating FBOs through CBPR methods can improve recruitment and retention of participants.

THE AFRICAN AMERICAN CHURCH

The African American church is an example of FBOs that are a central resource for public health in communities.[23] Recognized as an autonomous social institution in African American communities, the church has strived to attend to the spiritual, mental, and physical needs of its members. African American FBOs often take the lead in addressing community needs and community health. In working for the advancement of the community in various avenues of life, African American pastors have served as teachers, social activists, preachers, and agents of health-related change.[24] Many African American FBOs have a health ministry with a primary function to provide, to congregation members, education and resources related to health. African American pastors often indicate their willingness and interest in improving the health of their congregations and in partnering with public health organizations and researchers.[25] The tradition of community-oriented service, exemplified by African American pastors and churches, is highly consistent with community health.[23]

African American FBOs have been successfully involved in many areas of health promotion, including cancer and blood pressure screenings, delivery of educational programs and seminars, and physical activity interventions. A recent review highlighting obesity and dietary or physical activity programs conducted in African American FBOs[26] identified 27 studies that were "faith-placed" or "faith-based." The term "faith-placed" denotes a health promotion program conducted in an FBO setting, but not including scripture or other religious components. In comparison, "faith-based" refers to the integration of religious components into a health promotion program that is held at an FBO. The authors found that 70% of the 27 studies demonstrated reductions in weight, 60% improved fruit and vegetable consumption, and 38% showed an increase in physical activity.[26] However, interventions that incorporated culturally relevant lay health advisors (LHAs) and were "faith-based" did not demonstrate significantly better outcomes. In many of the studies, a dose-response relationship was evident in that participants who attended more sessions had better outcomes. Although FBOs are promising avenues for health promotion programs, there is variability in the success of programs to improve health outcomes and to be sustainable in the FBO over time.

There are several examples of CBPR programs that improved health outcomes in FBO settings. Holt and colleagues implemented CBPR studies in FBOs to improve cancer screening in African Americans.[27-29] These studies involved the use of educational materials developed with extensive engagement from community leaders and members, along with pilot testing in the community. Further, the programs were implemented by community health advisors (CHAs) recruited from FBOs. Developing educational screening programs (for breast, prostate, and colorectal cancer) using CBPR principals resulted in three evidence-based cancer communication interventions that improved cancer screening and knowledge. Integrating CBPR principals also promotes sustainability by establishing long-term partnerships. Holt and colleagues are currently testing implementation approaches using CBPR tenets to provide cancer education to additional churches and individuals.[30]

Another successful CBPR partnership resulted in a faith-based weight loss program.[31] The CBPR partnership was created from a 13-year collaboration between academic researchers and various community organizations across North Carolina. The WORD (Wholeness, Oneness, Righteousness, Deliverance) Leadership team consisting of academic researchers, pastors, church board representatives, and congregation members from three African American churches in rural North Carolina that implemented a community health assessment showing weight was the main concern. Formative focus groups with community members were conducted to develop a faith-based weight loss program with input from the WORD Leadership team. The resulting 8-week intervention was evaluated in a quasi-experimental study that found significant improvements in weight controlling for baseline body mass index (BMI), education, and age.

Capacity for Health Promotion

One area that has received recent attention is the organizational capacity of FBOs to implement health promotion programs. Organizational capacity is defined as having the needed resources, staffing, education, time, and infrastructure to deliver health promotion programs.[32] The motivation to deliver such programs, or readiness,[33] is a contextual factor in church-based health promotion. Similar to other community organizations, FBOs have a wide range of capacity and readiness.

Taking FBO organizational capacity and readiness into consideration when implementing a health promotion program contributes to the matching of intervention programs to baseline capacity and readiness levels. Many health promotion programs, such as the Diabetes Prevention Program,[34] are long in duration and complex to deliver, and require a high level of church capacity for success.

If a church has low capacity, they may be more successful delivering health promotion programs of shorter duration, such as healthy cooking classes or educational seminars while they invest resources to build capacity. Capacity and readiness are likely to be associated with program success in terms of implementation and outcomes. For work with FBOs, capacity and readiness are useful constructs that can be measured with instruments tailored for use in these settings. Currently, much of the literature and instrumentation on capacity and readiness is rooted in an organizational or business context, which speaks to the opportunity for working in multidisciplinary teams.

Summary and Future Directions

In summary, there has been much research on connections between religion/spirituality and health, and many, but not all studies have found a positive association with various health outcomes. With regard to health promotion interventions, FBOs are promising for reaching people, including low-income and ethnic minority populations. There have now been many CBPR studies conducted successfully in partnership with FBOs, providing examples of evidence-based interventions to improve health and to address health disparities. A remaining challenge is that, with few exceptions, many of these interventions establish an evidence base but are not being disseminated further. Since researchers may not know how to disseminate evidence-based interventions that they develop and evaluate,[35] and since FBO leadership often does not know where to access such interventions,[36] there are opportunities for the field of dissemination/implementation research to make a greater impact along the translational continuum. There is also a role for technology to disseminate more broadly evidence-based interventions to FBOs.[37] In the context of the translational continuum, there is a need to consider ways to pair FBOs with evidence-based interventions, while taking into account their baseline capacities including strengths and challenges, such as limited resources and overcommitted volunteers,[36] as well as their need for technical assistance. Finally, to enhance sustainability, the potential of evidence-based health promotion in FBOs will be maximized to the extent that it is institutionalized into the routine operations of the organizations.

References

1. Thoresen, C.E. and Harris, A.H. "Spirituality and Health: What's the Evidence and What's Needed?" *Annals of Behavioral Medicine* 24 (2002): 3–13.
2. Miller, W.R. and Thoresen, C.E. "Spirituality, Religion, and Health: An Emerging Research Field." *American Psychologist* 58 (2003): 24–35.
3. Powell, L. and Shahabi, L. "Religion and Spirituality: Linkages to Physical Health." *American Psychologist* 58 (2003): 36–52.

4. Oman, D., Kurata, J.H., Strawbridge, W.J. and Cohen, R.D. "Religious Attendance and Cause of Death over 31 Years." *International Journal of Psychiatry in Medicine* 32 (2002): 69–89.

5. Chida, Y., Steptoe, A., and Powell, L.H. "Religiosity/Spirituality and Mortality: A Systematic Quantitative Review." *Psychotherapy and Psychosomatics* 78 (2009): 81–90.

6. Feinstein, M., Liu, K., Ning, H., Fitchett, G., and Lloyd-Jones, D.M. "Burden of Cardiovascular Risk Factors, Subclinical Atherosclerosis, and Incident Cardiovascular Events Across Dimensions Of Religiosity: The Multi-Ethnic Study of Atherosclerosis." *Circulation* 121 (2010): 659–66.

7. Koenig, H.G., King, D.E. and Carson, V.B. *Handbook of Religion and Health*, 2nd ed. New York: Oxford University Press, 2012.

8. Koenig, H.G., McCullough, M.E. and Larson, D.B. *Handbook of Religion and Health*. New York: Oxford University Press, 2001.

9. Ellison, C.G. and Hummer, R.A. *Religion, Families, and Health: Population-Based Research in the United States.* New Brunswick, NJ: Rutgers University Press, 2010.

10. Holt, C.L., Roth, D.L., Clark, E.M. and Debnam, K. "Positive Self-Perceptions as a Mediator of Religious Involvement and Health Behaviors in a National Sample of African Americans." *Journal of Behavioral Medicine* 37 (2014): 102–12.

11. Holt, C.L., Roth, D.L., Huang, J. and Clark, E.M. "Gender Differences in the Roles of Religion and Locus of Control on Alcohol Use and Smoking Among African Americans." *Journal of Studies on Alcohol and Drugs* 76 (2015): 482–92.

12. Oman, D. and Thoresen, C.E. "Does Religion Cause Health? Differing Interpretations and Diverse Meanings." *Journal of Health Psychology* 7 (2002): 365–80.

13. Koenig, H.G., Larson, D.B. and Larson, S.S. "Religion and Coping with Serious Medical Illness." *Annals of Pharmacotherapy* 35 (2001): 352–59.

14. Holt, C.L., Wang, M.Q., Clark, E.M., Williams, B.R. and Schulz, E. "Religious Involvement and Physical and Emotional Functioning Among African Americans: The Mediating Role of Religious Support." *Psychology and Health* 28 (2013): 267–83.

15. Holt, C.L., Clark, E.M., Debnam, K.J. and Roth, D.L. "Religion and Health in African Americans: The Role of Religious Coping." *American Journal of Health Behavior* 38 (2014): 190–9.

16. Holt, C., Schulz, E., Williams, B., Clark, E. and Wang, M. "Social Support as a Mediator of Religious Involvement and Physical and Emotional Functioning in a National Sample of African-Americans." *Mental Health Religion and Culture* 17 (2014): 421–5.

17. Holt, C., Clark, E.M. and Roth, D. "Positive and Negative Religious Beliefs Explaining the Religion-Health Connection Among African Americans." *Int J Psychol Relig* 24 (2014): 311–31.

18. Holt, C., Clark, E., Wang, M., Williams, B. and Schulz, E. "The Religion-Health Connection Among African Americans: What Is the Role of Social Capital?" *J Commun Appl Soc Psychol* 25 (2015): 1–8.

19. Chaves, M., Anderson, S., Byassee, J. *American Congregations at the Beginning of the 21st Century: A Report from the National Congregations Study.* Durham, NC: Department of Sociology, Duke University, 2009.

20. Zech, C. "Understanding Denominational Structures: Churches as Franchise Organization." *International Journal of the Economics of Business* 10 (2003): 323–35.

21. Parrill, R. and Kennedy, B.R. "Partnerships for Health in the African American Community: Moving Toward Community-Based Participatory Research." *Journal of Cultural Diversity* 18 (2011):150–4.

22. Peterson, J., Atwood, J.R. and Yates, B. "Key Elements for Church-Based Health Promotion Programs: Outcome-Based Literature Review." *Public Health Nursing* 19 (2002): 401–411.

23. Levin, J.S. "The Role of the Black Church in Community Medicine." *Journal of the National Medical Association* 76 (1984): 477–83.

24. Levin, J. "Roles for the Black Pastor in Preventive Medicine." *Pastoral Psychology* 76 (1986): 477–83.

25. Holt, C.L. and McClure, S.M. "Perceptions of the Religion-Health Connection Among African American Church Members." *Qualitative Health Research* 16 (2006): 268–81.

26. Lancaster, K.J., Carter-Edwards, L., Grilo, S., Shen, C. and Schoenthaler, A.M. "Obesity Interventions in African American Faith-Based Organizations: A Systematic Review." *Obesity Reviews* 15 Suppl 4 (2014): 159–76.
27. Holt, C.L. and Klem, P.R. "As You Go, Spread the Word: Spirituality Based Breast Cancer Education for African American Women. *Gynecologic Oncology* 99 Suppl 1 (2005): S141–2.
28. Holt, C.L., Wynn, T.A., Litaker, M.S., Southward, P., Jeames, S. and Schulz, E. "A Comparison of a Spirituality-Based and a Non-Spirituality Based Educational Intervention for Informed Decision Making for Prostate Cancer Screening Among Church-Attending African American Men." *Urologic Nursing* 29 (2009): 249–58.
29. Holt, C.L., Litaker, M.S., Scarinci, I.C., et al. "Spiritually-Based Intervention to Increase Colorectal Cancer Screening Among African Americans: Screening And Theory-Based Outcomes from a Randomized Trial." *Health Education and Behavior* 40 (2013): 458–68.
30. Holt, C.L., Tagai, E.K., Scheirer, M., et al. "Translating Evidence-Based Interventions for Implementation: Experiences from Project HEAL in African American Churches. *Implementation Science* 9 (2014): 66.
31. Kim, K., Linnan, L., Campbell, M.K., Brooks, C., Koenig, H. and Wiesen, C. "The WORD (Wholeness, Oneness, Righteousness, Deliverance): A Faith-Based Weight-Loss Program Utilizing a Community-Based Participatory Research Approach." *Health Education and Behavior* 35 (2008):634–50.
32. Rabin, B.A. and Brownson, R.C. *Developing the Terminology for Dissemination and Implementation Research.* New York: Oxford University Press, 2012.
33. Weiner, B.J., Amick, H. and Lee, S.Y. "Conceptualization and Measurement of Organizational Readiness for Change: A Review of the Literature in Health Services Research and Other Fields." *Medical Care Research and Review* 65 (2008): 379–436.
34. Diabetes Prevention Program Research Group. "10-year Follow-up of Diabetes Incidence and Weight Loss in the Diabetes Prevention Program Outcomes Study." *Lancet* 374 (2009): 1677–86.
35. Kreuter, M.W. and Bernhardt, J.M. "Reframing the Dissemination Challenge: A Marketing and Distribution Perspective." *American Journal of Public Health* 99 (2009): 2123–7.
36. Graham-Phillips, A., Holt, C., Mullins, C., Slade, J., Savoy, A. and Carter, R. "Health Ministry and Activities in African American Faith-Based Organizations: A Qualitative Examination of Facilitators, Barriers, and Use of Technology." (2015). (Submitted for publication.)
37. Santos, S.L., Tagai, E.K., Wang, M.Q., Scheirer, M.A., Slade, J.L. and Holt, C.L. "Feasibility of a Web-Based Training System for Peer Community Health Advisors in Cancer Early Detection Among African Americans." *American Journal of Public Health* 104 (2014): 2282–9.

7

Special Issues in Conducting Community-Based Participatory Research Studies with Ethnic and Racial Minorities

MARIA E. FERNANDEZ, PHD, NATALIA I. HEREDIA, MPH, LORNA H. MCNEILL, PHD, MPH, MARIA EUGENIA FERNANDEZ-ESQUER, PHD, YEN-CHI L. LE, PHD, AND KELLY G. MCGAUHEY, BS

Introduction

In this chapter, we describe considerations for conducting community-based participatory research (CBPR) with members of racial and ethnic minority communities. We first discuss the origin of CBPR and why it is a relevant process for many of these groups. We then describe important issues related to culture and cultural humility of CBPR researchers working with racial and ethnic minority groups. While it was not possible to discuss all groups and highlight considerations for each, we chose examples of CBPR work with the primary racial/ethnic groups in the United States and provide examples of considerations based not only on race/ethnicity but also on other relevant factors. Finally, we highlight common themes and recommendations.

RECONNECTING WITH A FAMILIAR PROCESS

While many individuals who identify as racial/ethnic minorities may have never been exposed to CBPR, it is useful to recognize that the origins of this process actually emerged in other countries. Community-based participatory research, as it is currently described and practiced, emerged over time, and we find its basis in Kurt Lewin's early action research.[1,2] This process included planning, action, and then reflection and problem-solving before further action.[3] Community-based participatory research was heavily influenced by Paulo Freire's seminal work, *Pedagogy of the Oppressed*.[4] Freire was one of the first to assert that research and science do not involve only observation and collection of objective facts but rather include an interplay between the objective facts and subjective perceptions.[4] Early originators of CBPR, such as Fals-Borda,[5] emphasized the potential of learning from the communities being studied and the need to empower the individuals in those communities and thereby create social justice. This and other assertions created space in the research paradigm of the time for community members, previously objects of study, to become part of the research and shape its progress.[6] This trajectory of CBPR actually emerged in Latin America, Asia, and Africa. Since many of the racial and ethnic minorities in the United States have cultural origins from those regions, the philosophy of CBPR may not be wholly unfamiliar to them.

Nevertheless, health-related research and the medical community in the United States, and in other countries, continue to rely primarily on traditional research methods, and so most racial/ethnic minorities living in the United States may not have engaged in CBPR. Additionally, as researchers schooled in Western research methods, we should take into account certain considerations related to history, culture, immigration status, and settings when undertaking CBPR with ethnic/racial minorities.

Regardless of the research group, it is important to avoid assumptions about characteristics of individuals or communities based on group membership. We believe that while it may be useful to understand cultural norms and general sociocultural tendencies (e.g., some minority groups such as Hispanics and Asian have more of a collectivist than individualist mentality),[7-9] there is also danger in assuming that groups will hold these beliefs or that the beliefs are relevant for the issue at hand. For example, assumptions that Hispanics have strong family ties (*familismo*) or have fatalistic beliefs (*fatalismo*) may bias researcher perspectives.[10,11] It may be far more important for a CBPR investigator to understand that recent immigrants often send money back to their families in their country of origin (remittance) and how this may contribute to stress and lack of resources.

In our own research, we have encountered problems when we assume that Hispanics have fatalistic beliefs about cancer. We discovered, through CBPR processes, that while Hispanics who live close to the border may believe that cancer leads to death (an outcome expectation based on lived experience), they did not hold to predeterminism (the belief that if they were meant to die from cancer, there was nothing they could do to prevent it).[10,12] Because of the potential problems with ascribing certain beliefs and cultural norms to populations and the danger of stereotyping, we have, herein, avoided this approach.

CULTURE AND CULTURAL HUMILITY

Critical issues related to conducting CBPR with racial/ethnic minority communities are consideration of culture and approaching the research with cultural humility.

Culture has been defined as "the way of life, especially the general customs and beliefs, of a particular group of people at a particular time."[13] Culture provides implicit and explicit guidelines that people use to interact with others and with the world around them.[14] Misunderstanding and misinterpretation can occur between cultures because of the differences in behaviors, attitudes, and symbols and the meanings people attach to words.[15]

Because of increasing racial/ethnic diversity in the United States, many researchers and authors have described the importance of cultural sensitivity in research. While CBPR contains processes that, if carried out appropriately, should lead to findings that have integrated cultural beliefs, practice, and perspectives, it is still useful to follow recommended guidelines for increasing cultural sensitivity. Many of these have focused on the importance of self-evaluation and reflection as a necessary process.[15]

Bennet and colleagues describe the developmental model of intercultural sensitivity, a framework for how we can increase competence and sophistication in our experience and navigate differences when they are identified.[16-18] The authors report that this process begins with three ethnocentric stages-denial, defense, and minimization. Here, one's own culture is seen as central to reality. The process continues with three ethnorelative stages, acceptance, adaptation, and integration, in which one's own culture is viewed in the context of other cultures.[19]

Airhihenbuwa and colleagues describe the PEN-3 model and posit that a requirement for working in another culture is to identify and embrace positive aspects of the culture.[20] They describe three cultural domains in understanding the selection of priority populations and influences on health. These domains are cultural empowerment, relationships and expectations, and cultural identity. In a later report, Ford and Airhihenbuwa describe an analytic framework called critical race theory that can be used to understand racism as a factor influencing health.[15,21-24] The theory describes the importance of considering the possible influence that race and racism have on health at multiple levels (individual, interpersonal, community, societal) and advocates understanding these from the perspectives of the racial/ethnic group.[15]

While the concepts of cultural sensitivity and cultural competence certainly intend to convey a sense of the importance of understanding, respecting, and even celebrating culture within racial/ethnic groups, it is useful to think about cultural competency as a process rather than an attainable goal. Researchers must move beyond gaining knowledge about culture and include self-assessment of attitudes and behaviors when conducting CBPR, particularly when individuals belong to different racial/ethnic groups than the researchers. Even when researchers are of the same racial/ethnic group as the subjects, differences in socioeconomic status (SES), education, community history, geographic region, and many other factors may require careful assessment of one's own beliefs and biases.

Because understanding and effectively interacting with racial/ethnic communities is a process, the concept of *cultural humility* may represent this perspective better than "cultural competence." Tervalon[25] and Tervalon and Murray-Garcia[26] introduced the concept of cultural humility; they believed that healthcare professionals did not receive adequate training to prepare them to treat multicultural patients, and they pointed out that a competency-based approach to understanding culture is inappropriate because it is not possible to be fully competent and fully understand another culture.[15,25–27] Hook and colleagues subsequently described this process-oriented approach as the "ability to maintain an interpersonal stance that is other-oriented (or open to the other) in relation to aspects of cultural identity that are most important to the [person]."[28, p.2] Researchers must also be aware of different roles and what they mean in terms of cultural and power differences.

The concept of cultural humility aligns well with basic principles and skills needed for good CBPR practice. To engage with ethnic/racial populations with cultural humility, researchers must understand their own biases and assumptions, cultural background, power dynamics, and their own roles in society. They must develop skills, attitudes, and processes that exhibit honesty, flexibility, transparency, respect, and self-reflection.[29] Because researchers often work with multiple racial/ethnic groups, their ability to work effectively across cultures can allow the perspectives, strengths, and experiences of many groups to create powerful community change.[15,30]

Aligned with the principles of CBPR, cultural humility supports mutually beneficial relationships and a goal of reducing or eliminating power imbalances in research. Three main components to cultural humility are described by Tervalon and Murray-Garcia[26] and later summarized by Waters and Asbill[31]: a lifelong commitment to self-evaluation and self-critique, fixing power imbalances, and developing partnerships with people and groups who advocate for others.[31] The first is based on the assumption that we are never finished learning about another culture (or even perhaps our own) and therefore should be open, flexible, and self-reflective. It also underscores the importance of recognizing and being able to acknowledge that we may not know important aspects of cultures and how and why culture can influence the research process.

The desire to fix power imbalances is closely aligned with principles of CBPR and emphasizes the fact that while the researcher may have knowledge and training that the community does not, the community has information and lived experiences that are essential to understanding its problems and their solutions. The third component is the intention to develop partnerships with people and groups who advocate for others in order to make lasting change in communities and systems.[26] This piece underscores the intent of cultural humility to move beyond personal assessment and respect for cultural differences to include working together to make sustainable changes that improve communities.

Bartholomew and colleagues[15] describe processes for preparing health promotion planners to work in multicultural settings. They underscore the importance of including community members in primary planning groups and in continuing the process of personal development to enable planners to work within and across cultures.[15] Bartholomew and colleagues also advises against stereotyping based on culture. There are large variations among and within ethnic and racial groups and incorrect assumptions about beliefs or behaviors can obscure facts and inhibit researchers' listening and learning, despite CBPR processes.

Since stereotyping or making assumptions about individuals and communities based on culture is not conducive to good CBPR, we have avoided including lists of "common cultural factors" for the groups we discuss below. Instead, we describe CBPR challenges, successes, and recommendations based on the literature and on our own work. We highlight experiences from research studies conducted with African Americans, Hispanics, Asians, and Native Americans, and specific lessons learned from each group. In many cases, there are common considerations across groups, such as the need to establish trust, as well as common recommendations for good CBPR practice.

CBPR with Hispanic Groups

There are many CBPR studies conducted with Hispanic/Latino populations,[32-39] and the approach is widely accepted as a way of better understanding health inequities and of discovering and developing intervention approaches to reduce them. Nevertheless, there are challenges, and, in certain groups, these challenges may be even more pronounced. We present the issues that CBPR researchers have identified as important when working with Hispanic populations. We then provide examples of successful CBPR efforts. These examples highlight common issues relevant across Hispanic subgroups and also identify unique considerations for doing CBPR with certain marginalized groups.

HISPANICS IN THE UNITED STATES

Hispanics constitute the largest ethnic minority group in the United States. There were 55.3 million in the country in 2014, 17.3% of the total US population.[40] About 25% of US Hispanics are millennials (ages 18–33), and about one-third of all Hispanics are younger than 18.[41] Hispanics represent a diverse group who trace their ancestry to more than 20 Spanish-speaking nations. According to Pew Research Center's 2011 American Community Survey, about 65% traced their origins to Mexico,[42] followed by 9.5% of US Hispanics who have origins in Puerto Rico, with another 3.7 million living in Puerto Rico.[42] Salvadorans are the third largest group, followed by Cubans, Dominicans, Guatemalans, Colombians, Spaniards, Hondurans, Ecuadorians, Peruvians, Nicaraguans, Venezuelans, and Argentineans.

The majority (65%) of US Hispanics are native born.[40] Immigrants (19.4 million in 2014) can face significant issues related to discrimination, low SES, and healthcare access that negatively influence health and quality of life.[40,43-47] Hispanics have higher birth weight and lower smoking rates than other groups;[48-50] however, they experience health disparities in other areas, such as teenage pregnancy, diabetes, cervical cancer, asthma, and obesity.[48,50-52] Additionally, Hispanics have lower rates of insurance coverage than other groups.[53]

The diversity of the US Hispanic population is important to CBPR investigators[54,55] because health problems, health risk behaviors, and cultural factors may vary according to the subgroup. Mexicans, for example, have higher rates of diabetes than other groups; Puerto Ricans smoke more than Mexicans.[56] These differences across groups may be as fundamental as how people refer to themselves.

Throughout this section, we will refer to this diverse population as *Hispanic*; however, this may not be the preferred term of all individuals who have ethnic affiliations with one or more Spanish-speaking country.[57] There has been long-standing debate, primarily among academicians, about the right terminology.[58,59] This may be among the very first issues to be understood and clarified when undertaking CBPR. While the research community usually refers to individuals that identify with an ancestry in a Spanish-speaking country as Hispanics or those originating from Latin America as Latinos, many US immigrant Hispanic populations identify themselves according to their country of origin (e.g., Mexican, Salvadoran, Cuban). Early discussions about how people see themselves is an important step in conducting CBPR among Hispanics.[60]

CONSIDERATIONS FOR CONDUCTING CBPR WITH HISPANIC POPULATIONS

Investigators who conduct research with these populations have reported that Hispanics experience numerous barriers specifically with CBPR participation, such as lack of trust, transportation, time, and language.[32,33] Other barriers to both research participation and healthcare use include lack of health insurance, cost, the lack of language-appropriate services or protocols, discrimination due to immigration status, and lack of transportation to access healthcare resources or attend research appointments.[34-37,61]

Building networks and trust within the Hispanic community is critical to carrying out a successful CBPR study. While this should be a goal for any CBPR effort, it may be a particularly important with Hispanic populations. Network building is likely more salient among recent immigrants, who might have experienced discrimination, or for research efforts on a stigmatized health problem such as HIV. To build trust, researchers and community members must cultivate relationships. Researchers should be present and seen by community members at times other than when data are being collected. Data collection should include consideration of culturally sensitive topics, like immigration status, and community members should be involved in selecting the research focus.[62-64] If community members are also data collectors, it could be important to have formal protocols on whether they should interview neighbors or acquaintances.[62] Further, selection of primary language and determination of jargon to be used are important considerations. When training community members to collect data, specialized curricula may be needed to make human subject training information accessible.[63] Researchers should also look for opportunities to offer services or other contributions to the community that might not be directly related to the research or data collection.[32]

As with other groups, it is important to establish partnerships with organizations that serve the Hispanic community in order to build the researcher-community relationship and heighten the study's credibility.[32–34,63] This may be even more important with the emergence of an anti-immigrant sentiment that can affect Hispanics' willingness to participate in research and may require more time to build trust and establish relationships within the community.[35,36]

An example of a partnership established to foster and support CBPR was Latinos in Network for Cancer Control (LINCC).[65–67] The LINCC partnership was supported through both a Cancer Prevention and Control Research Network funded by the US Centers for Disease Control and Prevention[66] and the National Cancer Institute (NCI) and an NCI Community Network Program Center.[65] It was established in 2002 and comprised 65 academic and community organizations, including 130 individuals, all focused on improving cancer control among Hispanics.[68] The researchers and community partners used CBPR methods to develop a collaborative cancer control research and practice agenda that led to new initiatives, funding, and research. A goal of this network was to accelerate use of evidence-based community cancer control interventions. Network members were involved in a participatory evaluation to assess LINCC function. It concluded that LINCC was able to create meaningful relationships among various Hispanic- and cancer-focused academic and community partners and achieve synergy to develop important products, such as interventions and training.[68] Importantly, the partnership led to new CBPR research conducted by the community and community-based organizations themselves.[69]

Rhodes and colleagues[36] describe a CBPR effort that illustrates challenges and successes and provides an example of the need to reach people where they live, work, and play. The aim of their study was to develop an intervention to reduce HIV and other STIs among Hispanic men who were recent immigrants.[36] They engaged men who belonged to a rural multicounty soccer league in North Carolina.

The researchers noted the challenges in networking and gaining trust partly because of the immigration status of participants (documented or undocumented). Participants and community leaders hesitated, at first, to participate in CBPR because they did not understand or trust the process and because of the anti-immigration sentiment in the larger community, which included anti-immigration rallies and targeted crime against Hispanics and Hispanic-serving groups.[70]

The researchers and community members worked together for more than 8 months to establish trust and expand the partnership. Rhodes and colleagues [36] describe a CBPR partnership that was characterized by informal decision-making and a fluid structure, which, the authors note, was unlike some CBPR reports.[71-74] They underscore the importance of resisting specific expectations about how partnerships should look and work and allowing the partnership to develop its own ways of functioning. The authors noted they acknowledged and prepared for tensions in the general community that could affect partnership functioning, such as stigma, discrimination, and anti-immigrant attitudes. Rhodes and colleagues attribute the success of their CBPR partnership to being community-initiated and having blended resources and perspectives from many partners, all of which allowed for colearning and collaborative development of an intervention.[36] The study also tapped into the soccer league, which proved to be an innovative and effective approach that relied on existing relationships and organizations that they would later expand.

Some Hispanic populations experience unique challenges and greater health disparities. Hispanics living along the Texas-Mexico border have among the highest rates of cervical cancer in the country and extremely high rates of diabetes.[75-78] This region is home to many migrant farmworkers, a group who have high levels of exposure to pesticides, sun and heat-induced illnesses, and work-related injuries.[79-81] Kilanowski (2014) reported that while CBPR considers the important social context and ecological factors influencing health, the method meets challenges among farmworkers.[82] There are approximately 3 million migrant and seasonal farmworkers in the United States, and about 72% are foreign born. Some, however, are reluctant to fully engage in CBPR efforts because of fear of deportation, which could result in severe consequences for individuals and families. Kilanowski suggests avoiding using full names or asking about immigration status and reassuring potential participants that their information will remain confidential. Also, CBPR investigators must be willing to travel to the farmworkers (including the fields where they are working) to gather data and conduct observation and be considerate of time schedules (of both children and adults) because participants may not be available during regular work hours. Mobility of some farmworkers, particularly migrants, may present a further challenge. The researcher must understand typical migration patterns, changes in schedules, and travel due to availability of work or other factors. When people travel back and forth between the United States and their home countries, research may also need to be continued in the home country to ensure a complete view of the population has been achieved.[62]

Despite these challenges, there have been many successful CBPR efforts with farmworkers and with border populations.[36,83-86] Key lessons from these efforts included the importance of identifying community strengths and resources as well as needs. For example, in a study to develop and evaluate breast and cervical cancer screening among Hispanic farmworkers, we found that strong community ties and stability in the *colonias* (typically semirural residential areas often lacking basic services) make them an excellent place for community members to convene and for us to carry out both the research and intervention components of the study.[84] Although many colonia residents were migrant farmworkers they considered the south Texas colonia their home, they return year after year and slowly built permanent residences there. Also, since immigrants typically go to where they have friends and family, colonias residents often have relatives who live close by. The availability of strong community ties and resources, such as community centers, were critical for program development and implementation decisions. The CBPR partnership also revealed that colonia residents were accustomed to and accepting of lay health workers (*promotoras*) who provide health education and facilitate access to healthcare services.[83,84]

Latino day laborers (LDLs) are another population of Hispanics who experience particular health challenges. These immigrant workers from Mexico and Central America often speak only Spanish and are routinely exposed to environmental, social, and psychological stressors that impact their ability to protect their health and well-being.[87,88] Their working conditions exacerbate these stressors, as they are constantly searching for short-term, usually low-wage work for which they have to adapt daily to different work contexts, demands, and job characteristics.[89] To address the needs of these LDL workers, researchers at the University of Texas Health Science Center School of Public Health, Center for Health Promotion and Prevention Research, partnered with the Fe y Justicia Workers Center (FYJWC), a local community-based organization dedicated to assisting low-wage workers to organize in order to improve their working conditions and defend their legal rights.

The partnership with FYJWC (formerly Houston Interfaith Workers Justice Center) developed over several years as a result of mutual interest in improving the lives and working conditions of LDLs. The relationship also developed as a result of working together in distributing personal protective equipment at the local day labor corners, the places where LDLs gather to wait for jobs. The FYJWC conducted the initial distribution of this equipment in 2008 after Hurricane Ike, and the Center for Health Promotion and Prevention Research team continued the work during a day labor corner survey conducted the same year.[90]

Working together on behalf of day laborers facilitated the development of a relationship based on common goals that solidified during a recently completed study entitled Vales+Tú: A Program to Prevent Injury Disparities Among Latino Day Laborers. The goals of this project were to identify environmental, social, and psychological factors that contribute to LDLs' workplace injuries and to undertake a pilot program on reducing hazardous work conditions. The broader conceptual framework on which this project is based considers the workplace practices of day laborers as embedded in a context of social and occupational inequalities where workers struggle to make a living and protect their health. Ameliorating these inequalities required the direct participation of day laborers to identify their own health and occupational problems and the potential solutions.

The academia-community partnership formed with FYJWC was based on a shared commitment to principles of participatory research and action. To promote their vision of inclusion and changes in workplace safety, the researchers at the Center for Health Promotion and Prevention Research extended their work by forming a community advisory board (CAB). The CAB included LDLs, community-based organizations, university researchers, city officials and community organizers working on behalf of Latino health and safety. The CAB called this partnership the Day Laborer Health Partnership. Members of the CAB were involved in all aspects of the research project from planning to dissemination of study results. The advisory board especially recognized the need to actively engage LDLs, as partners not clients, in all aspects of the research process. Thus, LDLs who were part of the local day labor corners were invited to be part of the research team. Through periodic training, the laborers increased their ability to advocate for their peers and to develop their skills as community researchers. Day laborers who were part of Vales+Tú shared responsibility for participant recruitment, data collection, program implementation, interpretation of results, and dissemination. Involving them as central to the research process strengthened their commitment to the project and their resolve to advocate for their community and to work collectively on behalf of LDL health and workplace safety.

Researchers who work with day laborers need to consider both their resiliency as Latino immigrant men and their vulnerability as temporary workers. They share with other Latino immigrants a life of hardship yet hope for a better future. However, while the lives of other Latino men stabilize over time with more steady work, the life of day laborers is chronically uncertain, as the start date and duration of the next job is seldom clear. This uncertainty translates into unstable living situations, troubled relationships, and constant stress that reduces their ability to improve their lives and the future of their children.

Building a relationship with community partners takes time and effort. However, this investment makes it easier for researchers and community members to work side by side, implementing the tasks required for a research project. In particular, involving day laborers in the research process anchors the goals of the project in more realistic expectations, congruent with their needs. Finally, researchers work with community organizations invested in social justice must be based on mutual support and a commitment to pursue common goals beyond the duration of a research project.

In building CBPR projects with LDLs, it is important to remember that they are part of a diverse and heterogeneous Hispanic community.[91-93] Close collaboration with community members and organizations is key to effectively building trust, the need for which is heightened in this community.[32-36] Culturally sensitive topics should be handled with care, community partner input sought, and careful explanation about the scope of the research given.[36,62-64] While particular consideration should be given to the subgroups who face specific challenges—farmworkers, LDLs, border populations—it is also important to be aware of the barriers presented by language, trust, financial and health resources, and transportation.[32,34-37,61,82]

The many CBPR efforts with Hispanic communities have resulted in both successful partnerships and programs and identified challenges. Lessons learned from these efforts can help us continue to improve CBPR with Hispanics as well as with other groups. It is only through these collaborative efforts that researchers and communities can come together to address health disparities in Hispanic populations including those who are particularly vulnerable.

CBPR Among African American Groups

Researchers have described challenges of conducting research in general and CBPR specifically with African American populations. Some authors describe a historical lack of trust in the African American community of researchers and medical research.[94,95] This distrust stems from previous unethical research, including the much-publicized Tuskegee Study of Untreated Syphilis, which withheld life-saving treatment from African Americans after penicillin had already become standard of care,[96] and the creation of the HeLa cervical cancer cell line without the knowledge or permission of the patient Henrietta Lacks or her family.[97] Although it is important for researchers to learn from these and other historical events, they should not assume either that African American community members will distrust the research or, if they do, that the distrust cannot be overcome.[98-100] Instead investigators should begin by acknowledging that history gives some African Americans reason to be wary of research and may influence their decisions to participate or to engage in efforts of collaborative planning for research.

In order to work successfully within the African American community, researchers must commit resources over a period of time to build the relationship and be respected by community members.[101,102] This respect often involves open communication about concerns and feelings over past injustices,[103,104] as well as understanding and accommodating cultural and individual preferences. For example, in their article on successful strategies for conducting research with low-income, African American populations, Adderley-Kelly and colleagues noted that it is important to address older African Americans formally, unless otherwise indicated by the individual.[101] They further noted that researchers can gain insight about these and other issues by talking, formally or informally, with community members thereby building cultural competence.[101]

Community-based participatory research is one method that can begin to bridge the lack of trust of research.[105] However, CBPR itself might be difficult for community members to understand in the way currently described in the literature.[106] Smith and colleagues have recently developed a set of guiding principles that build on the existing CBPR structure[107] but that resonate with African Americans because they use cultural phrases and language from music. These are the seven guiding principles: We are family; It takes a village; Come as you are; Just stand; Health, Wholeness, and Healing; Go tell it to the mountain; and We shall overcome, someday.[106]

Effective CBPR studies have suggested using neighborhood spaces and engaging with community leaders to increase participation and begin to build and regain the community's trust. Researchers should not assume direct or immediate access to conduct research with members of these communities but must work hard to identify partners with similar values, goals, or missions or must build on existing relationships.[101,108] Beyond using familiar spaces and building partnerships with community leaders, researchers should demonstrate their willingness to listen to the community's voice and share decision-making power by forming a CAB.[101] Whether cultivating partnerships or convening a CAB, researchers must ensure that there are community members and leaders who can bring their experiences and expertise to the table to ensure that the different segments of the African American community are heard.[109]

REACHING PEOPLE WHERE THEY ARE

Community-based participatory research with racial and ethnic communities requires the successful development of relationships. Rather than expecting community members to attend meetings and engage in research activities at medical centers or in university settings, researchers should try to reach people where they live and work, such as in community centers, beauty salons, and churches. For example, the North Carolina BEAUTY and Health Project first established a relationship with the community and then collaboratively developed the idea and assessed feasibility for a health promotion program in hair salons, an important institution in the African American community. The research team (including community members) gauged interest of African American salons and their cosmetologists to be a part of health promotion activities. They worked with those who were interested to determine the most relevant health concerns and what behavioral changes were needed to improve them. The project was successful in training the cosmetologists to deliver health promotion activities and positively impacting their customers.[110,111]

Another effective CBPR effort, the Dan River Partnership for a Healthy Community, involved several projects that were collaboratively developed after first conducting three needs assessments within the community.[112] Subsequently, one of these projects included a community garden with primarily African American youth who lived in public housing.[113]

As described in chapter 6, African American churches are a central part of communities,[94,114,115] having a high percentage of the African American community who attend church services, having stable memberships, and representing individuals of high, middle, and low SES.[94,116,117] Partnerships with African Americans churches have resulted in many successful health promotion and prevention programs and outcomes, like increasing physical activity,[118–120] increasing fruit and vegetable intake,[119,121–124] and increasing cancer-screening behaviors such as colorectal cancer screening.[125,126]

Some argue that partnership with African American churches could positively influence community members' perspective of the researchers.[94] Researchers must recognize, however, that these partnerships require time and effort to cultivate as community leaders and organizations may be unfamiliar with research, perhaps distrustful of university or academic centers, and have competing priorities that demand their attention and time. A first step would be to identify community leaders within the church and discuss the purpose of the research with them, determining how it may fit in with community concerns and interests. Once a relationship is established, the research agenda is created collaboratively so that researchers, church leaders, and members can work together to seek funding for relevant issues. Often, however, researchers approach church leaders and members who already have an interest in the target health behavior or outcome but they often approach them after already having received funding for a particular health or social issue.[127] In this case, it is important for researchers and church leaders and members to come to a shared vision for the research process and outcomes.[15,128] This aligns with the CBPR principles (discussed in chapter 1) of shared decision-making, power sharing among partners, and including community partners in all phases of the research, including the identification of health priorities.[107]

In line with the CBPR principles, researchers working with African American churches should involve members in all steps of the research process, especially the design phase.[94] This ensures that the intervention is more than simply a church-placed intervention where the church is merely the setting for the intervention, but rather that the church is truly a collaborative partner.[102] Researchers should be prepared to describe how the research would benefit the church members, in order for pastors and church leaders to find the research acceptable.[108] Thus if an intervention or education service is not part of the planned research (e.g., recruitment for a cohort or other observational study), there may need to be adjustments to assure church members there is some tangible, direct benefit.

Describing and coming to an agreement during the design phase of the research is important because it will delineate the scope and depth of the interactions (including data collection, analysis, intervention, reporting) that may or may not be acceptable to church leaders. Researchers should always be sensitive to their partner's needs and the limitation those needs may have on the topics addressed. Investigators should be aware that the collaboration with African American churches could limit the content that is taught, if certain topics areas are inappropriate in the context,[127] and may necessitate that interventions or curricula include spiritual references or religious themes.[94,129]

To facilitate input from church leaders and members, researchers could hold sessions during the design phase to introduce all proposed components and content, allowing discussion to ensure that changes could be made before the program is implemented.[94] This early and ongoing participation would be crucial to establishing trust within the church[130,131] and ensure that the curriculum and intervention is suitable for the community.[132]

During the development and implementation of an intervention, researchers should build on such church assets and resources as the communication structure.[127,131] This may include social networks within the church (such as phone trees) that could be used for recruitment, intervention delivery, or dissemination of findings.[127] Since church members often view the pastor or other leaders as trusted sources and approach them for guidance and information, leaders may serve as effective deliverers of important health messages.[94] Church leaders, representatives, and researchers should work together to ensure that the intervention is not overly burdensome. For example, intervention programming or other research could be held at the church, be scheduled along with existing activities,[131] and be flexible enough to adjust from group to individual sessions if individuals are unable to attend,[133] and data collection should be reduced to only that which is necessary.[108]

Before study implementation, research staff and involved church leaders will likely need training.[127] Research staff will want to take time to learn the culture of the church so that they can approach the CBPR effort with an attitude of cultural humility.[94] Researchers and church leaders and members should work together to determine who will collect the data and who will deliver the intervention. Some research teams find that training community members for these tasks works best as they can more easily connect with and relate to participants.[108,133–135] This approach may have some challenges related to funding that may limit dedicated staff for the research and competing time commitments among community members or volunteers. Further, community members may need continuous support from research staff to deliver the intervention. For example, they may need help dealing with participants' concerns over fellow church members seeing their private information.[134,136]

As a specific research study within a large collaboration comes to a close, researchers should once again consider program sustainability. For example, if community members and church leaders had been trained to deliver the intervention or collect data, there may be momentum to continue delivering health education.[94] Researchers could also donate the program materials and equipment to the congregation.[94] When looking to expand the program, researchers could use the larger church networks, perhaps capitalizing on relationships between pastors of different churches that could allow a program to expand beyond one church.[127] To continue the partnership, researchers could help churches identify other funding sources and build their grant-writing skills so they could apply for new funding.[94]

EXAMPLE OF CBPR IN AFRICAN AMERICAN CHURCHES

An example of a successful research-community partnership is one developed between the University of Texas MD Anderson Cancer Center in Houston and the Project CHURCH network of African American churches. Project CHURCH was initiated in December 2008 with an African American church (Church A) that had more than 15,000 members and had previous collaborations with MD Anderson Cancer Center. Project Church expanded expanded in 2012, and two new African American churches were created (Churches B and C with ~5,000 members each). The churches were all located in a similar geographical area, though church members lived throughout five counties in the greater Houston area.

To build a strong foundation for the partnership, researchers approached church leaders with the idea for a research collaboration but not a specific study. Research staff spent the first year discussing questions and concerns about the motivations for a potential study and products, attending church worship services and activities, helping church members seek out health services in the community, and providing cancer control programming, such as speakers, as requested by the churches. Although the churches' focus puts health in line with their mission, research itself was not specified, so building a deep bidirectional partnership that included aspects of service delivery was important to allow research to proceed. After a strong foundation was built, the partnership launched a mutually agreed on cohort study to understand intrapersonal, interpersonal, institutional, community, and public policy cancer risk factors that could contribute to racial/ethnic disparities in cancer-related outcomes. The CABs (one at each church), comprising researchers and church members who were compensated, were also a central part of Project CHURCH. The CABs helped to develop and advise on all research procedures, protocols, materials, questionnaires, and content. For example, the content of the questionnaire was negotiated each year with the CAB, when necessary introducing new constructs of interest to the group and removing old ones. The instruments included not only common questions but also items of interest to the specific church, such as questions on survivorship for one church that had a significant number of cancer survivors.

Data collection was initiated in 2008 and concluded in 2013, with a final cohort size of 2,338 representing the three churches. Using churches' established communication structures, researchers communicated details of the study and recruited participants. This included communicating to the congregation during services, posting information on church media (website, newsletter, flyers), and using interpersonal communication within church networks. To make study participation more convenient and provide a more familiar setting for participants, Church A provided a permanent office space within the church. All research staff were African American and received training in cultural competence with faith-based organizations. After data collection was complete, Project CHURCH research staff communicated the results to the study participants and the church congregations as a whole. Apart from professional academic publications, this was achieved through newsletters that also included other health information, an annual report that included CAB-reviewed content, and individual feedback based on survey responses (based on CAB recommendations).

Given that the initial study was not an intervention but rather a cohort study, Project CHURCH provided cancer risk and prevention information as requested, structured cancer prevention program activities (e.g., smoking cessation classes, fitness activities such as salsa dancing), and services to help connect church members to needed healthcare. As the partnership progressed and research funding became available, cancer prevention interventions were developed and implemented to address health concerns identified in the research studies. For example, through cohort data, the researchers found that some 80% of participants were overweight or obese. We implemented the Healthy Habits Study, to determine whether counseling could improve diet and physical activity in overweight African American adults.

Project CHURCH is a good example of the CBPR process within an African American community. It was successful because activities aligned with the seven principles of CBPR, described earlier. Special considerations for conducting CBPR in African American churches, such as addressing the concerns of congregation members, providing tangible services requested by the community, and seeking CAB input and approval for all study-related items, led to a productive and ongoing collaborative process. Currently, MD Anderson Cancer Center researchers continue to be extensively involved with church partners. They have included student trainees, particularly from Project CHURCH churches themselves, and provided them with applied, hands-on research experience opportunities that help develop and enhance their understanding of cancer health disparities. The research team has also established an Ancillary Studies Committee to review requests for new proposed research with the Project CHURCH cohort and ensure the research proposed is relevant to African Americans and benefits the cohort.

Considerations of history, trust, respect, and culture are essential when conducting CBPR with African American or any racial/ethnic minority groups. Successful CBPR efforts have engaged the community in areas where they live, work, receive services, and worship. The CBPR experience and studies described above demonstrate the mutual benefit that can emerge from carefully conducted and collaborative research.

CBPR Among Asian Americans

Asians were the fastest growing ethnic minority group in the United States between 2000 and 2010.[137] In fact, by 2050, 1 in 10 persons living in the United States will be Asian American. The designation "Asian American" embraces a variety of Asian subgroups; the largest are Chinese, followed by Asian Indians, Filipinos, Vietnamese, Korean, and Japanese.[137] Although the Asian American population has experienced significant growth, health disparities remain. These disparities are masked by the small sample size of most research studies of this population and the tendency of national datasets to aggregate the different ethnic subgroups.[138,139]

Although Asian Americans are often called the model minority and share similar cultural traits, such as allocentrism, there are differences among Asian subgroups. This heterogeneity includes differences in income, family unit and household size, insurance coverage, and education, as well as other sociodemographic characteristics.[140] For example, Chinese Americans tend to be more educated and have higher income than Vietnamese Americans. The subgroups also differ in their health behaviors, health outcomes, and healthcare utilization.[140]

HEALTH RISKS AND BEHAVIORS

The health problems and risk factors that disproportionately affect Asian Americans include cancer, diabetes, hepatitis B, depression, and tobacco-related illnesses.[140] Asians and Pacific Islanders are the *only* US racial/ethnic populations to experience cancer as the leading cause of death.[138] Asian Americans have a 60% higher prevalence of diabetes than non-Hispanic Whites[141] and the highest hepatitis B infection rates compared with other ethnicities.[142] Although 30% of Asian American girls in grades 5–12 reported more depression symptoms than their non-Asian counterparts,[143] Asian American children are less likely to receive mental healthcare.[144] Asian American women over 65 have the highest suicide rates among US women in that age group.[145] Adult Asian American men have the highest smoking rates.[146]

Compared with all other US women, Asian American women are the least likely to have ever undergone mammography, even though breast cancer is among the most commonly diagnosed cancers in this group.[147]

Asian Americans face many barriers to healthcare including lack of insurance, lack of acculturation, limited English proficiency,[148] and their own cultural norms. Approximately 14.6% of Asian Americans are uninsured.[149] Less-acculturated Asian women with access barriers to care are less likely to be screened for breast cancer.[150] As seen with other subgroups, there can be a lack of trust in research and individuals who may not belong to their racial/ethnic group.

BARRIERS TO RESEARCH PARTICIPATION AND UTILIZATION OF HEALTHCARE

Previous work has shown that there may be several factors that influence use of the healthcare system that may also influence participation in CBPR efforts that are related to healthcare. These may include preference for Eastern medicine in these communities, cultural beliefs about not looking for asymptomatic ailments, and the stigma if friends and family were to find out about certain disease diagnoses.[151,152] If the goal of the research or intervention is to deliver a health or educational service, researchers should consider the Asian American subgroup and other characteristics, such as gender, when understanding influences on use and acceptability of the intervention or service. For example, among Vietnamese women the gender of the physician rather than the ethnicity was a major determinant for requesting or approving cancer-screening services.[153,154]

Another factor that specifically affects participation in research by undocumented Asian American immigrants is the false belief that a signed research consent form becomes a document that could lead to deportation. This points to a lack of understanding of the consent and confidentiality procedures and how study information is used.[139] Researchers could help alleviate this issue by using CBPR processes to understand and generate solutions on how to best communicate and respond to concerns among undocumented populations who may have this concern.

There are important considerations to be taken into account and openly discussed with the community throughout the design and development of CBPR. Researchers must be aware that language barriers could be a deterrent to participation[155] and that linguistic and social isolation may discourage potential participants from becoming involved in or frequenting community events or organizations.[155,156] Other common barriers reported by Asian Americans are time constraints, family commitment, and transportation difficulties.[155] These should be considered during intervention design and data collection procedures to minimize the burden. Potential solutions are to have participation opportunities during lunch breaks, evenings, and weekends and offering childcare during research participation.

Some authors argue that there are cultural considerations that if taken into account could improve participation. For example, because collective decision-making is a core value for several Asian cultures, addressing health issues as a family matter rather than as a personal issue can be an effective approach for engaging Asian communities, especially if the target audience are women or elderly.[151,157–159]

Planning and implementing CBPR with Asian American communities may include considerations of cultural practices and beliefs. To improve participation in CBPR researchers may want to consider the following strategies:

1. working with community-based organizations and groups,
2. using community or lay health workers from the communities of interest,
3. using culturally appropriate materials and language,
4. employing multiple recruitment methods, including social networks to recruit family members and friends, flyers, and broadcast media,[160,161]

5. scheduling community partner meetings, focus groups, and research participation events outside business hours, and
6. planning for program sustainability.

Researchers may benefit from working with community groups, establishing and then maintaining long-standing partners in the community, gaining insight from community members, and developing a CAB. Having a community partner intro-duce the researcher and the project to the community may increase acceptance and participation. Partnering with community-based organizations (CBOs) that primarily serve Asian communities can facilitate entry into a community and increase trust. Often, CBOs are trusted by the community members they serve and therefore may help recruit and attract participants to the CBPR process.[138,161] In return, researchers could offer to help the CBOs with their program evalua-tions, which they often must provide to their funders. The CBO would then ben-efit from the expertise of researchers, who could help build capacity within the organization to conduct their own evaluations in the future or even compete for additional sources of funding to conduct independent research that the CBO is interested in.[162] This collaboration may help in recruitment and reach as well as sustainability and future research. Mutual knowledge transfer and training in the planning phase would provide the CBO with basic research concepts,[157] services, or education that CBOs, themselves, may not be able to provide.

EXAMPLES OF SUCCESSFUL CBPR

'Imi Hale Native Hawaiian Cancer Awareness, Research and Training Network is an example of an Asian American–focused CBPR.[157] This network was nation-ally funded through the National Cancer Institute of the US National Instittes of Health (NIH) and was the only network of its kind based in a CBO rather than an academic or medical center. 'Imi Hale staff were primarily Native Hawaiians, while their Community Council members included various professionals from throughout the Hawaiian islands, and the Scientific Council comprised academ-ics, half of whom were Native Hawaiian. In line with the CBPR principle of capac-ity building, 'Imi Hale worked with several Native Hawaiian Heath Care Systems, providing them with funding for their outreach staff. 'Imi Hale also provided training in community outreach and mobilization, cultural competency, research, health education, grant writing, manuscript writing, and program evaluation to all network members. For their part, Native Hawaiian Heath Care Systems helped recruit participants and test educational materials. To continue the collaborative research process with the Native Hawaiian community, 'Imi Hale aimed to build their cancer research skills. This iterative process was time and labor intensive, consisting of many cycles of seeking and incorporating community feedback on general research directions and then on the cultural relevancy of materials.

The 'Imi Hale network also provided training and opportunities for Native Hawaiians to work on the research study and be involved in all important decisions, including how funds were spent. This collaborative network, led by and for Native Hawaiians, was able to build community capacity to write scientific papers, provide cancer education, mobilize, and other skills, as well as increase the availability of Native Hawaiian–specific educational materials.

As with other groups, successful CBPR efforts with Asian American communities require understanding of opportunities and challenges and appropriate application of the CBPR process. Community-based participatory research has great potential to help increase understanding of the unique and varied health needs of Asian Americans including disaggregating information about Asians and better understanding and attending to the needs of individual subgroups that comprise the Asian American community in the United States.

CBPR Among Native Americans

American Indians and Alaskan Natives (AIAN) are a diverse group with a long experience of systematic discrimination, health and wealth disparities, and poverty.[163-168] According to the Office for Minority Health, US Department of Health and Human Services, in 2012, AIAN households had a median household income nearly $20,000 lower than the median household income for non-Hispanic White families.[169] AIAN communities often exist in geographically isolated areas with heightened environmental health risks, food insecurity, and disproportionally high rates of unemployment.[163,165,166-170] Leading causes of morbidity and mortality among AIAN include diabetes, heart disease, accidents, stroke, substance abuse and related diseases, and sudden infant death syndrome. Health disparities are in diabetes rates, infant mortality, stomach and liver cancer, liver disease, strokes, and death due to hepatitis C.[169] Skinner and Masuda's 2013 study on health in a Canadian AIAN community found that local AIAN youth recognized pests and inadequate waste disposal as health priorities.[168] A report filed in 2007 for Healthy People 2010 also found increasing disparities in air pollution in AIAN communities.[171]

Given these disparities, there is a need for resources and research in AIAN communities to tackle these issues and find interventions or other solutions to address them. Conventional research methods have been deemed ineffective and biased, since they lack cultural sensitivity, insider knowledge, and tangible benefit for the Native American community.[163] Community-based participatory research is a common approach used by researchers working with AIAN communities because its principles are thought to mitigate the effects of historical injustice and power imbalance sometimes seen with conventional methods.[163,165,170,172-174] When AIAN voices, culture, and methods are central, CBPR may be considered as a decolonizing research method.[175] Another term is "tribal participatory research," which focuses on empowering the AIAN community as well as on issues of social justice and change.[165] However, AIAN CBPR projects may have less federal funding and are generally more descriptive, with fewer interventions and less dissemination, compared with CBPR in multiple or unspecified races.[176]

Researchers working with AIANs are likely aware that tribal nations are sovereign. As such, then may have their own form of institutional review board to approve research with human subjects, contractual ownership of data and authority over its use, or protocols for approving publications that result from research.[166,167,170,174,177,178] As with other ethnic and racial minority groups, creating a CAB is key to ensure that any research or intervention is culturally sensitive and acceptable. The CAB members could include such key community figures such as tribal elders, chiefs, or council members.[163,166,167] Further sharing or transferring power within the CBPR framework could be paying AIAN research team members or treating CAB members as academic partners.[166,167,170] In other cases, it may be more appropriate for the AIAN community or leaders to be the primary grant holders.[177]

Along with using CBPR guiding principles to build relationships and set the groundwork within the community, consideration should be given to culturally competent methods and data collection. The use of Western theoretical models must be carefully considered in AIAN CBPR research. When Simonds and Christopher undertook CBPR on provider–patient interactions within the Crow nation, the PRECEDE-PROCEED theoretical model, though previously agreed on by CAB members, ran counter to Crow culture and so hampered rather than helped the research process.[179] The Crow value stories as whole entities, so fragmenting them by separating stories into themes for analysis cause them to lose meaning and context. Based on this experience, the researchers recommend that AIAN CBPR partnerships take steps to ensure that research remains decolonizing and respectful of AIAN cultural diversity. This can be accomplished by discussing worldviews, recognizing that decolonization is an ongoing process, and continuing to critically evaluate theories and methods throughout the research process to determine and maintain their fit within the cultural context. Seeing that the PRECEDE-PROCEED model would not work, Simonds and Christopher developed a new model based on Crow cultural values and symbology, which grounded analysis in a culturally meaningful way.[175]

To ensure culturally relevant data collection, qualitative methods may be more appropriate for the communication styles and social norms of many Native American groups.[163] Photovoice, a process that allows community members to visually record their community's assets to promote dialogue about community issues,[180] is a common data collection technique used in AIAN communities because it is thought to be culturally competent and able to create greater power parity.[172,174,179,181] Apart from photovoice specifically, culturally competent data collection or dissemination may include holding these procedures in or integrating them with a community event.[164,167,168,172,174] Depending on the protocols determined by the sovereign AIAN group, the entire tribal community—not just

CAB members—may own the intellectual property generated by research, with provisions for participants to review transcripts and request changes and to have the right to hear research results first and request resolutions for conflicting data interpretations.[163,164,167,170,172,177,178] In some situations, knowledge about the AIAN group may be perceived as belonging to its members specifically and not something to be shared with outsiders.[178] Even if data ownership is not specified, it could be good practice to disseminate findings to the AIAN community first. For example, when the Huu-Ay-Aht First Nation partnered with researchers to evaluate the use of photovoice, they used a series of community potluck meals to ensure community members were successfully appraised of the project's progress and findings in a timely manner.[172] Additionally, any resulting publications may also need to be reviewed and approved by CAB or the AIAN leaders.[166,174,177]

STEPS FOR CONDUCTING CBPR RESEARCH IN AIAN

The first step in any AIAN CBPR project should be to contact tribal leadership, as this acknowledges sovereignty and helps researchers learn who controls permission to approach tribal members and whether the tribe has its own review board.[166,167,170,174,177,178] If tribal leaders approve a CBPR partnership, researchers should consider council members, chiefs, or elders for CAB membership.[163,166,167] Funding sources may include payment for AIAN staff or it may be awarded directly to the AIAN council with researchers as subcontractors.[166,167,170,177] A formal, written agreement should be made involving data use, analysis and ownership, and publication rights; this may include provisions for data or biological samples to be housed in the AIAN community, for participants to review interview transcripts, or for the community to review findings and request reinterpretation.[163,164,167,170,172,177,178] In addition to steps regularly taken for CBPR, the CAB should discuss whether Western theories and methods fit with the local AIAN worldview and engage in a continuing discussion on cultural competence of the methods.[175] Photovoice may help to center AIAN perspectives.[172,174,179,181] In addition to honoring the data ownership agreement, progressive data findings may be disseminated regularly to the community at large if the CAB members or tribal leadership so desire.[172,178] Manuscripts should be reviewed by the CAB members and, possibly, the AIAN leadership before publication.[166,174,177]

LESSONS LEARNED

An advantage of CBPR, when used to its strengths in this setting, is that it allows for the cultural differences between AIAN and Western research cultures to generate data and to create unique, viable solutions for distinctive, diverse AIAN cultures. Given the high level of health disparities faced by AIAN populations, the need for culturally relevant interventions to help close those gaps is evident.[163,165–171,175]

Used as a decolonizing method to center in-group knowledge, CBPR may have a greater ability to help than traditional Western research approaches, but CBPR projects must increasingly focus on intervention and dissemination, not merely description.[163,165,170,172-176]

Summary

This chapter described considerations for conducting CBPR with racial/ethnic minority groups and provided both recommendations and examples of effective CBPR efforts. The literature on CBPR with minorities has highlighted several important factors that influence the success of CBPR. While some of these are specific to certain groups, many, such as trust, fear of deportation (among immigrant groups), the need to work with trusted community organizations, and a focus on empowerment and sustainability, are important considerations across all groups.

Openness and flexibility of researchers, a common recommendation for all CBPR practice, may be particularly important when working with racial/ethnic minorities. As illustrated above in the example of research with the Crow Nation, CBPR researchers must be willing to revise not only data collection approaches but also analytic strategies if they run counter to cultural norms.

The importance of establishing partnerships with CBOs or other groups who can advocate for the community and make lasting change was another common theme. These partnerships provide mutual support and understanding with the common goal of improving health and quality of life beyond the period of the research project. Researchers conducting CBPR with racial/ethnic communities must recognize that only with the combined knowledge and experiences of researchers and communities can CBPR efforts truly be successful and result in the reduction of health disparities.

Perhaps one of the most important considerations for conducting research with racial/ethnic minority communities is the importance of approaching CBPR with an attitude of cultural humility. This should include researcher self-assessment of attitudes and behaviors that may influence interactions, understanding, and interpretation of findings. It is a commitment to continue learning and recognition that one is never fully "competent" in another culture. Therefore the willingness to develop oneself as a CBPR researcher that has the skills, attitudes, and processes that display self-reflection, flexibility, honesty, transparency, and respect is a prerequisite of such an approach.

Continuing to learn from our successes as well as our failures in collaborative CBPR efforts with racial/ethnic minority communities can help improve both the experience of CBPR for researchers and communities alike, and most importantly, can lead to decreased disparities, and increased health and quality of life for minority communities.

References

1. Lewin, K. *Resolving Social Conflicts*. Washington, DC: American Psychological Association 1948.
2. Lewin, K. "Action Research and Minority Problems." *Journal of Social Issues* 2.4 (1946): 34–46.
3. Lazarus, S., Duran, B., Caldwell, L. and Bulbulia, S. "Public Health Research and Action: Reflections on Challenges and Possibilities of Community-Based Participatory Research, Public Health—Social and Behavioral Health, Prof. Jay Maddock (Ed.), ISBN: 978-953-51-0620-3, InTech, Available from: http://www.intechopen.com/books/public-health-social-and-behavioral-health/public-health-research-andaction-reflections-on-challenges-and-possibilities-of-community-based-par
4. Freire, P. *Pedagogy of the Oppressed*, trans. M. B. Ramos. New York: Continuum, 1970.
5. Fals-Borda, O. and Rahman, M.A. *Action and Knowledge: Breaking the Monopoly with Participatory Action-Research*. New York: Apex, 1991.
6. Wallerstein, N. and Duran, B. "The Theoretical, Historical, and Practice Roots of CBPR." *Community-Based Participatory Research for Health: From Process to Outcomes* 2 (2008): 25–46.
7. McLaughlin, L.A. and Braun, K.L. "Asian and Pacific Islander Cultural Values: Considerations for Health Care Decision Making." *Health and Social Work* 23.2 (1998): 116–26.
8. Schwartz, S.J., Weisskirch, R.S., Hurley, E.A., et al. "Communalism, Familism, and Filial Piety: Are They Birds of a Collectivist Feather?" *Cultural Diversity and Ethnic Minority Psychology* 16.4 (2010): 548.
9. Gaines, Jr., S.O., Marelich, W.D., Bledsoe, K.L., et al. "Links Between Race/Ethnicity and Cultural Values as Mediated by Racial/Ethnic Identity and Moderated by Gender." *Journal of Personality and Social Psychology* 72.6 (1997): 1460.
10. Fernandez, M.E., Wippold, R., Torres-Vigil, I., et al. "Colorectal Cancer Screening Among Latinos from US Cities Along the Texas-Mexico Border." *Cancer Causes and Control* 19.2 (2008): 195–206.
11. Abraido-Lanza, A.F., Viladrich, A., Florez, K.R., Cespedes, A., Aguirre, A.N. and De La Cruz, A.A. "Fatalismo Reconsidered: A Cautionary Note for Health-Related Research and Practice with Latino Populations." *Ethnicity and Disease* 17.1 (2007): 153.
12. Fernandez, M.E., Palmer, R.C. and Leong-Wu, C.A. "Repeat Mammography Screening Among Low-Income and Minority Women: A Qualitative Study." *Cancer Control* 12 Suppl 2 (2005): 77–83.
13. "Culture." *Cambridge Dictionary* (2016). <http://dictionary.cambridge.org/dictionary/english/culture> (accessed July 9, 2016).
14. Helman, C. *Culture, Health and Illness: An Introduction for Health Professionals*. Oxford: Butterworth-Heinemann, 1997.
15. Bartholomew Eldredge, L.K., Markham, C., Ruiter, R.A.C., Fernandez, M.E., Kok, G. and Parcel, G. *Planning Health Promotion Programs: An Intervention Mapping Approach* (4th ed.). San Francisco: Jossey Bass; 2016.
16. Bennett, J.M. "Cultural Marginality: Identity Issues in Intercultural Training." In *Education for the Intercultural Experience* (2nd ed.), ed. R.M. Paige. Yarmouth, ME: Intercultural Press, 1993; pp. 109–35.
17. Bennett, J. "Developing Intercultural Competence: For International Education Faculty and Staff." *2011 Association of International Education Administrators Conference*. 2011, February 22.
18. Bennett, M.J. "Towards Ethnorelativism: A Developmental Model of Intercultural Sensitivity." In *Education for the Intercultural Experience* (2nd ed.), ed. R.M. Paige. Yarmouth, ME: Intercultural Press, 1993; pp. 21–71.
19. Bennett, J.M. and Bennett, M.J. "Developing Intercultural Sensitivity: An Integrative Approach to Global and Domestic Diversity." In *Handbook of Intercultural Training* (3rd ed.), ed. D. Landis, J.M. Bennett and M.J. Bennett. Thousand Oaks, CA: Sage, 2004; pp. 147–65.
20. Airhihenbuwa, C.O. "On Being Comfortable with Being Uncomfortable: Centering an Africanist Vision in Our Gateway to Global Health." *Health Education and Behavior* 34.1 (2007): 31–42.

21. Ford, C.L. and Airhihenbuwa, C.O. "Critical Race Theory, Race Equity, and Public Health: Toward Antiracism Praxis." *American Journal of Public Health* 100 Suppl 1 (2010): S30–5.

22. Valdes, F., Culp, J.M. and Harris, A. *Crossroads, Directions and a New Critical Race Theory.* Philadelphia, PA: Temple University Press, 2002.

23. Delgado, R. and Stefancic, J. *Critical Race Theory.* New York: New York University Press, 2001.

24. Bonilla-Silva, E. *Racism Without Racists: Color-Blind Racism and the Persistence of Racial Inequality in the United States.* Lanham, MD: Rowman & Littlefield, 2006.

25. Tervalon, M. "Components of Culture in Health for Medical Students' Education." *Academic Medicine* 78.6 (2003): 570–6.

26. Tervalon, M. and Murray-Garcia, J. "Cultural Humility Versus Cultural Competence: A Critical Distinction in Defining Physician Training Outcomes in Multicultural Education." *Journal of Health Care for the Poor and Underserved* 9.2 (1998): 117–25.

27. Levi, A. "The Ethics of Nursing Student International Clinical Experiences." *Journal of Obstetric, Gynecologic, and Neonatal Nursing* 38.1 (2009): 94–9.

28. Hook, J.N., Davis, D.E., Owen, J., Worthington, E.L., Jr. and Utsey, S.O. "Cultural Humility: Measuring Openness to Culturally Diverse Clients." *Journal of Counseling Psychology* 60.3 (2013): 353.

29. Hixon, A.L. "Beyond Cultural Competence." *Academic Medicine* 78.6 (2003): 634.

30. "Community Tool Box: Adapting Community Interventions for Different Cultures and Communities." *University of Kansas* (2016). <http://ctb.ku.edu/en/table-of-contents/analyze/choose-and-adapt-community-interventions/cultural-adaptation/main> (accessed July 9, 2016).

31. Waters, A. and Asbill, L. "Reflections on Cultural Humility." *American Psychological Association* (2013). <http://www.apa.org/pi/families/resources/newsletter/2013/08/cultural-humility.aspx> (accessed July 9, 2016).

32. Eakin, E.G., Bull, S.S., Riley, K., Reeves, M.M., Gutierrez, S. and McLaughlin, P. "Recruitment and Retention of Latinos in a Primary Care-Based Physical Activity and Diet Trial: The Resources for Health Study." *Health Education Research* 22.3 (2007): 361–71.

33. Garcia, C.M., Gilchrist, L., Campesino, C., Raymond, N., Naughton, S. and de Patino, J.G. "Using Community-Based Participatory Research to Develop a Bilingual Mental Health Survey for Latinos." *Progress in Community Health Partnerships* 2.2 (2008): 105–20.

34. Shattell, M.M., Hamilton, D., Starr, S.S., Jenkins, C.J. and Hinderliter, N.A. "Mental Health Service Needs of a Latino Population: A Community-Based Participatory Research Project." *Issues in Mental Health Nursing* 29.4 (2008): 351–70.

35. Martinez, I.L., Carter-Pokras, O. and Brown, P.B. "Addressing the Challenges of Latino Health Research: Participatory Approaches in an Emergent Urban Community." *Journal of the National Medical Association* 101.9 (2009): 908–14.

36. Rhodes, S.D., Hergenrather, K.C., Montano, J., et al. "Using Community-Based Participatory Research to Develop an Intervention to Reduce HIV and STD Infections Among Latino Men." *AIDS Education and Prevention* 18.5 (2006): 375–89.

37. Larkey, L.K., Gonzalez, J.A., Mar, L.E. and Glantz N. "Latina Recruitment for Cancer Prevention Education via Community Based Participatory Research Strategies." *Contemporary Clinical Trials* 30.1 (2009): 47–54.

38. Rios-Ellis, B., Espinoza, L., Bird, M., et al. "Increasing HIV-Related Knowledge, Communication, and Testing Intentions Among Latinos: Protege tu Familia: Hazte la Prueba." *Journal of Health Care for the Poor and Underserved* 21.3 (2010): 148–68.

39. Shetgiri, R., Kataoka, S.H., Ryan, G.W., Askew, L.M., Chung, P.J. and Schuster, M.A. "Risk and Resilience in Latinos: A Community-Based Participatory Research Study." *American Journal of Preventive Medicine* 37.6 (2009): S217–24.

40. Stepler, R. and Brown, A. *Statistical Portrait of Hispanics in the United States.* Washington, DC: Pew Research Center, 2016.

41. Patten, E. *The Nation's Latino Population Is Defined by Its Youth.* Washington, DC: Pew Research Center, 2016.

42. Lopez, M.H., Gonzalez-Barrera, A. and Cuddington, D. *Diverse Origins: The Nation's 14 Largest Hispanic-Origin Groups.* Washington, DC: Pew Research Center, 2013.

43. Bustamante, A.V., Fang, H., Garza, J., et al. "Variations in Healthcare Access and Utilization Among Mexican Immigrants: The Role of Documentation Status." *Journal of Immigrant and Minority Health* 14.1 (2012): 146–55.

44. Rodriguez, M.A., Bustamante, A.V. and Ang, A. "Perceived Quality of Care, Receipt of Preventive Care, and Usual Source of Health Care Among Undocumented and Other Latinos." *Journal of General Internal Medicine* 24.3 (2009): 508–13.

45. Perez-Escamilla, R., Garcia, J. and Song, D. "Health Care Access Among Hispanic Immigrants: ¿Alguien está escuchando?[Is Anybody Listening?]." *NAPA Bulletin* 34.1 (2010): 47–67.

46. Ayon, C. *Economic, Social, and Health Effects of Discrimination on Latino Immigrant Families.* Washington, DC: Migration Policy Institute, 2015, September.

47. McCarthy, J. *Immigrant Status Tied to Discrimination Among Hispanics.* Gallup, 2015, August 20.

48. Centers for Disease Control and Prevention. "CDC Health Disparities and Inequalities Report-United States, 2011." *MMWR: Morbidity and Mortality Weekly Report* 60 (2011): 1–113.

49. Acevedo-Garcia, D., Soobader, M.-J. and Berkman, L.F. "The Differential Effect of Foreign-Born Status on Low Birth Weight by Race/Ethnicity and Education." *Pediatrics* 115.1 (2005): e20–30.

50. Centers for Disease Control and Prevention. "Health Disparities Experienced by Hispanics—United States." *MMWR: Morbidity and Mortality Weekly Report* 53.40 (2004): 935–7.

51. Vega, W.A., Rodriguez, M.A. and Gruskin, E. "Health Disparities in the Latino Population." *Epidemiologic Reviews* 31.1 (2009): 99–112.

52. Siegel, R., Naishadham, D. and J emal, A. "Cancer Statistics for Hispanics/Latinos, 2012." *CA: A Cancer Journal for Clinicians* 62.5 (2012): 283–98.

53. DaNavas-Walt, C., Proctor, B.D. and Smith, J.C. "Income, Poverty, and Health Insurance Coverage in the United States: 2010." Washington, DC: US Census Bureau, 2011.

54. Brown, A. and Lopez, M.H. *Mapping the Latino Population, By State, County, and City.* Washington, DC: Pew Research Center, 2013, August 29.

55. Guzman, B. *The Hispanic Population, 2000. Census 2000 Brief.* US Census Bureau, 2001.

56. Ai, A.L., Appel, H.B., Huang, B. and Lee, K. "Overall Health and Healthcare Utilization Among Latino American Women in the United States." *Journal of Women's Health* 21.8 (2012): 878–85.

57. Guzman, B. and McConnell, E.D. "The Hispanic Population: 1990–2000 Growth and Change." *Population Research and Policy Review* 21.1–2 (2002): 109–28.

58. Hayes-Bautista, D.E. "Identifying 'Hispanic' Populations: The Influence of Research Methodology upon Public Policy." *American Journal of Public Health* 70.4 (1980): 353–6.

59. Hayes-Bautista, D.E. and Chapa, J. "Latino Terminology: Conceptual Bases for Standardized Terminology." *American Journal of Public Health* 77.1 (1987): 61–8.

60. Mahtani, M. "What's in a Name? Exploring the Employment of 'Mixed Race' as an Identification." *Ethnicities* 2.4 (2002): 469–90.

61. Cristancho, S., Garces, D.M., Peters, K.E. and Mueller, B.C. "Listening to Rural Hispanic Immigrants in the Midwest: A Community-Based Participatory Assessment of Major Barriers to Health Care Access and Use." *Qualitative Health Research* 18.5 (2008): 633–46.

62. Parrado, E.A., McQuiston, C. and Flippen, C.A. "Participatory Survey Research Integrating Community Collaboration and Quantitative Methods for the Study of Gender and HIV Risks Among Hispanic Migrants." *Sociological Methods and Research* 34.2 (2005): 204–39.

63. Kim, S., Flaskerud, J.H., Koniak-Griffin, D. and Dixon, E.L. "Using Community-Partnered Participatory Research to Address Health Disparities in a Latino Community." *Journal of Professional Nursing* 21.4 (2005): 199–209.

64. Foster, J. and Stanek, K. "Cross-Cultural Considerations in the Conduct of Community-Based Participatory Research." *Family and Community Health* 30.1 (2007): 42–9.

65. National Cancer Institute. "Community Networks Program (CNP) Program Information." *National Cancer Institute*, 2015, February 17. <http://www.cancer.gov/about-nci/organization/crchd/disparities-research/cnpc> (accessed July 12, 2016).

66. Harris, J.R., Brown, P.K., Steven, C., et al. "The Cancer Prevention and Control Research Network." *Preventing Chronic Disease* 2.1 (2005). Available from: URL: http://www.cdc.gov/pcd/issues/2005/jan/04_0059.htm.

67. Cancer Prevention and Control Research Network. *Cancer Prevention and Control Research Network* (2016). <cpcrn.org> (accessed July 12, 2016).

68. Corbin, J.H., Fernandez, M.E. and Mullen, P.D. "Evaluation of a Community-Academic Partnership Lessons from Latinos in a Network for Cancer Control." *Health Promotion Practice* 16.3 (2015): 345–53.

69. Fernandez, M.E., Melvin, C.L., Leeman, J., et al. "The Cancer Prevention and Control Research Network: An Interactive Systems Approach to Advancing Cancer Control Implementation Research and Practice." *Cancer Epidemiology, Biomarkers and Prevention* 23.11 (2014): 2512–21.

70. Yeoman, B. "Hispanic Diaspora." *Mother Jones* 25.4 (2000): 34–40. Foundation for National Progress.

71. Metzler, M.M., Higgins, D.L., Beeker, C.G., et al. "Addressing Urban Health in Detroit, New York City, and Seattle Through Community-Based Participatory Research Partnerships." *American Journal of Public Health* 93.5 (2003): 803–11.

72. Veazie, M.A., Teufel-Shone, N.I., Silverman, G.S., et al. "Building Community Capacity in Public Health: The Role of Action-Oriented Partnerships." *Journal of Public Health Management and Practice* 7.2 (2001): 21–32.

73. Viswanathan, M., Ammerman, A., Eng, E., et al. *Community-Based Participatory Research: Assessing the Evidence: Summary"* In AHRQ Evidence Report Summaries. Rockville, MD: AHRQ Publications, 2004.

74. Israel, B.A., Schulz, A.J., Parker, E.A. and Becker, A.B. "Community-Based Participatory Research: Policy Recommendations for Promoting a Partnership Approach in Health Research." *Education for Health* 14.2 (2001): 182–97.

75. Byrd, T.L., Peterson, S.K., Chavez, R. and Heckert, A. "Cervical Cancer Screening Beliefs Among Young Hispanic Women." *Preventive Medicine* 38.2 (2004): 192–7.

76. Hanis, C.L., Ferrell, R.E., Barton, S.A., et al. "Diabetes Among Mexican Americans in Starr County, Texas." *American Journal of Epidemiology* 118.5 (1983): 659–72.

77. Diaz-Apodaca, B.A., Ebrahim, S., McCormack, V., De Cosio, F.G., and Ruiz-Holguin, R. "Prevalence of Type 2 Diabetes and Impaired Fasting Glucose: Cross-Sectional Study of Multiethnic Adult Population at the United States-Mexico Border." *Revista Panamericana de Salud Publica* 28.3 (2010): 174–81.

78. Coughlin, S.S., Richards, T.B., Nasseri, K., et al. "Cervical Cancer Incidence in the United States in the US-Mexico Border Region, 1998–2003." *Cancer* 113 Suppl 10 (2008): 2964–73.

79. Das, R., Steege, A., Baron, S., Beckman, J. and Harrison, R. "Pesticide-Related Illness Among Migrant Farm Workers in the United States." *International Journal of Occupational and Environmental Health* 7.4 (2001): 303–12.

80. Hansen, E. and Donohoe, M. "Health Issues of Migrant and Seasonal Farmworkers." *Journal of Health Care for the Poor and Underserved* 14.2 (2003): 153–64.

81. Fleischer, N.L., Tiesman, H.M., Sumitani, J., et al. "Public Health Impact of Heat-Related Illness Among Migrant Farmworkers." *American Journal of Preventive Medicine* 44.3 (2013): 199–206.

82. Kilanowski, J.F. "Challenges in Community-Based Research with Latino Migrant Farmworker Children and Families." *Journal of Pediatric Health Care* 28.5 (2014): 461–5.

83. Fernandez, M.E., Savas, L.S., Carmack, C.C., et al. "A Randomized Controlled Trial of Two Interventions to Increase Colorectal Cancer Screening Among Hispanics on the Texas-Mexico Border." *Cancer Causes and Control* 26.1 (2015): 1–10.

84. Fernandez, M.E., Gonzales, A., Tortolero-Luna, G., et al. "Effectiveness of Cultivando la Salud: A Breast and Cervical Cancer Screening Promotion Program for Low-Income Hispanic Women." *American Journal of Public Health* 99.5 (2009): 936–43.

85. Reininger, B.M., Barroso, C.S., Mitchell-Bennett, L., et al. "Process Evaluation and Participatory Methods in an Obesity-Prevention Media Campaign for Mexican Americans." *Health Promotion Practice* 11.3 (2010): 347–57.

86. Reininger, B.M., Mitchell-Bennett, L., Lee, M., et al. "Tu Salud, ¡Si Cuenta!: Exposure to a Community-Wide Campaign and Its Associations with Physical Activity and Fruit and Vegetable Consumption Among Individuals of Mexican Descent." *Social Science and Medicine* 143 (2015): 98–106.

87. de Castro, A.B., Fujishiro, K., Sweitzer, E. and Oliva, J. "How Immigrant Workers Experience Workplace Problems: A Qualitative Study." *Archives of Environmental and Occupational Health* 61.6 (2006): 249–58.

88. Negi, N.J. "Identifying Psychosocial Stressors of Well-Being and Factors Related to Substance Use Among Latino Day Laborers." *Journal of Immigrant and Minority Health* 13.4 (2011): 748–55.

89. Buchanan, S.N., Nickels, L. and Morello, J. "Occupational Health Among Chicago Day Laborers: An Exploratory Study." *Archives of Environmental and Occupational Health* 60.5 (2005): 276–80.

90. Fernandez-Esquer, M.E., Fernandez-Espada, N., Atkinson, J.A. and Montano, C.F. "The Influence of Demographics and Working Conditions on Self-Reported Injuries Among Latino Day Laborers." *International Journal of Occupational and Environmental Health* 21.1 (2015): 5–13.

91. Cho, Y., Frisbie, W.P., Hummer, R.A. and Rogers, R.G. "Nativity, Duration of Residence, and the Health of Hispanic Adults in the United States." *International Migration Review* 38.1 (2004): 184–211.

92. Etzioni, A. "Inventing Hispanics: A Diverse Minority Resists Being Labeled." *Brookings Review* 20.1 (2002): 10–3.

93. Gonzalez Burchard, E., Borrell, L.N., Choudhry, S., et al. "Latino Populations: A Unique Opportunity for the Study of Race, Genetics, and Social Environment in Epidemiological Research." *American Journal of Public Health* 95.12 (2005): 2161–8.

94. Campbell, M.K., Hudson, M.A., Resnicow, K., Blakeney, N., Paxton, A. and Baskin, M. "Church-Based Health Promotion Interventions: Evidence and Lessons Learned." *Annual Review of Public Health* 28 (2007): 213–34.

95. George, S., Duran, N. and Norris, K. "A Systematic Review of Barriers and Facilitators to Minority Research Participation Among African Americans, Latinos, Asian Americans, and Pacific Islanders." *American Journal of Public Health* 104.2 (2014): e16–31.

96. Rockwell, D.H., Yobs, A.R. and Moore, M.B. "The Tuskegee Study of Untreated Syphilis: The 30th Year of Observation." *Archives of Internal Medicine* 114.6 (1964): 792–8.

97. Skloot, R. *The Immortal Life of Henrietta Lacks.* New York: Crown, 2010.

98. Katz, R.V., Russell, S.L., Kegeles, S.S., et al. "The Tuskegee Legacy Project: Willingness of Minorities to Participate in Biomedical Research." *Journal of Health Care for the Poor and Underserved* 17.4 (2006): 698.

99. Shavers, V.L., Lynch, C.F. and Burmeister, L.F. "Knowledge of the Tuskegee Study and Its Impact on the Willingness to Participate in Medical Research Studies." *Journal of the National Medical Association* 92.12 (2000): 563.

100. Buseh, A.G., Stevens, P.E., Millon-Underwood, S., Townsend, L. and Kelber, S.T. "Community Leaders' Perspectives on Engaging African Americans in Biobanks and Other Human Genetics Initiatives." *Journal of Community Genetics* 4.4 (2013): 483–94.

101. Adderley-Kelly, B. and Green, P.M. "Strategies for Successful Conduct of Research with Low-Income African American Populations." *Nursing Outlook* 53.3 (2005): 147–52.

102. Parrill, R. and Kennedy, B.R. "Partnerships for Health in the African American Community: Moving Toward Community-Based Participatory Research." *Journal of Cultural Diversity* 18.4 (2011): 150–4.

103. Wallerstein, N.B. and Duran, B. "Using Community-Based Participatory Research to Address Health Disparities." *Health Promotion Practice* 7.3 (2006): 312–23.

104. Corbie-Smith, G. "The Continuing Legacy of the Tuskegee Syphilis Study: Considerations for Clinical Investigation." *American Journal of the Medical Sciences* 317.1 (1999): 5–8.

105. Dancy, B.L., Wilbur, J., Talashek, M., Bonner, G. and Barnes-Boyd, C. "Community-Based Research: Barriers to Recruitment of African Americans." *Nursing Outlook* 52.5 (2004): 234–40.

106. Smith, S.A., Whitehead, M.S., Sheats, J.Q., Ansa, B.E., Coughlin, S.S. and Blumenthal, D.S. "Community-Based Participatory Research Principles for the African American Community." *Journal of the Georgia Public Health Association* 5.1 (2015): 52–6.

107. Israel, B.A., Schulz, A.J., Parker, E.A. and Becker, A.B. "Review of Community-Based Research: Assessing Partnership Approaches to Improve Public Health." *Annual Review of Public Health* 19.1 (1998): 173–202.

108. Ammerman, A., Corbie-Smith, G., St George, D.M., Washington, C., Weathers, B. and Jackson-Christian, B. "Research Expectations Among African American Church Leaders in the PRAISE! Project: A Randomized Trial Guided by Community-Based Participatory Research." *American Journal of Public Health* 93.10 (2003): 1720–7.

109. Bharmal, N., Kennedy, D., Jones, L., et al. "Through Our Eyes: Exploring African-American Men's Perspective on Factors Affecting Transition to Manhood." *Journal of General Internal Medicine* 27.2 (2012): 153–9.

110. Linnan, L.A., Ferguson, Y.O., Wasilewski, Y., et al. "Using Community-Based Participatory Research Methods to Reach Women with Health Messages: Results from the North Carolina BEAUTY and Health Pilot Project." *Health Promotion Practice* 6.2 (2005): 164–73.

111. Linnan, L.A. and Ferguson, Y.O. "Beauty Salons: A Promising Health Promotion Setting for Reaching and Promoting Health Among African American Women." *Health Education and Behavior* 34.3 (2007): 517–30.

112. Zoellner, J., Motley, M., Wilkinson, M.E., Jackman, B., Barlow, M.L. and Hill, J.L. "Engaging the Dan River Region to Reduce Obesity: Application of the Comprehensive Participatory Planning and Evaluation Process." *Family and Community Health* 35.1 (2012): 44–56.

113. Grier, K., Hill, J.L., Reese, F., et al. "Feasibility of an Experiential Community Garden and Nutrition Programme for Youth Living in Public Housing." *Public Health Nutrition* 18.15 (2015): 2759–69.

114. Eng, E., Hatch, J. and Callan, A. "Institutionalizing Social Support Through the Church and into the Community." *Health Education Quarterly* 12.1 (1985): 81–92.

115. Jackson, R.S. and Reddick, B. "The African American Church and University Partnerships: Establishing Lasting Collaborations." *Health Education and Behavior* 26.5 (1999): 663–74.

116. Lugo, L., Stencel, S., Green, J., et al. *"US Religious Landscape Survey: Religious Affiliation-Diverse and Dynamic."* 2008. Available from http://www.pewforum.org/files/2013/05/report-religious-landscape-study-full.pdf (accessed July 15, 2016).

117. Baskin, M.L., Resnicow, K. and Campbell, M.K. "Conducting Health Interventions in Black Churches: A Model for Building Effective Partnerships." *Ethnicity and Disease* 11.4 (2001): 823–33.

118. Thomson, J.L., Goodman, M.H. and Tussing-Humphreys, L. "Diet Quality and Physical Activity Outcome Improvements Resulting from a Church-Based Diet and Supervised Physical Activity Intervention for Rural, Southern, African American Adults: Delta Body and Soul III." *Health Promotion Practice* 16.5 (2015): 677–88.

119. Baruth, M. and Wilcox, S. "Multiple Behavior Change Among Church Members Taking Part in the Faith, Activity, and Nutrition Program." *Journal of Nutrition Education and Behavior* 45.5 (2013): 428–34.

120. Duru, O.K., Sarkisian, C.A., Leng, M. and Mangione, C.M. "Sisters in Motion: A Randomized Controlled Trial of a Faith-Based Physical Activity Intervention." *Journal of the American Geriatric Society* 58.10 (2010): 1863–9.

121. Campbell, M.K., Denmark-Wahnefried, W., Symons, M., et al. "Fruit and Vegetable Consumption and Prevention of Cancer: The Black Churches United for Better Health Project." *American Journal of Public Health* 89.9 (1999): 1390–6.
122. Resnicow, K., Jackson, A., Blissett, D., et al. "Results of the Healthy Body Healthy Spirit Trial." *Health Psychology* 24.4 (2005): 339–48.
123. Resnicow, K., Jackson, A., Wang, T., et al. "A Motivational Interviewing Intervention to Increase Fruit and Vegetable Intake Through Black Churches: Results of the Eat for Life Trial." *American Journal of Public Health* 91.10 (2001): 1686–93.
124. Resnicow, K., Campbell, M., Carr, C., et al. "Body and Soul: A Dietary Intervention Conducted Through African-American Churches." *American Journal of Preventive Medicine* 27.2 (2004): 97–105.
125. Campbell, M.K., James, A., Hudson, M.A., et al. "Improving Multiple Behaviors for Colorectal Cancer Prevention Among African American Church Members." *Health Psychology* 23.5 (2004): 492–502.
126. Erwin, D.O., Spatz, T.S., Stotts, R.C. and Hollenberg, J.A. "Increasing Mammography Practice by African American Women." *Cancer Practice* 7.2 (1999): 78–85.
127. Berkley-Patton, J., Thompson, C.B., Martinez, D.A., et al. "Examining Church Capacity to Develop and Disseminate a Religiously Appropriate HIV Tool Kit with African American Churches." *Journal of Urban Health* 90.3 (2013): 482–99.
128. Green, L.W. and Kreuter, M.W. *Health Program Planning: An Educational and Ecological Approach* (4th ed.). New York: McGraw-Hill, 2005.
129. Lightfoot, A.F., Taggart, T., Woods-Jaeger, B.A., Riggins, L., Jackson, M.R. and Eng, E. "Where Is the Faith? Using a CBPR Approach to Propose Adaptations to an Evidence-Based HIV Prevention Intervention for Adolescents in African American Faith Settings." *Journal of Religion and Health* 53.4 (2014): 1223–35.
130. Corbie-Smith, G., Ammerman, A.S., Katz, M.L., et al. "Trust, Benefit, Satisfaction, and Burden: A Randomized Controlled Trial to Reduce Cancer Risk Through African-American Churches." *Journal of General Internal Medicine* 18.7 (2003): 531–41.
131. Davis, D.S., Goldmon, M.V. and Coker-Appiah, D.S. "Using a Community-Based Participatory Research Approach to Develop a Faith-Based Obesity Intervention for African American Children." *Health Promotion Practice* 12.6 (2011): 811–22.
132. Harmon, B.E., Adams, S.A., Scott, D., Gladman, Y.S., Ezell, B. and Hebert, J.R. "Dash of Faith: A Faith-Based Participatory Research Pilot Study." *Journal of Religion and Health* 53.3 (2014): 747–59.
133. Nicolaidis, C., Wahab, S., Trimble, J., et al. "The Interconnections Project: Development and Evaluation of a Community-Based Depression Program for African American Violence Survivors." *Journal of General Internal Medicine* 28.4 (2013): 530–8.
134. Dodani, S. "Community-Based Participatory Research Approaches for Hypertension Control and Prevention in Churches." *International Journal of Hypertension* 2011 (2011): 273120.
135. Boltri, J.M., vis-Smith, M., Zayas, L.E., et al. "Developing a Church-Based Diabetes Prevention Program with African Americans Focus Group Findings." *Diabetes Educator* 32.6 (2006): 901–9.
136. Young, S., Patterson, L., Wolff, M., Greer, Y. and Wynne, N. "Empowerment, Leadership, and Sustainability in a Faith-Based Partnership to Improve Health." *Journal of Religion and Health* 54.6 (2015): 2086–98.
137. Hoeffel, E.M., Rastogi, S., Kim, M.O. and Shahid, H. *The Asian Population: 2010.* 2010 Census Briefs. US Census Bureau, 2012.
138. Cook, W.K., Weir, R.C., Ro, M., et al. "Improving Asian American, Native Hawaiian, and Pacific Islander Health: National Organizations Leading Community Research Initiatives." *Progress in Community Health Partnerships* 6.1 (2012): 33–41.
139. Kwan, P.P., Briand, G., Lee, C., et al. "Use of a Community-Based Participatory Research Approach to Assess Knowledge, Attitudes, and Beliefs on Biospecimen Research Among Pacific Islanders." *Health Promotion Practice* 15.3 (2014): 422–30.

140. Barnes, P.M., Adams, P.F. and Powell-Griner, E. *Health Characteristics of the Asian Adult Population: United States, 2004–2006.* US Department of Health & Human Services, Centers for Disease Control and Prevention, National Center for Health Statistic, 2008.

141. McNeely, M.J. and Boyko, E.J. "Type 2 Diabetes Prevalence in Asian Americans Results of a National Health Survey." *Diabetes Care* 27.1 (2004): 66–9.

142. President's Advisory Commission on Asian Americans and Pacific Islanders. *Addressing Health Disparities: Opportunities for Building a Healthier America.* The White House, 2003.

143. Schoen, C., Davis, K., Collins, K.S., Greenberg, L., Des Roches, C. and Abrams, M. *The Commonwealth Fund Survey of the Health of Adolescent Girls.* Report No. 252. New York, NY: The Commonwealth Fund, 1997.

144. Ku, L. and Matani, S. "Left Out: Immigrants' Access to Health Care and Insurance." *Health Affairs* 20.1 (2001): 247–56.

145. Office of Minority Health. *Mental Health and Asian Americans.* US Department of Health and Human Services, 2013 September 18. <http://minorityhealth.hhs.gov/omh/browse.aspx?lvl=4&lvlID=54> (accessed July 15, 2016).

146. President's Advisory Commission on Asian Americans and Pacific Islanders. *Addressing Health Disparities: Opportunities for Building a Healthier America.* The White House, 2003.

147. Gomez, S.L., Tan, S., Keegan, T.H. and Clarke, C.A. "Disparities in Mammographic Screening for Asian Women in California: A Cross-Sectional Analysis to Identify Meaningful Groups for Targeted Intervention." *BMC Cancer* 7.1 (2007): 1.

148. Ryan, C. *Language Use in the United States: 2011.* American Community Survey Reports. Washington, DC: US Census Bureau, 2013.

149. DaNavas-Walt, C., Proctor, B.D., Smith, J.C. *Income, Poverty, and Health Insurance Coverage in the United States: 2010.* Current Population Reports, Consumer Income. Washington, DC: US Census Bureau, 2011.

150. Pourat, N., Kagawa-Singer, M., Breen, N. and Sripipatana, A. "Access Versus Acculturation: Identifying Modifiable Factors to Promote Cancer Screening Among Asian American Women." *Medical Care* (2010): 1088–96.

151. Nguyen-Truong, C.K., Lee-Lin, F., Leo, M.C., et al. "A Community-Based Participatory Research Approach to Understanding Pap Testing Adherence Among Vietnamese American Immigrants." *Journal of Obstetric, Gynecological and Neonatal Nursing* 41.6 (2012): E26–40.

152. Ma, G.X., Gao, W., Tan, Y., Chae, W.G. and Rhee, J. "A Community-Based Participatory Approach to a Hepatitis B Intervention for Korean Americans." *Progress in Community Health Partnerships* 6.1 (2012): 7–16.

153. Lam, T.K., McPhee, S.J., Mock, J., et al. "Encouraging Vietnamese-American Women to Obtain Pap Tests Through Lay Health Worker Outreach and Media Education." *Journal of General Internal Medicine* 18.7 (2003): 516–24.

154. Nguyen, T.T., McPhee, S.J., Gildengorin, G., et al. "Papanicolaou Testing Among Vietnamese Americans: Results of a Multifaceted Intervention." *American Journal of Preventive Medicine* 31.1 (2006): 1–9.

155. Katigbak, C., Foley, M., Robert, L. and Hutchinson, M.K. "Experiences and Lessons Learned in Using Community-Based Participatory Research to Recruit Asian American Immigrant Research Participants." *Journal of Nursing Scholarship* 48.2 (2016): 210–8.

156. Nguyen, T.T., McPhee, S.J., Bui-Tong, N., et al. "Community-Based Participatory Research Increases Cervical Cancer Screening Among Vietnamese-Americans." *Journal of Health Care for the Poor and Underserved* 17 Suppl 2 (2006): 31–54.

157. Braun, K.L., Tsark, J.U., Santos, L., Aitaoto, N. and Chong, C. "Building Native Hawaiian Capacity in Cancer Research and Programming: A Legacy of 'Imi Hale." *Cancer* 107 Suppl 8 (2006): 2082–90.

158. Nguyen, A.B. and Belgrave, F.Z. "Suc Khoe La Quan Trong Hon Sac Dep! Health is Better Than Beauty! A Community-Based Participatory Research Intervention to Improve Cancer Screening Among Vietnamese Women." *Journal of Health Care for the Poor and Underserved* 25.2 (2014): 605–23.

159. Dong, X., Chang, E.-S., Wong, E. and Simon, M. "Working with Culture: Lessons Learned from a Community-Engaged Project in a Chinese Aging Population." *Aging Health* 7.4 (2011): 529–37.

160. Dong, X., Chang, E.S., Wong, E., Wong, B., Skarupski, K.A. and Simon, M.A. "Assessing the Health Needs of Chinese Older Adults: Findings from a Community-Based Participatory Research Study in Chicago's Chinatown." *Journal of Aging Research* 2010 (2011): 124246.

161. Chesla, C.A., Chun, K.M., Kwan, C.M., et al. "Testing the Efficacy of Culturally Adapted Coping Skills Training for Chinese American Immigrants with Type 2 Diabetes Using Community-Based Participatory Research." *Research in Nursing and Health* 36.4 (2013): 359–72.

162. Ma, G.X., Toubbeh, J.I., Su, X. and Edwards, R.L. "ATECAR: An Asian American Community-Based Participatory Research Model on Tobacco and Cancer Control." *Health Promotion Practice* 5.4 (2004): 382–94.

163. Baldwin, J.A., Johnson, J.L. and Benally, C.C. "Building Partnerships Between Indigenous Communities and Universities: Lessons Learned in HIV/AIDS and Substance Abuse Prevention Research." *American Journal of Public Health* 99 Suppl 1 (2009): S77–82.

164. English, K.C., Wallerstein, N., Chino, M., et al. "Intermediate Outcomes of a Tribal Community Public Health Infrastructure Assessment." *Ethnicity and Disease* 14.3 Suppl 1 (2004): S61–9.

165. Fisher, P.A. and Ball, T.J. "Tribal Participatory Research: Mechanisms of a Collaborative Model." *American Journal of Community Psychology* 32.3–4 (2003): 207–16.

166. Jernigan, V.B., Jacob, T. and Styne, D. "The Adaptation and Implementation of a Community-Based Participatory Research Curriculum to Build Tribal Research Capacity." *American Journal of Public Health* 105 Suppl 3 (2015): S424–32.

167. Oetzel, J., Wallerstein, N., Solimon, A., et al. "Creating an Instrument to Measure People's Perception of Community Capacity in American Indian Communities." *Health Education and Behavior* 38.3 (2011): 301–10.

168. Skinner, E. and Masuda, J.R. "Right to a Healthy City? Examining the Relationship Between Urban Space and Health Inequity by Aboriginal Youth Artist-Activists in Winnipeg." *Social Science and Medicine* 91 (2013): 210–8.

169. *Profile: American Indian/Alaska Native.* US Department of Health and Human Services, Office of Minority Health 2016, February 3. <http://minorityhealth.hhs.gov/omh/browse.aspx?lvl=3&lvlID=62> (accessed July 10, 2016).

170. Organ, J., Castleden, H., Furgal, C., Sheldon, T. and Hart, C. "Contemporary Programs in Support of Traditional Ways: Inuit Perspectives on Community Freezers as a Mechanism to Alleviate Pressures of Wild Food Access in Nain, Nunatsiavut." *Health and Place* 30 (2014): 251–9.

171. Garcia, T., Keppel, K. and Hallquist, S. *Healthy People 2010 Snapshot for the American Indian or Alaska Native Population: Progress Toward Targets, Size of Disparities, and Changes in Disparities.* Centers for Disease Control and Prevention, 2014.

172. Castleden, H. and Garvin, T. "Modifying Photovoice for Community-Based Participatory Indigenous Research." *Social Science and Medicine* 66.6 (2008): 1393–405.

173. Jetter, K.M., Yarborough, M., Cassady, D.L. and Styne, D.M. "Building Research Capacity with Members of Underserved American Indian/Alaskan Native Communities: Training in Research Ethics and the Protection of Human Subjects." *Health Promotion Practice* 16.3 (2015): 419–25.

174. Shea, J.M., Poudrier, J., Thomas, R., Jeffery, B. and Kiskotagan, L. "Reflections from a Creative Community-Based Participatory Research Project Exploring Health and Body Image with First Nations Girls." *International Journal of Qualitative Methods* 12.1 (2013): 272–93.

175. Simonds, V.W. and Christopher, S. "Adapting Western Research Methods to Indigenous Ways of Knowing." *American Journal of Public Health* 103.12 (2013): 2185–92.

176. Pearson, C.R., Duran, B., Oetzel, J., et al. "Research for Improved Health: Variability and Impact of Structural Characteristics in Federally Funded Community Engaged Research." *Progress in Community Health Partnerships* 9.1 (2015): 17–29.

177. Johansson, P., Knox-Nicola, P. and Schmid, K. "The Waponahki Tribal Health Assessment: Successfully Using CBPR to Conduct a Comprehensive and Baseline Health Assessment of Waponahki Tribal Members." *Journal of Health Care for the Poor and Underserved* 26.3 (2015): 889–907.

178. Harding, A., Harper, B., Stone, D., et al. "Conducting Research with Tribal Communities: Sovereignty, Ethics and Data-Sharing Issues." *Environmental Health Perspectives* (2011): 11–24.

179. Gray, N., Ore de, B.C., Farnsworth, A. and Wolf, D. "Integration of Creative Expression into Community-Based Participatory Research and Health Promotion with Native Americans." *Family and Community Health* 33.3 (2010): 186–92.

180. Wang, C. and Burris, M.A. "Photovoice: Concept, Methodology, and Use for Participatory Needs Assessment." *Health Education and Behavior* 24.3 (1997): 369–87.

181. Jardine, C.G. and James, A. "Youth Researching Youth: Benefits, Limitations and Ethical Considerations Within a Participatory Research Process." *International Journal of Circumpolar Health* 71 (2012): 1–9.

8

Community-Based Participatory Research Studies Involving Immigrants

LISA M. VAUGHN, PHD AND FARRAH JACQUEZ, PHD

Compared with other nations, the United States hosts the largest number of immigrants, and numbers continue to increase particularly in nontraditional migration areas such as the Midwest. Although immigrants to the United States are heterogeneous in terms of cultural and religious background, education, skill levels, migration experiences, and legal status, they are more likely to experience inequities in access to and utilization of healthcare and disparities in health. US immigrants are at high risk for social determinants of ill health and are likely to experience immigration-related stressors that negatively affect their health and well-being. Most research about immigrant health has been conducted using traditional, empirical approaches, and immigrants have not been involved as partners in the research process. Community-based participatory research (CBPR) is well suited for partnering with immigrants in the research process and offers benefits for both immigrant community members and researchers. In this chapter, we highlight five exemplar studies in which CBPR was conducted with immigrants and conclude with a CBPR case study that partnered with Latino immigrants in Cincinnati, Ohio.

In this chapter, we illustrate why CBPR is a particularly advantageous framework for involving immigrants. Specifically, we provide an overview of the research literature about immigrants and health disparities, review the benefits of CBPR as they relate to immigrants, and examine a range of CBPR studies that have involved them. We conclude with a case study of a CBPR project with Latino immigrants in Cincinnati, Ohio.

US Immigrant Populations and Health Disparities

In 2015, 244 million people (3.3% of the world's population) lived outside their country of origin.[1] This number is expected to continue expanding in many countries.[2] Of all nations, the United States hosts the largest number of immigrants/foreign-born (i.e., people without US citizenship at birth, including naturalized citizens, lawful permanent residents, refugees and asylees, persons on certain temporary visas, and those who are unauthorized),[3,4] and immigrant populations continue to increase.[5] In the United States, many non-traditional destination areas have seen growth compared to previous immigrant settlement in "gateway" cities.[6-8] As of 2013, the total US immigrant population was 41.3 million, which was 13% of the total 316 million residents.[3] Over half of all US immigrants come from Latin America, and almost 30% are from Asia.[9] The estimated number of unauthorized immigrants living in the United States varies, but, for the last 10 years, estimates are in the range of 11–12 million.[3,10,11] US immigrants occupy the spectrum of educational and skill levels. On the high end, immigrants make up at least 25% of all US physicians, 24% of workers in science and engineering, and 47% of scientists with doctoral degrees.[12] On the low end of this continuum are immigrants who have educational levels below that of the average US citizen and who tend to occupy low-skilled jobs in agriculture, service industries, and construction. For example, about 75% of all US farm workers and almost 100% of people working in fresh fruit and vegetable production are legal or undocumented immigrants.[12]

Although immigrants to the United States are heterogeneous in terms of cultural and religious background, education, skill levels, migration experiences, and legal status, they are more likely to experience inequities in access to and utilization of healthcare[9] and disparities in health.[13] They report a lower quality of healthcare[14] relative to the native population. Although data are lacking for individual groups, most immigrant populations in the United States are at higher risk for social determinants of ill health, such as poverty, low educational levels, substandard housing, unemployment or underemployment, uncertain legal status, financial barriers (e.g., difficulty in obtaining a small business loan or home mortgage), exposure to violence during migration and in their US neighborhoods after arrival, food insecurity, language barriers, transportation issues, family separation and diminished social support, fear of deportation, and discrimination.[15-18]

Nevertheless, immigrants generally have better infant, child, and adult health; higher life expectancy; and lower disability and mortality rates in comparison to those born in the United States.[9] This is often referred to as the "immigrant health paradox."[19] Explanations include the idea that immigrants may be healthier than those who remain in their native countries, engage in lower health risk behaviors in the United States, have a more positive outlook on life, and have higher levels of family and social support.[9,19,20] Depending on time in the United States, however, immigrants tend to have a decline in their overall health and lose their mortality advantage.[9] For instance, the longer immigrants reside in the United States, the more likely they are to have increased tobacco, alcohol, and drug use[21] and to be at increased risk for obesity, diabetes, and cancer, all linked to an unhealthy American diet.[22–24]

Immigrant-Specific Stressors

Immigrants are likely to experience immigration-related stressors that negatively affect their health and well-being. For instance, immigrants may experience acculturative stress (i.e., stress occurring from adaptation to a new culture) when adjusting to US norms and societal expectations; such stress can be compounded by language, financial, and isolation barriers.[25] Some immigrants have undergone challenging and traumatic journeys to the United States or, in their native country, experienced traumatic events such as war, torture, terrorism, famine, or natural disasters, which may have influenced their decision to migrate. These premigration and migratory journey experiences can lead to posttraumatic stress disorder and to a high risk for other mental health concerns.[18]

In the US immigrant groups, there are a wide range of mental health issues, many related to the stress of immigration itself, family circumstances, acculturation, and the social determinants of health.[15] Mental health problems include anxiety, depression, posttraumatic stress disorder, substance abuse, and a higher prevalence of thoughts of suicide and severe mental illness.[12] Some subgroups of immigrants (e.g., refugees; lesbians; gay, bisexual, and transgendered persons; and older adults) are particularly vulnerable to stressors that negatively affect their mental health.[12] In addition, prevention and treatment of mental illness can be challenging because immigrants may manifest physical complaints and symptoms rather than an underlying mental health concern, or not seek mental health care due to stigmatization of mental illness in their native countries.[26,27]

Additional stressors may arise when immigrants encounter difficulties as they attempt to seek physical and mental healthcare. Immigrants may not be aware of available health and wellness resources, and accessible services and resources may not be culturally sensitive or linguistically appropriate.[12,27–30] Further, access to healthcare may be restricted due to logistical barriers such as transportation, finances, distance, lack of health insurance, ineligibility due to immigration status, or lack of interpreters.[12,27–30] Undocumented immigrants may be fearful of the potential for identification and subsequent deportation if they seek services.[12,28,29]

As a result of the accumulation of traumatic events, health risks, and stressors that immigrants may face, they can be susceptible to toxic stress, an endemic problem that has biological consequences and detrimental effects on learning, behavior, and physical and mental health across their life spans.[31] Toxic stress is the mechanism by which poverty, discrimination, maltreatment, and other adversities lead to health, educational, and income disparities.[31,32] Acculturation, discrimination, hostility, and immigration status can contribute to increased levels of toxic stress among immigrants.[15,33]

Traditional Research Studies and Immigrant Health

Similar to research with other vulnerable populations, most studies on immigrant health have been conducted using traditional, empirical approaches in which data are collected *from* immigrants, interventions are designed *for* immigrants, and outcomes resulting from research are *about* immigrants.[34] Traditionally, immigrants have not been involved as partners in the research process but rather have been the distant "subjects" of primarily researcher- or institution-driven inquiries to diagnose problems and design interventions. Although this trajectory of traditional research has been helpful in establishing and documenting the extent of health disparities for immigrants and delineating baselines of health risk across immigrant populations, immigrants have rarely been engaged in the research process, from defining the research topic or question to disseminating the results in ways that are most relevant for the community. In regard to research, immigrants can be hard to reach, and they can be unintentionally stigmatized by research findings. Thus, it is necessary that they become involved in the research process.[12,35,36] Furthermore, traditional approaches to research with immigrants tend to consider broad ethnic classifications as homogeneous groups and thus promote a "one size fits all" for research that can miss the contextual and cultural nuances and the assets, resources, and strengths distinctive to individual immigrant groups or subgroups. Needed to improve immigrant health is a partnership approach, such as CBPR, which is collaborative, is focused on shared decision-making, and has relevance for immigrant communities. Community-based participatory research values immigrants' knowledge by positioning immigrant community members as experts about their health and communities and as "doers" who are empowered to enact social change toward eradicating health disparities.[37,38] Community-based participatory research is recognized for its utility in reducing health disparities primarily due to the inclusion of those communities most directly affected by the disparity in identifying problems and potential solutions.[37,39]

Research Benefits of CBPR That Involves Immigrants

Community-based participatory research is well suited for partnering with immigrants in the research process. In their CBPR case study describing a project about restaurant workers' health and safety in San Francisco's Chinatown, Chang and colleagues[40] outline eight advantages of using a CBPR framework with urban immigrant communities:

> (1) helping ensure that the research question comes from, or is of genuine importance to, the local community; (2) increasing trust

and credibility with the community, which can in turn improve participation in research; (3) enhancing the cultural acceptability of study instruments, often improving their validity; (4) improving the design and implementation of interventions, thus increasing the likelihood of success; (5) improving data interpretation; (6) identifying and using new channels for dissemination; (7) helping translate the findings into action that will benefit the community; and (8) building individual and community capacity and leaving behind a community better able to evaluate and address other health and social issues of local concern.[40, p.1027]

Overview of CBPR Studies Involving Immigrants

An increasing number of research studies have used CBPR to explore complex health issues among immigrants. We recently conducted a review of 161 peer-reviewed articles published between 1985 and March 31, 2016, in which CBPR was conducted in partnership with immigrants.[41] All of the 161 articles were published after 2002, with a notable increase in publications in 2010 and afterward. The articles included in the analysis covered a wide range of health-related issues, with the most prevalent being chronic health conditions (e.g., hypertension, asthma, diabetes), health promotion/education (parenting, accessing medical care), and sexual health (sexually transmitted disease protection, condom use). Most (70%) of the articles involved Latino immigrants living in the United States. Here, we highlight five articles from this review that illustrate the diverse methods, populations, and benefits of CBPR studies involving immigrants and provide a case study of our own CBPR project involving Latino immigrants.

1. *Bangladeshi health promoters in New York.* Patel and colleagues[42] collaborated with Bangladeshi community health promoters to conduct a door-to-door community survey about health needs among 167 Bangladeshi immigrant women living in Bronx, NY. The researchers partnered with a South Asian community-based organization that selected and trained six Bangladeshi community members to serve as health promoters for the project. To garner trust and support, the community organization and community health workers first conducted an awareness campaign and performed outreach in the Bangladeshi community to prepare residents for and provide information about the upcoming survey. The survey results revealed health risks, including depression, overweight/obesity, type 2 diabetes, hypertension, and lack of physical exercise and preventive screenings such as Pap smears. The survey participation rate was >90%, illustrating the partnership's ability to access

a hard-to-reach community for participation in research. The linguistic and cultural barriers of Bangladeshi immigrant women had the potential to hinder their participation in research; however, the CBPR approach overcame the traditional obstacles to research participation and engaged a recent and fast-growing immigrant community in the United States.

2. *Environmental justice for Vietnamese nail salon workers.* Quach and colleagues[43] partnered with the California Healthy Nail Salon Collaborative, comprising community advocates, public health professionals, health providers, and environmental activists, in evaluating workplace exposure to chemical solvents among Vietnamese nail salon workers. The community-academic partnership collaborated to develop the study instruments, protocols, recruitment process, and interpretation of results. For guidance on recruitment and survey development, researchers organized a community advisory committee of Vietnamese salon owners and workers. In a survey of 80 Vietnamese nail salon workers from 20 salons in California, researchers found higher than guideline-recommended levels for toluene, methyl methacrylate, and total volatile organic compounds, all of which can contribute to headaches, breathing problems, and other health symptoms reported by salon workers. By partnering with the Vietnamese immigrant population, researchers were able to recruit salon workers and generate data that could be used by community partners to advocate for environmental justice.

3. *Immigrants and refugees researching tuberculosis.* In a study to understand perceptions of tuberculosis (TB) among immigrants and refugees at an adult education center, Wieland and colleagues[44] worked with community partners and conducted, at the center, focus groups with 83 diverse immigrant and refugee learners and staff. The groups were attended by a substantial proportion of learners with high-risk characteristics for TB and latent TB infection because of emigration from countries where TB is endemic. Through an established CBPR community–academic partnership, 28 adult education center learners, community members, and academic partners were recruited to be trained in 20 hours of focus group moderation and 4 hours of CBPR. Thematic analysis of the focus group data revealed challenges related to TB control and prevention, misperceptions about how TB is transmitted; lack of understanding about latent TB; barriers to TB testing and medication use; and feelings of secrecy, fear, isolation, and shame related to TB. Learners and staff of the center were also involved in designing the focus group questions, thematically analyzing the data, and disseminating the results at a World TB Day event. Use of a CBPR framework for this project improved the quality of data and the overall research process by involving community members of the target population and trusted staff at the adult education center in each step of the research process including the research design, data collection, interpretation of data, and dissemination of results.

4. *Haitian refugees promoting reproductive health.* Barbee, Kobetz, and colleagues[45] used a CBPR approach to implement a community-based intervention for cervical cancer screening in Little Haiti, an ethnic enclave of Haitians in Miami, Florida. Given the strong sociocultural barriers to Pap screening in Haitian women, the researchers determined whether pairing self-sampling (collecting specimens at home) for human papillomavirus (HPV) with Haitian community health workers is a culturally acceptable method for cervical cancer screening among a sample of 246 Haitian immigrant women living in Little Haiti. Community-based participatory research was used to assess the cultural acceptability of a particular data collection method, self-sampling, and the effectiveness of a community-based intervention, community health workers, to address an identified health disparity for Haitian immigrant women.

5. *Somali refugees studying sexual health.* In a study designed to understand the views of Somali men toward female genital cutting and women's childbirth experiences in a refugee community in Arizona, Johnson-Agbakwu et al.[46] built a CBPR partnership with key stakeholders within the target Somali refugee community. Collaborating through the established partnership, the researchers incorporated community leaders' insights about Somali cultural values into the data collection strategies and worked with familiar and well-respected male community members as facilitators and interpreters. Since the topic addressed sensitive health and gender issues, use of CBPR allowed for an increase in trust and willingness to participate in research within the Somali community.

Case Study: Latinos Unidos por la Salud

As an example of the CBPR process with immigrants and its potential to improve research quality, we present here our community-academic partnered research team, Latinos Unidos por la Salud. Cincinnati, Ohio, is a nontraditional migration area that does not have a long history of Latino residents. In the past 10 years, however, there has been exponential growth in the Latino population. The local healthcare infrastructure is faced with the challenge of meeting the distinctive linguistic and cultural needs of a new immigrant population. Through our long-standing partnership with Latino community organizations and advocacy groups, we knew that Latino immigrants were having difficulty accessing high-quality healthcare; however, we had no data to guide interventions. Local healthcare surveys and hospital records did not provide representative samples of Latino immigrants (particularly those who are undocumented). Highly publicized immigration raids and statewide policies restricting employment and driving privileges for undocumented immigrants made many local Latino families reluctant to be active in their communities. We learned from our Latino-serving partner organizations that Latinos feared interactions with social systems that could result in immigration investigations; even documented immigrants were afraid to put their friends and families at risk. Because of these factors, we identified strategies to engage Latino immigrants in research so that interventions could be designed to address disparities in healthcare access, quality, and outcomes.

Over the past two decades, the National Institutes of Health has emphasized that successful recruitment of minorities into health research is necessary to address health disparities. Despite the directive, empirically validated strategies to recruit minorities are rarely described in the literature. To reach the "hidden population" of immigrant Latinos in our nontraditional migration area and to collaborate with them in the research process, we worked with community partners to create Latinos Unidos por la Salud (LU-Salud), a team of academic researchers and seven immigrant Latina women who worked together to collect, analyze, and disseminate data about healthcare experiences of Latino immigrants in Cincinnati. Conceived through a CBPR lens, the project was funded by a $20,000 Clinical and Translational Science Award funded by Greater Cincinnati. During monthly meetings on Sunday afternoons, in which meals were served, childcare was provided, and transportation costs were reimbursed, the Latina women and the academic partners made decisions about research questions, survey design, participant recruitment, and data collection strategies. Academic partners led training on survey administration and focus group facilitation; community partners shared expertise on the Latino immigrant experience in our area that was necessary for understanding how to recruit participants.

Various logistical realities served as challenges to shared decision-making. Because we needed funding to compensate the community partners before getting them involved, the original grant application was written by the academic partners and therefore did not equitably include community and academic input. As a result, the funding was in the hands of the academic partners. We attempted to overcome this disparity by having the entire team make decisions about how to spend the money. For example, we had an intense discussion about how the community partners would be compensated for their work in administering surveys. We created a pay structure ensuring that we collected the minimum amount of surveys we needed (200) but created incentives for reaching a higher goal of 500 surveys. The community partners wanted to reserve funding to have a celebration when we reached the goal of 500 surveys. Despite our efforts to share decision-making about money, when academic partners are giving the money and the community partners are receiving it, an uneven power dynamic exists.

Despite the challenges, LU-Salud has demonstrated that partnering with community members who are typically marginalized in the research process improves research quality. Over the course of a year, the Latina community partners of LU-Salud administered over 500 surveys and facilitated four focus groups with Latino immigrants to interpret the survey results. Together, we disseminated the results of the project in both Spanish and English to local Latino-serving organizations and stakeholders. After finishing the first funded phase of the partnership, we secured another small grant to conduct a concept-mapping project for developing intervention strategies to target the Latino health priorities identified in the survey. Based on the results of the concept mapping, we found that our Latino immigrant partners wanted an intervention targeting stress and that they valued community-based, interactive strategies to address health issues. We secured another grant from our regional United Way to develop and validate a stress intervention for Latino immigrants in our area. LU-Salud has now expanded to include 20 Latino immigrant partners who are serving as *promotores* in our pilot stress-intervention project. In the next phase of the partnership, we plan to expand the stress intervention to a broader sample and demonstrate that such an intervention developed by community and academic partners is feasible and efficacious in nontraditional migration areas.

To demonstrate the potential for CBPR with immigrants to improve research quality, we now provide an evaluation of the degree to which LU-Salud capitalized on the eight advantages of using CBPR as described by Chang and colleagues.[40]

1. *Helping ensure that the research question comes from, or is of genuine importance to, the local community.* In our nontraditional destination area, we knew, from working with Latino-serving social service agencies, that Cincinnati did not have the linguistically and culturally appropriate infrastructure to support immigrant Latinos. Although we speculated that Latino immigrants were having healthcare challenges, we did not have data regarding use, barriers, or perceptions of quality. By sharing decision-making with Latino immigrant partners, we were able to focus our survey research questions and intervention targets on issues experienced by the Latino community. At times, that required adjusting course to adapt to new information identified through community research efforts. For example, although we began our partnership with LU-Salud with the idea of focusing on healthcare navigation and overcoming barriers to healthcare access, through surveys, focus groups, and concept mapping, Latino immigrants prioritized stress and social support as the primary concern. As such, we are now piloting a stress intervention project with LU-Salud members serving as *promotores*.

2. *Increasing trust and credibility with the community, which can in turn improve participation in research.* Gaining trust and credibility with the Cincinnati immigrant Latino community was essential to investigate health disparities in our city. Although, prior to our work, various regional organizations had performed surveys that included Hispanic populations, there were no data describing the health and healthcare experiences of Latino immigrants in Cincinnati. The community partners' input ensured that our data collection procedures were culturally and contextually appropriate. The community partners have collected all data in community settings, which has improved engagement in research. For example, in our project, 516 immigrant Latinos

participated in the survey, making it the largest survey of Latino immigrants ever completed in our city.

3. *Enhancing the cultural acceptability of study instruments, often improving their validity.* The community partners of LU-Salud have been and are involved in the development of research protocols, including surveys and focus group guides. We create instruments in Spanish and later translate them into English for dissemination. When we do use existing measures, community partners consider the wording and language level of each item. Because these partners collect the data, they have power to veto or adjust questions or discussion topics that they believe are not contextually appropriate.

4. *Improving the design and implementation of interventions, thus increasing the likelihood of success.* Academic and community partners of LU-Salud have designed an intervention that meets the prioritized health needs of our local Latino immigrant community. Specifically, we have been able to reflect the community's perspective in the target and the process of our intervention. After the survey project revealed areas identified by the community as the most noteworthy health problems for Latinos, we conducted a concept mapping study in which a sample of more than 200 stakeholders generated strategies to address these areas.[47] Through concept mapping, community stakeholders prioritized stress as the most feasible and potentially relevant target for intervention. In addition, community stakeholders emphasized the need for community-based interventions that relied on peer support and education. Armed with community priorities, the academic members of the research team identified an empirically validated model of stress intervention delivered by promotores to Latino immigrants in a nontraditional destination area,[48] which could serve as a model. We are currently delivering a stress intervention that builds on previous reports but is culturally tailored for our local context.

5. *Improving data interpretation.* Collaboration with community members was valuable in understanding research results in context and to plan and develop action strategies. For example, following the survey, we held "data interpretation sessions" or focus groups in which we presented the survey results and asked Latino immigrants to assist in interpreting the findings. Community and academic members of LU-Salud cofacilitated these groups. Gaining the community's perspective of the data deepened our understanding of the reasons why healthcare utilization patterns of Latino immigrants differed from other Cincinnati residents. Latino immigrants described experiencing, during healthcare visits, discrimination based on language and lack of health insurance coverage. They also described variations in the quality of interpreters at clinics throughout the region, which gave perspective into why some community clinics were overutilized.[49]

6. *Identifying and using new channels for dissemination.* We disseminated the work of LU-Salud into academic outlets and into community settings that have the potential to affect the practices of local healthcare systems. For example, we held a community forum at the partnering pediatric medical center (Cincinnati Children's Hospital Medical Center) in which both academic and community members of LU-Salud made presentations to more than 70 attendees. Spanish-speaking team members were provided with headset-based interpretation, and their presentations were translated into English for the audience. The forum provided an opportunity for the community partners to serve as experts for a primarily academic and healthcare professional audience and to explain our research from the community perspective. We also presented the results of our research to Latino-serving social service and advocacy organizations, which have used the data to guide their own intervention planning. We provided one-page handouts of our results in Spanish and English for distribution by local Latino organizations. By sharing decision-making with Latino immigrant partners, we identified the community outlets that would be most appropriate for dissemination.

7. *Helping translate the findings into action that will benefit the community.* In addition to the stress intervention project described above, findings from the LU-Salud survey are being translated into action in order to affect health concerns in the local Latino immigrant community. For instance, to address the 30% uninsured rate in Latino children identified in our survey, a local Latino-serving agency conducted a project to identify and address barriers to accessing health insurance for Latino children. As a result of their project based on LU-Salud's work, the agency is planning to distribute informational materials about obtaining children's health insurance in hospital/maternity/ob-gyn waiting rooms, to conduct educational sessions for Latina women's groups, and to provide audiovisual educational material to address literacy barriers that were associated with lack of insurance.

8. *Building individual and community capacity and leaving behind a community better able to evaluate and address other health and social issues of local concern.* LU-Salud is not project-based, but is a long-term partnership between Latino immigrants and academic research partners. We also regularly partner with local Latino-serving organizations in an advisory capacity and help disseminate results directly into the community. We believe that, in our city, the long-term partnership has contributed to an adjustment in the culture of health for Latino immigrants. The community members of LU-Salud have been recruited to work in other grant-funded projects and are regularly asked to give their perspective on Latino health issues in our area. In addition, LU-Salud has served as a bridge among several local agencies and Latino-focused groups in terms of connecting resources, networking, advising, and collaborating to address issues of concern for Latinos.

Conclusion

Given the continued growth of US immigrant populations, the pervasiveness of health inequities, and the barriers to healthcare faced by immigrants, CBPR is particularly suited to address immigrant health disparities through involvement of immigrants in the research process. Specifically, the use of a CBPR approach allows for bidirectional communication, enhanced trust, shared leadership and ownership, and mutual benefits in the research process between academics and immigrant communities. Furthermore, the quality and rigor of research are improved by participant engagement, contextually relevant research questions, externally valid data interpretation, and culturally valid measurement instruments and techniques. The results of immigrant-partnered research are more widely disseminated and have greater potential for real-world impact and sustainable actions.

For conducting CBPR with immigrants, the following guidelines should be considered:

1. Immigrants are not homogeneous even when they are from the same country of origin. Due to differences in education, jobs, income, age/generation, gender, documentation status, religion, sexuality, length of time in the United States, and other psychosocial factors, individual immigrants have nuanced contextual and cultural circumstances affecting their lives. Depending on the goals of the research study, the involvement of a diverse group of immigrant stakeholders from a particular community is likely to enhance the research outcomes. Community leaders, gatekeepers, and staff of social service agencies provide perspectives. But to ensure that interventions are contextually appropriate for the most vulnerable populations, researchers should consider including recently immigrated, undocumented, and/or low-income immigrants in the partnership.

2. The immigration process is complex and can include multiple stressors that affect immigrant health and well-being. Immigrants come to and live in the United States under a wide variety of circumstances. Some flee their countries because of war, persecution, and/or extreme poverty. Immigrants may have experienced trauma either in their country of origin or during the migration. Because of their status and potential language barriers, immigrants may face discrimination and prejudice. Some US immigrants are undocumented, which can contribute to fear, isolation, and chronic anxiety. Although immigrants have different levels of vulnerability, CBPR is appropriate for research with immigrants because it gives voice to the spectrum of experiences and thereby builds on their strengths and addresses the barriers for individual immigrants.

3. Members of the academy and immigrant populations can differ in ways that serve as obstacles to collaboration, including language, documentation status,

and education level. These differences can instill disengagement or even distrust by immigrant populations, which contributes to the lack of representation of immigrants in research. As such, CBPR researchers, in collaboration with immigrants, should take the approach of long-term partnerships. Traditionally, researchers have tended to gather data without a previous relationship and/or topic of importance to the particular community. This "drive-by" or "helicopter" approach to research may unintentionally cause harm or contribute to further distrust and to the sense that immigrants exist to be used for their data. In order to overcome the differences in language and life experiences between researchers and immigrants, CBPR researchers should consider innovative and creative methods of data collection that help answer complex research questions and are a better fit for immigrant groups (e.g., an arts-based method may offer ways to respond that are not limited by verbal or written language).

References

1. *United Nations Population Fund—Migration.* 2016. <http://www.unfpa.org/migration#>
2. *World Migration in Figures.* 2013. <http://www.oecd.org/els/mig/World-Migration-in-Figures.pdf>
3. Zong, J. and Batalova, J. "Frequently Requested Statistics on Immigrants and Immigration in the United States." *Migration Policy Institute.* 2015. <http://www.migrationpolicy.org/article/frequently-requested-statistics-immigrants-and-immigration-united-states>
4. *Migration Policy Institute Tabulations of U.S. Department of Homeland Security, Office of Immigration Statistics, Yearbook of Immigration Statistics (Various Years).* 2016. <http://www.dhs.gov/files/statistics/publications/yearbook.shtm>
5. *FAIR.* 2013. <http://www.fairus.org/issue/rising-immigrant-admissions-to-the-united-states>
6. Ellis, M., Wright, R. and Townley, M. "The Allure of New Immigrant Destinations and the Great Recession in the United States." *International Migration Review* 48.1 (2014): 3.
7. Singer, A. *The Rise of New Immigrant Gateways.* Washington, DC: Center on Urban and Metropolitan Policy, Brookings Institution, 2004.
8. Singer, A. "Contemporary Immigrant Gateways in Historical Perspective." *Daedalus* 142.3 (2013): 76–91.
9. Singh, G.K., Rodriguez-Lainz, A. and Kogan, M.D. "Immigrant Health Inequalities in the United States: Use of Eight Major National Data Systems." *Scientific World Journal* 2013 Oct 27;2013:512313. doi:10.1155/2013/512313. eCollection 2013.
10. *Estimates of the Unauthorized Population for States.* 2016. <http://data.cmsny.org/state.html>
11. Passel, J.S. and Cohn, D. "Unauthorized Immigrant Population Stable for Half a Decade." *Pew Research Center* (2015). <http://www.pewresearch.org/fact-tank/2015/07/22/unauthorized-immigrant-population-stable-for-half-a-decade/>
12. *Psychology of Immigration 101.* 2016. <http://www.apa.org/topics/immigration/immigration-psychology.aspx>
13. Dey, A.N. and Lucas, J.W. "Physical and Mental Health Characteristics of US-and Foreign-Born Adults, United States, 1998–2003." *Centers for Disease Control* (2006). <http://www.cdc.gov/nchs/data/ad/ad369.pdf>

14. Saha, S., Arbelaez, J.J. and Cooper, L.A. "Patient-Physician Relationships and Racial Disparities in the Quality of Health Care." *American Journal of Public Health* 93.10 (2003): 1713–9.

15. Linton, J.M., Choi, R. and Mendoza, F. "Caring for Children in Immigrant Families: Vulnerabilities, Resilience, and Opportunities." *Pediatric Clinics of North America* 63.1 (2016): 115–30.

16. Kirmayer, L.J., Narasiah, L., Munoz, M., et al. "Common Mental Health Problems in Immigrants and Refugees: General Approach in Primary Care." *Canadian Medical Association Journal* 183, no. 12 (2011): E959–67.

17. Bigby, J. *Cross-Cultural Medicine.* Philadelphia: American College of Physicians Press, 2003.

18. Pumariega, A.J., Rothe, E. and Pumariega, J.B. "Mental Health of Immigrants and Refugees." *Community Mental Health Journal* 41.5 (2005): 581–97.

19. Markides, K.S. and Rote, S. "Immigrant Health Paradox." *Emerging Trends in the Social and Behavioral Sciences: An Interdisciplinary Searchable, and Linkable Resource.* Wiley, 2015. http://onlinelibrary.wiley.com/book/10.1002/9781118900772

20. Kandula, N.R., Kersey, M. and Lurie, N. "Assuring the Health of Immigrants: What the Leading Health Indicators Tell Us." *Annual Review of Public Health* 25 (2004): 357–76.

21. Nguyen, H.H. "Acculturation in the United States." In *The Cambridge Handbook of Acculturation Psychology*, ed. S.L. David and J.W. Berry. New York: Cambridge University Press, 2006.

22. Li, F.P. and Pawlish, K. "Cancers in Asian Americans and Pacific Islanders: Migrant Studies." *Asian American and Pacific Islander Journal of Health* 6.2 (1997): 123–9.

23. Kandula, N.R., Diez-Roux, A.V., Chan, C., et al. "Association of Acculturation Levels and Prevalence of Diabetes in the Multi-Ethnic Study of Atherosclerosis (MESA)." *Diabetes Care* 31.6 (2008): 1621–8.

24. Koya, D.L. and Egede, L.E. "Association Between Length of Residence and Cardiovascular Disease Risk Factors Among an Ethnically Diverse Group of United States Immigrants." *Journal of General Internal Medicine* 22.6 (2007): 841–6.

25. Vaughn, L.M. and Holloway, M. "West African Immigrant Families from Mauritania and Senegal in Cincinnati: A Cultural Primer on Children's Health." *Journal of Community Health* 35.1 (2010): 27–35.

26. Kirmayer, L.J. "Cultural Variations in the Clinical Presentation of Depression and Anxiety: Implications for Diagnosis and Treatment." *Journal of Clinical Psychiatry* 62 (2001): 22–30.

27. Saechao, F., Sharrock, S., Reicherter, D., et al. "Stressors and Barriers to Using Mental Health Services Among Diverse Groups of First-Generation Immigrants to the United States." *Community Mental Health Journal* 48.1 (2012): 98–106.

28. Vaughn, L.M. and Jacquez, F. "Characteristics of Newly Immigrated, Spanish-Speaking Latinos Who Use the Pediatric Emergency Department: Preliminary Findings in a Secondary Migration City." *Pediatric Emergency Care* 28.4 (2012): 345–50.

29. Clough, J., Lee, S. and Chae, D.H. "Barriers to Health Care Among Asian Immigrants in the United States: A Traditional Review." *Journal of Health Care for the Poor and Underserved* 24.1 (2013): 384–403.

30. Li, J., Maxwell, A.E., Glenn, B.A., et al. "Healthcare Access and Utilization Among Korean Americans: The Mediating Role of English Use and Proficiency." *International Journal of Social Science Research* 4.1 (2016): 83–97.

31. Lupien, S.J., McEwen, B.S., Gunnar, M.R. and Heim, C. "Effects of Stress Throughout the Lifespan on the Brain, Behaviour and Cognition." *Nature Reviews Neuroscience* 10.6 (2009): 434–45.

32. Shonkoff, J.P., Garner, A.S., Siegel, B.S., et al. "The Lifelong Effects of Early Childhood Adversity and Toxic Stress." *Pediatrics* 129.1 (2012): e232–46.

33. Romero, S. and Williams, M.R. "The Impact of Immigration Legislations on Latino Families: Implications for Social Work." *Advances in Social Work* 14.1 (2013): 229–46.

34. Chang, C., Salvatore, A.L., Lee, P.T., et al. "Adapting to Context in Community-Based Participatory Research: 'Participatory Starting Points' in a Chinese Immigrant Worker Community." *American Journal Of Community Psychology* 51.3-4 (2013): 480–91.

35. Newell, C.J. and South, J. "Participating in Community Research: Exploring the Experiences of Lay Researchers in Bradford." *Community, Work and Family* 12.1 (2009): 75–89.
36. Vaughn, L.M., Jacquez, F., Zhen-Duan, J., et al. "Improving Research Quality and Reaching a Hidden Population Through an Immigrant Community Research Team." *Action Research* (Under review).
37. Israel, B.A., Coombe, C.M., Cheezum, R.R., et al. "Community-Based Participatory Research: A Capacity-Building Approach for Policy Advocacy Aimed at Eliminating Health Disparities." *American Journal of Public Health* 100.11 (2010): 2094–102.
38. Israel, B.A., Schulz, A.J., Parker, E.A. and Becker, A.B. "Community-Based Participatory Research: Policy Recommendations for Promoting a Partnership Approach in Health Research." *Education for Health* 14.2 (2001): 182–97.
39. Wallerstein, N.B., Yen, I.H. and Syme, S.L. "Integration of Social Epidemiology and Community-Engaged Interventions to Improve Health Equity." *American Journal of Public Health* 101.5 (2011): 822.
40. Chang, C., Minkler, M., Salvatore, A.L., Lee, P.T., Gaydos, M. and Liu, S.S. "Studying and Addressing Urban Immigrant Restaurant Worker Health and Safety in San Francisco's Chinatown District: A CBPR Case Study." *Journal of Urban Health: Bulletin of the New York Academy of Medicine* 90.6 (2013): 1026–40.
41. Vaughn, L.M., Jacquez, F., Lindquist-Grantz, R., Parsons, A. and Melink, K. "Immigrants as Research Partners: A Review of Immigrants in Community-Based Participatory Research (CBPR)." *Journal of Immigrant and Minority Health* (2016). doi:10.1007/s10903-016-0474-3.
42. Patel, V.V., Rajpathak, S. and Karasz, A. "Bangladeshi Immigrants in New York City: A Community Based Health Needs Assessment of a Hard to Reach Population." *Journal of Immigrant and Minority Health* 14.5 (2012): 767–73.
43. Quach, T., Gunier, R., Tran, A., et al. "Characterizing Workplace Exposures in Vietnamese Women Working in California Nail Salons." *American Journal of Public Health* 101.S1 (2011): S271–6.
44. Wieland, M.L., Weis, J.A., Yawn, B.P., et al. "Perceptions of Tuberculosis Among Immigrants and Refugees at an Adult Education Center: A Community-Based Participatory Research Approach." *Journal of Immigrant and Minority Health* 14.1 (2012): 14–22.
45. Barbee, L., Kobetz, E., Menard, J., et al. "Assessing the Acceptability of Self-Sampling for HPV Among Haitian Immigrant Women: CBPR in Action." *Cancer Causes and Control: CCC* 21.3 (2010): 421–31.
46. Johnson-Agbakwu, C.E., Helm, T., Killawi, A. and Padela, A.I. "Perceptions of Obstetrical Interventions and Female Genital Cutting: Insights of Men in a Somali Refugee Community." *Ethnicity and Health* 19.4 (2013): 440–57.
47. Vaughn, L.M., Jacquez, F., Marschner, D. and McLinden, D. "Using Concept Mapping to Visualize Latino Immigrants' Strategies for Health Interventions." *International Journal of Public Health* (In press).
48. Green, M.A., Perez, G., Ornelas, I.J., et al. "Amigas Latinas Motivando el ALMA (ALMA): Development and Pilot Implementation of a Stress Reduction Promotora Intervention." *Californian Journal of Health Promotion* 10 (2012): 52.
49. Vaughn, L.M., Jacquez, F., Marschner, D., et al. "Healthcare Utilization and Barriers to Care Among Latino Immigrants in a New Migration Area." *International Journal of Public Health* (2016) 61: 837. doi:10.1007/s00038-016-0838-4.

9

Applying a Community-Based Participatory Research Approach to Address Determinants of Cardiovascular Disease and Diabetes Mellitus in an Urban Setting

TOBIA HENRY AKINTOBI, PHD, MPH, KISHA B. HOLDEN, PHD, MSCR,

LATRICE ROLLINS, PHD, MSW, RODNEY LYN, PHD, MPH, HARRY J.

HEIMAN, MD, MPH, PAMELA DANIELS, PHD, MBA, GLENDA WRENN,

MD, ALLYSON S. BELTON, MPH, PETER BALTRUS, PHD, SHANICE

BATTLE, MPH, AND LASHAWN M. HOFFMAN

While the scientific evidence demonstrates that individually focused interventions designed to decrease cardiovascular disease (CVD) and diabetes risk can be impactful, individuals and families reside within social and physical environments/communities that may serve as barriers or facilitators of healthy lifestyles. This chapter details an established community-based participatory research (CBPR) model designed to reduce risk for CVD and type 2 diabetes mellitus (DMII) among underserved and vulnerable African Americans through policy, systems, and environmental improvement in a Metropolitan Atlanta community. To comprehensively employ CBPR processes to the community health needs assessment (CHNA), lessons learned over a 15-year collaboration led by a community-majority board were employed and included a mixed-method community health needs assessment led by community residents. To move beyond mapping and documenting health disparities, the CHNA results were prioritized toward the identification of community and evidence-based initiatives in response. Reducing the future burden of DMII and CVD depends on the success of both "top-down" national/state initiatives and "bottom-up" targeted CBPR approaches that bring together transdisciplinary teams that not only address health disparities but also employ policy, systems, and environment changes that advance health equity.

Introduction

The 2013 Centers for Disease Control and Prevention (CDC) Health Disparities and Inequalities Report[1] offers a comprehensive "assessment that highlights health disparities and inequalities across a wide range of diseases, behavioral risk factors, environmental exposures, social determinants, and health-care access by sex, race and ethnicity, income, education, disability status, and other social characteristics." In the report, Meyer et al.[1, p.184] concluded that "reducing disparities requires national leadership to engage a diverse array of stakeholders; facilitate coordination and alignment among federal departments, agencies, offices, and nonfederal partners; champion the implementation of effective policies and programs; and ensure accountability." The majority of such initiatives are "top-down" and do not incorporate the leadership and guidance from those living in communities that represent both the burdens and potential solutions central to understanding and addressing obstinate health disparities. When extreme differences in health/health outcomes are significantly associated with social disadvantages, the differences can be labeled as health inequities; and in most cases these differences (1) are systematic and avoidable; (2) are facilitated and exacerbated by circumstances in which people live, work, and contend with illness; and (3) may be intensified by political, economic, and/or social influences.[2] It is imperative that public health professionals, researchers, clinicians and health policy makers embrace lead roles and multidisciplinary teams that include community leaders to bridge the gap between the rich and the poor concerning health issues, by promoting health equity and setting guidelines for global health initiatives. In order to address health inequities, social justice must be expanded to reach people on a larger scale which is more inclusive and less exclusive.

While the scientific evidence demonstrates that individually focused interventions can be impactful, individuals and families reside within social and physical environments/communities that may serve as barriers or facilitators of healthy lifestyles. Health risk factors not only cluster within individuals and families but are also influenced by social, economic, and structural factors that impact health-promoting lifestyles. The concentration of disadvantage that often permeates urban, low-income, underserved, vulnerable, and racial/ethnic minority neighborhoods may restrict resident opportunities to engage in healthy behaviors that reduce risk for chronic diseases such as diabetes and cardiovascular disease (CVD). Thus, a direct negative impact on the health of these communities may ensue. This chapter details the national prevalence and epidemics of CVD and DMII, correlates of risk factors for these diseases, and limitations of using a siloed approach to address CVD and DMII. Most importantly, we present the application of an established CBPR approach to an evidence-based, culturally tailored model designed to reduce risk for CVD and DMII among underserved and vulnerable African Americans through policy, systems, and environmental improvement.

Background

CARDIOVASCULAR DISEASE AND DIABETES EPIDEMICS

Cardiovascular Disease

Cardiovascular disease refers to the class of diseases that impair functioning of the heart and blood vessels. Over the past several decades, the incidence and prevalence of CVD has increased globally. Between 1990 and 2005, CVD mortality rates increased globally from 14.4 million to 17.5 million. Over 13.3 million of these deaths were caused by stroke (cerebrovascular disease) and heart attack (coronary heart disease) combined. In 2012, the 17.5 million deaths due to CVD made it the leading cause of noncommunicable disease mortality worldwide.[3] In the United States, CVDs are the leading cause of death for both men and women, accounting for over 600,000 deaths each year.[4]

Correlates of Cardiovascular Disease and Diabetes

Cardiovascular disease is closely linked to another common chronic condition— DMII. Caused by insulin resistance or the body's failure to produce enough insulin, DMII is currently the seventh leading cause of death in the United States.[4] In 2012, 1.5 million deaths were attributed to diabetes worldwide.[3] According to the CDC, about 75% of people with DMII die from CVD, specifically heart disease and stroke.[5-6] Together, heart disease and stroke lead to death and disability more often than any other cause of death for those diagnosed with DMII. Further, the risk of heart disease and stroke after a DMII diagnosis is more than double compared to those with no DMII diagnosis.[7]

The relationship between diabetes and CVD is characterized by the interactions of several modifiable risk factors for both diseases. For instance, obesity and hypertension are modifiable risk factors for CVD, but are also associated with insulin resistance.[7] Physical inactivity is a modifiable risk factor for both CVD and DMII. Having diabetes causes elevated blood glucose, which is a risk factor for CVD in persons both with and without diabetes.[8]

Economic Impacts

In addition to causing preventable deaths and a compromised quality of life, CVD has a significant economic toll on society. In 2011, CVD and stroke accounted for an estimated $320.1 billion in direct medical costs in the United States, which included hospital and nursing home visits, medications and home healthcare as well as visits with doctors and other healthcare professionals.[9] Lost future productivity, an indirect cost associated with CVD morbidity and mortality, was estimated at $124.5 billion in the same year.[9]

Type 2 diabetes mellitus also contributes to a significant proportion of US healthcare costs. Diabetes accounts for billions in direct medical costs and indirect costs associated with missed workdays, reduced productivity at work and at home, reduced employment from prolonged disability, and premature mortality. Between 2007 and 2012, diabetes costs in the United States increased from over $174 billion to $245 billion; representing $176 billion for direct medical costs and $69 billion in reduced productivity.[12,14,16,20] After adjusting for age and sex differences, those with diagnosed diabetes had medical expenditures estimated at 2.3 times higher than those without diabetes.[12,14,16]

Racial/Ethnic Disparities

Racial and ethnic minorities in the United States experience disproportionately higher morbidity and mortality rates for CVD and DMII.[1,14,20] Mortality and disability due to CVD and complications of uncontrolled diabetes are 1.5 to 2.5 times higher in African Americans than their White counterparts.[1] Similar disparities exist among American Indian and Alaska Natives. Minority populations, especially in the South, are at higher risk for having undetected or poorly treated risk factors such as hypertension and overweight/obesity. Figure 9.1 illustrates CVD-related mortality rates among African Americans and Whites aged 35–64 years

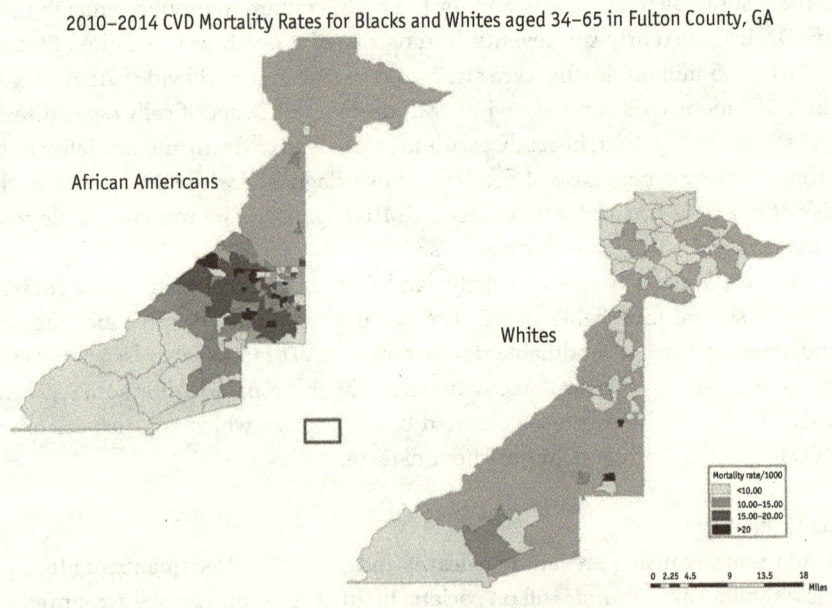

Figure 9.1 2010–2014 CVD Mortality Rates for Blacks and Whites aged 34–65 in Fulton County, GA. Map created by Lilly Immergluck from data provided by special agreement with the Georgia Department of Public Health (2016). Funded by a grant from the American Heart Association.

in census tracts in Fulton County, Georgia. Predominately African American census tracts have higher rates than those that are predominately Whites. The gray areas of the map are census tracts with less than 5 CVD deaths (such areas are censored by Georgia's Department of Public Health). The lack of overlap of areas with sufficient data between African Americans and Whites is reflective of racial segregation of the two groups. As in many other urban areas of the United States, in Fulton County, Georgia, African Americans and Whites largely live in different places that may be differentially shaping their lifestyles, access to healthcare, and ultimately the cause and timing of their deaths.

Fifty-four percent of Georgia adults do not exercise regularly (i.e., 30 or more minutes of moderate physical activity five or more days per week) and 25.1% do not exercise at all.[15,21] In Fulton County, 53.5% of adults ages 18 years and older do not meet the recommended level of physical activity, and 19.3% are inactive.[16] In addition, more than 75% of Georgia adults do not consume the recommended daily servings of five or more fruits and vegetables; 69.5% of adults ages 18 years and older in Fulton County do not meet this dietary standard for healthy eating. The majority of adults 18 years of age and older in Georgia are overweight and obese (65.8%). The rate of overweight and obesity among Fulton County adults is 53.7%.[22-23] Given the dramatic income inequality between north and south Fulton County and the disparate socioeconomic conditions, the rate of overweight and obesity are likely to be much higher in South Fulton County.[17]

Risk Factors

BEHAVIORAL

Some of the modifiable risk factors for CVD are behavioral and may lead to DMII and other related medical conditions. These include tobacco use, poor dietary habits, sedentary lifestyle, and excessive alcohol use. Cigarette smoking contributes to the build-up of plaque in arterial walls and increases the risk of blood clotting. Diets high in cholesterol, saturated fat, and sodium have been associated with increased incidence of CVD.[18] Sedentary lifestyles and excess body fat both increase risk for heart disease by adversely affecting other risk factors such as blood pressure, triglycerides, and cholesterol levels. Excessive alcohol use also contributes to plaque build-up while increasing blood pressure and triglyceride levels.[25] Almost half of US adults over 20 years of age have at least one of the following three risk factors: uncontrolled hypertension, uncontrolled cholesterol, or current smoking.[24]

STRUCTURAL

A number of policy, social, and environmental-level barriers to healthy eating and adequate physical activity have been identified among African Americans. These barriers include lack of access to healthy and affordable foods; ready access to fast foods; lack of knowledge about healthy food and beverage choices; culture; eating patterns developed during their youth; food preferences (e.g., energy dense, poor nutritional value "comfort foods"); family and other responsibilities that lead to lack of time and energy to shop for and cook healthy foods; and family influences.[16,24-25] In addition, the prevalence of physical inactivity is higher among African Americans with lower levels of education and income.[26] There are also several barriers that affect an individual's ability to participate in physical activity. These barriers include physical limitations; embarrassment; lack of motivation; family responsibilities and lack of childcare; inadequate social support; social norms; and lack of safety (e.g., neighborhood crime).[8,16,27,28]

RELEVANCE OF POLICY, SYSTEMS, AND ENVIRONMENTAL CHANGE APPROACHES

Public health efforts to accelerate chronic disease prevention and reduce health disparities and inequities are increasingly focused on policy, systems, and environmental (PSE) approaches. Leading agencies and organizations including the CDC, National Institutes of Health (NIH), Institute of Medicine (IOM), Robert Wood Johnson Foundation (RWJF), and American Public Health Association (APHA) have called for increased efforts at the state and local levels to advance such approaches. Changing policies and environments to promote active living and healthy eating requires cooperation among diverse sectors. The CDC has highlighted the importance of coordination among multiple sectors as a key to successful efforts. The IOM has emphasized the importance of engaging the nonhealth sectors in changing policies and environments to address chronic disease.[29-31] The APHA is strongly promoting a collaborative approach to improve health by incorporating health considerations into decision-making across sectors and policy areas.[32]

LIMITATIONS OF EXISTING COMMUNITY-CLINICAL LINKAGES

Studies confirm that incremental lifestyle changes, such as modest weight loss through healthy eating and increases in physical activity, can help keep those most at risk, including people with prediabetes, from developing diabetes, or delay diabetes onset.[29,30] If 50% of persons with prediabetes were to make healthy lifestyle changes, this could result in a potential reduction of 6,000 cases of diabetes in Atlanta each year.[18,19,31] By 2025, this change would result in a reduction of approximately 96,700 cases of diabetes and a cumulative savings of about $6.2 billion.[34] Similarly, 7,500 fewer people would develop end-stage renal disease by 2025.[20] Despite this potential improvement, even people who have regular contact with a primary care provider often experience challenges in adopting healthier lifestyles. For many, knowledge gained through the clinical encounter is challenged by community level factors that prevent full adoption of provider recommendations for a healthier lifestyle.

MENTAL HEALTH CORRELATES

According to recent data, the prevalence of depression is higher among individuals with chronic diseases, including diabetes and CVD (Figure 9.2). It is estimated that the prevalence of depression is 27% in patients with diabetes and 16%–23% in patients with CVD.[33] Individuals who are depressed are 1.6 times more likely to develop CVD than individuals who do not have depressive symptoms.[34-36] Studies indicate that depression can lead to eating disorders including food overconsumption[38] and poor quality of nutrition intake. Moreover, mental illness is related to lower levels of physical activity;[37,39,40] and severe symptoms of depression can predict a decline in engagement of physical activity,[39] which may increase risk for obesity. Individuals diagnosed with posttraumatic stress disorder (PTSD) have been reported to have an increased risk of hypertension and other CVDs.[40-41] Miller et al.[42] found that exposure to stressors at an early age contribute greatly to an individual's susceptibility to CVD and other chronic diseases later on in life. Other research has shown that individuals with diabetes and a co-occurring substance abuse problem have poorer clinical outcomes and are less adherent to treatment than diabetics without a substance abuse problem.[43]

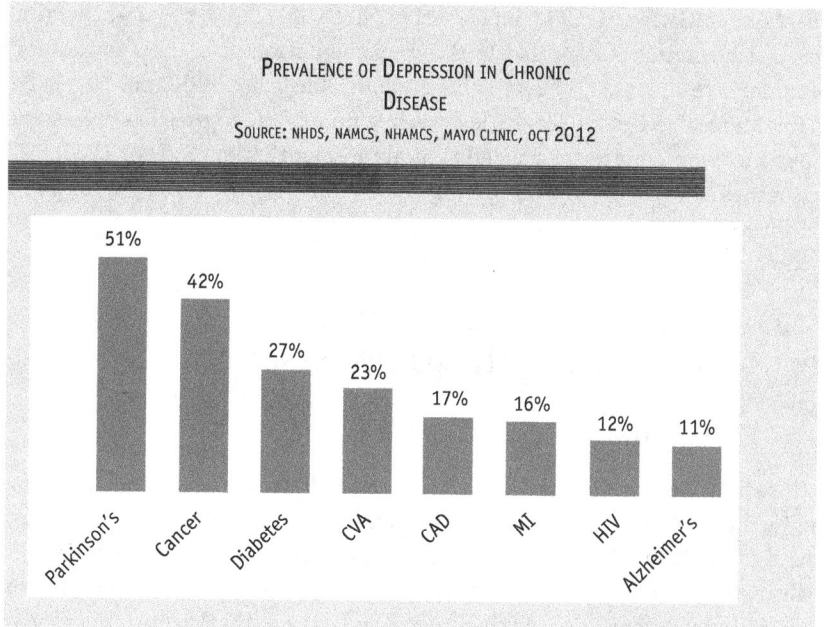

Figure 9.2 Prevalence of depression in chronic disease. Chronic Diseases. National Center for Chronic Disease Prevention and Health Promotion. Division of Population Health. Issue Brief No. 2.

Intervention Approaches for Addressing DMII and CVD

Randomized controlled trials (such as the Diabetes Prevention Program) of group and lifestyle interventions for DMII and CVD have been found to be effective in high-risk obese, minority, and underserved populations.[43-45] Translation of these approaches into primary care were found to be effective in some settings[45] but were only moderately successful in urban, predominantly African American patients.[46] In the BPTEACH Trial,[47] patient education combined with physician education was found to be more effective for CVD risk reduction than usual care.

The use of interventions that include community-clinical linkages may extend the reach and effectiveness of clinical interventions and provide cost savings,[44,55,56] especially when the interventions are culturally tailored and appropriate for people with varying levels of health literacy.[45,48-49] Community-engaged interventions for CVD and DMII often include community health workers and healthcare advocates.[46,50-53] Systematic reviews of team-based care have identified this approach as effective, although there is a need to examine the effectiveness of interventions that combine this approach with CBPR.[54]

Community-based participatory research interventions often provide results that resonate beyond study participants. For example, the Neighborhoods on the Move initiative, a CVD intervention, both increased physical activity in a high-risk community and led to the implementation of 60 new initiatives by community residents.[55] If sustainable and portable, this CBPR approach is helpful for addressing health disparities.[52] While non-CBPR approaches are essential in patients who require specialized clinical intervention for CVD or DMII, CBPR approaches are effective for mitigating risk factors in both at-risk groups and the general population.

Framing the Local Context Through Community-Based Participatory Research

THE PREVENTION RESEARCH CENTER

Both national and state DMII and CVD patterns have been validated, confirmed, and further delineated among Metropolitan Atlanta residents by the Morehouse School of Medicine Prevention Research Center (MSM PRC) and its Community Coalition Board (CCB). The MSM PRC is part of a network of 26 academic research centers funded by the CDC to achieve local and national health objectives focused on gaining knowledge of the best methodologies for solving the nation's health problems. Guided by the theme Risk Reduction and Early Detection in African American and Other Minority Communities: Coalition for Prevention Research, the center conducts research; implements and evaluates demonstration projects;

trains health professionals and community residents: and disseminates research findings.

THE COMMUNITY-BASED PARTICIPATORY RESEARCH FRAMEWORK

The MSM PRC is grounded in CBPR, through which it conducts research in partnership *with* and not *on* the community. The CBPR approach emphasizes community-academic partnership and shared leadership in the planning, implementation, evaluation, and dissemination of interventions.[55-57] The involvement of the community in all stages of the research ensures that the research outcomes are relevant to, owned, and sustained by the community. The CBPR approach also emphasizes public health problems of local relevance and multilevel perspectives that recognize and attend to the social determinants of health and disease.

A COMMUNITY-DRIVEN INFRASTRUCTURE

The CCB is composed of leaders and representatives from neighborhoods, academic institution partners, and social service agencies. The CCB governance structure ensures that neighborhood representatives are always in the majority and that the chair, vice chair, and secretary seats are filled by neighborhood representatives.[58-63] Further, in any vote that pits neighborhoods against academics and agency members, the neighborhood members always maintain the majority of votes. The CCB members review and prioritize critical needs, dialogue about appropriate solutions, and vote during bimonthly meetings. To ensure an evidence-based approach for developing and implementing research and training programs that are aligned with community priorities, CHNAs are conducted by the MSM PRC staff, the CCB and partnering communities at least every 2 years.[60,64-65] The MSM PRC core research and other projects are strategically developed and implemented in response to priorities identified through the CHNA process.

RESEARCH PARTNER COMMUNITIES

The MSM PRC's research partner communities (RPCs) have a total population of 55,757 with 89.3% of residents identified as African American/Black. Almost 41% of African American households within the neighborhood planning units (NPUs) live below the poverty level.[64-66] The Georgia Institute of Technology and the City of Atlanta Planning Department developed a neighborhood health (NH) and quality of life indicator among the 25 City of Atlanta NPUs.[67] The indicator is composed of access to nutritious foods; neighborhood walkability; diabetes morbidity; hypertensive heart disease morbidity; esophageal, renal, and uterine cancer morbidity; and years of potential life lost. All RPCs are characterized among least healthy according to indicator rankings (Figure 9.3). The NPUs were also

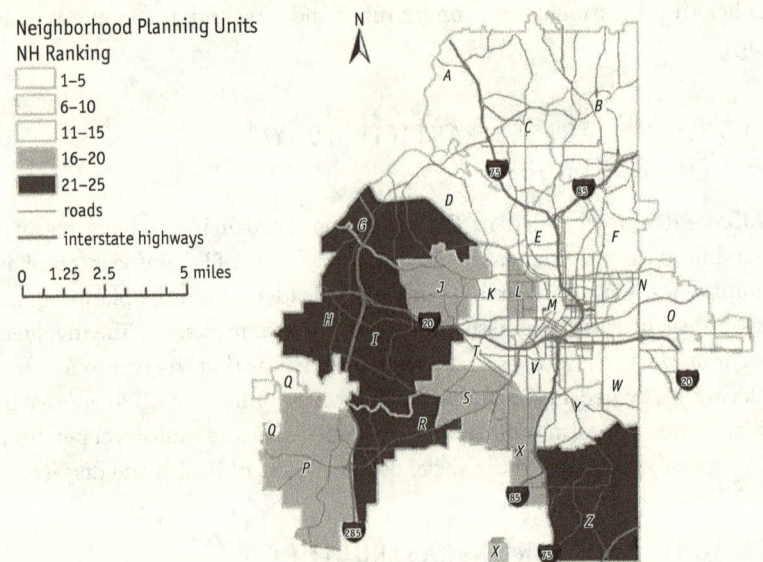

Figure 9.3 Neighborhood planning units NH ranking. Lee, A., Leous, A., Botchwey, N., Guhathakurta, S., & Kennedy, J. (2012). *Quality of Life and Health in Atlanta*. Paper presented at the 2012 Georgia Planning Association Meeting, Columbus, GA.

ranked in a socioeconomic conditions (SEC) scale. All RPCs are in the low SEC category representing increased risk associated with established social determinants of health.[67]

COMMUNITY HEALTH NEEDS ASSESSMENT

The RPCs included in the 2013 CHNA were Metropolitan Atlanta NPUs V, X, Y, and Z, consisting of 23 census tracts. The NPUs are citizen advisory councils that make recommendations to the mayor and City Council on zoning, land use, and other planning issues. Each City of Atlanta NPU contains 5–10 well-defined neighborhoods. Each NPU elects officers and holds monthly public meetings to discuss relevant and timely issues of importance to its residents (e.g., city zoning, economic and civic development).[64] This well-established, preexisting neighborhood-driven leadership structure has been the foundation for the community-led and policy-driven infrastructure of the MSM PRC CCB since its inception in 1998.

Methodology

To comprehensively employ CBPR processes to the CHNA, several steps were taken to build on lessons learned over the 15-year collaboration. First, in response to changing community contexts and communication channels, the Data Monitoring and Evaluation subcommittee, co-led by a CCB member and staff person, reviewed and revised the previously administered CHNA survey questions, wording, and themes. The draft survey was then pilot-tested among community residents through a focus group to identify issues related to respondent burden, consistency with survey goals, and culturally relevant language. The MSM PRC staff and students and CCB members were trained in uniform participant recruitment and survey administration at regularly occurring community events.

A three-pronged approach to recruitment and collection of primary data was then employed. First, survey respondents were recruited by CCB members, postcard flyers, radio broadcasts, neighborhood meetings, Facebook announcements, and community e-mail listservs. The CCB members identified these approaches as ideal mechanisms to recruit and collect data in the local community. The second approach featured training CCB members to disseminate surveys to residents within their respective NPUs. The third approach enlisted the use of electronic and social media, through providing an online link to the survey to residents using e-mail listservs and the MSM PRC Facebook page.

Data Sources
The CHNA consisted of both primary and secondary data sources. Secondary data included, but were not limited to, incidence and prevalence rates for leading causes of morbidity and mortality through multiple sources (i.e., Georgia Department of Health, state, county, city, and local governments, community-serving organizations, partner agencies and institutions). Primary data consisted of surveys of residents aged 18 years or older. Through use of both open- and closed-ended questions, participants were asked to detail their community- and individual-level health concerns, their determinants, and corresponding solutions. In addition, participants were asked about strategies for disseminating health information in their communities.

Results
The top three Black-White health disparities identified through secondary data sources are among the leading causes of morbidity and mortality in these communities (Table 9.1). They are aligned with CHNA priorities and include CVD and DMII.

Table 9.1 **Age-Adjusted Rates of CVD and Diabetes Morbidity and Mortality Among Blacks and Whites per 100,000, Fulton County, GA, 201176**

Disease/Health Condition	Morbidity		Mortality	
	White	Black	White	Black
Major Cardiovascular Diseases	693.5	1486.2	230.5	293.1
Diabetes	65.2	290.7	7.5	33.8

Three hundred sixty-one community residents in RPCs completed CHNA surveys (primary data). The most frequently cited health concerns included high blood pressure, diabetes, and overweight/obesity. Challenges related to mental, emotional, and behavioral health were cited among the top 10 areas of need. The NPUs included in this project are located in census tracts delineated by the highest number of emergency room visits per 1,000 persons. Among the common causes identified for these concerns were "stores without fresh fruits and vegetables," "access and knowledge of healthy foods," and "lack of affordable and healthy food and exercise options."

Moving from the CHNA to Action

To move beyond mapping and documenting health disparities, the CHNA results were discussed with the CCB at a strategic planning retreat. It was agreed that all potential research, training, service, and health initiatives should be aligned with the health condition priorities identified through the CHNA. Further, CCB members agreed that health interventions and strategies should be sought that catalyzed action and advocacy toward advancing health equity. The MSM PRC has strategically leveraged results of its CHNA to systematically review and prioritize interventions through its CCB governance structure and guide and advance implementation of its core research. All projects are ideally reviewed during the development of grant application(s), and vetted and approved or rejected by the CCB prior to final submission. A project review committee appointed by the board chair reviews project proposals and makes implementation suggestions/recommendations to the full board prior to beginning the research in partnering communities.

In 2014, a CDC funding opportunity announcement presented a potential opportunity to be responsive to the CHNA findings through a focus on increasing access to environments that promote physical activity and access to healthy foods through a community coalition. The section that follows details the proposed model.

Framing the Solution Through a Transdisciplinary, Multilevel Model

The Transforming Metropolitan Atlanta Communities through Prevention, Primary Care Linkages and Policy Improvement Model (Figure 9.4) uses a CBPR approach that increases support for policy, systems, and environmental (PSE) level change, and improves clinic-community linkages to decrease CVD and DMII risk and improve mental and behavioral health. This community-centered approach is guided by the MSM PRC CCB, through which health priorities, implementation strategies and their assessment have guided Metropolitan Atlanta neighborhood residents since 1999 (Figure 9.4).

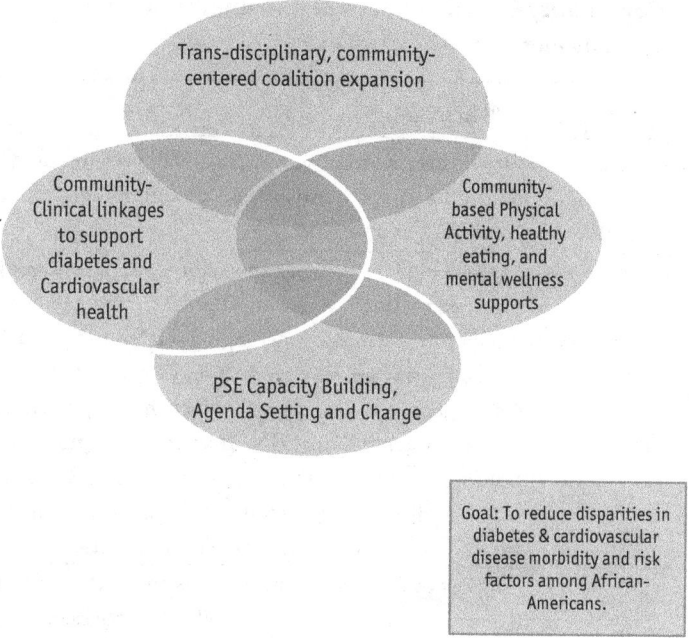

Figure 9.4 The transforming metropolitan Atlanta communities through prevention, primary care linkages and policy improvement model.

COMMUNITY-BASED PARTICIPATORY APPROACH (CBPA)

The establishment of a governing body that ensures a CBPA can be challenging when (1) academicians have not previously been guided by neighborhood experts about the evolution of a community's context, (2) community members have not led discussions regarding their health priorities, and/or (3) academic and neighborhood experts have not historically worked together as a single body with established rules guiding roles and function. As mentioned above, neighborhood representatives on the CCB are always in the majority in number and leadership but are complemented by other stakeholders from multiple sectors (e.g., local governance, health, community coalition board, urban planning, work sector), unified under a common agenda of enhancing community health and integrated care in their most vulnerable local communities (Table 9.2).

POLICY, SYSTEMS AND ENVIRONMENT PRIORITIES

Policy, systems, and environmental approaches central to this model include access to healthful foods and environments conducive to physical activity. These strategies are response to interventions promoted by the Community Prevention Services Task Force, which recommends strategies that combine diet and physical

Table 9.2 **Community Coalition Board Leadership, Support, and Engagement**

Activity Key Element	CCB Activities
Implementation	Bimonthly review of progress at CCB meetings. May modify or reject approaches to ensure community relevance, credibility, and validity
Communication	Serve as subject matter experts on PSE topic development for presentations, workshops, webinars, and Web/social media content and/or messaging related to the Coalition's efforts. Coauthor manuscripts and written documents, e.g., journal articles, bulletins, fact sheets; present findings and promotes the Coalition at scientific, community, and policy-driven presentations, on radio and TV, and through other media and social media outlets; disseminates research findings and health materials in communities served
Evaluation	Support evaluation efforts by assisting in the development of surveys for appropriate data collection; participating in data collection; presenting evaluation findings; providing input from the CCB and assisting in programmatic decision-making based on evaluation findings that impact the PRC and/or the CCB. A subgroup of 3–4 CCB members constitute a project review committee who meet quarterly with Coalition leadership to assess the progress, outcomes, and impact of its work and provide critical feedback to foster community accountability and optimum community engagement

activity promotion programs for people at increased risk of DMII based on strong evidence of effectiveness in reducing new-onset diabetes.

INCREASING HEALTHFUL FOOD ACCESS

This effort focused on corner stores as community sites for food access. Corner stores have been strong partners in efforts to improve access to healthy foods in urban communities. This initiative sought to increase the available inventory of healthful foods and beverages in the target communities by recruiting 21 corner stores to participate in a Healthy Corner Store Initiative. This approach is informed by the work of The Food Trust, a nationally recognized nonprofit leader in this area. The Food Trust and the City of Philadelphia's Department of Public Health have successfully partnered to implement an array of programs focused on increasing the healthy food inventory and educating consumers in corner stores in that city. The Food Trust found that partnering with corner stores is an effective strategy to improve healthy food access in underserved communities. They also reported that corner store owners are willing to introduce healthy inventories, but they need support and simple steps to follow.[67] Specific activities implemented to advance the Healthy Corner Store Initiative and assess its impact included: identification and mapping of existing corner stores in the target community; observation and documentation of store use patterns by patrons; introduction of the Healthy Corner Store Initiative and recruitment of store managers/owners; provision of guidance and training for store personnel on choosing, handling, displaying, and pricing products; development of in-store marketing materials to promote healthy products; outreach and engagement to residents and other stakeholders to build awareness and demand for healthy foods; delivery of technical assistance to participating stores to track progress, troubleshoot challenges, and build rapport and community connections; and implementation of intercept surveys with corner store customers prior to and following inventory changes to assess purchasing behaviors.

INCREASING OPPORTUNITIES FOR PHYSICAL ACTIVITY

Though there are numerous approaches to increasing opportunities for physical activity, this initiative focused on the promotion, development, and implementation of Complete Streets. The Safe and Complete Streets Act, proposed in the US Congress in 2011, defines complete streets as roadways that safely accommodate all travelers, particularly public transit users, bicyclists, pedestrians, motorists, and freight vehicles to enable all travelers to use the roadways safely and efficiently. Roadways designed using the Complete Streets approach may include one or a combination of evidence-based components. Over 625 regional and local jurisdictions and 27 states have adopted Complete Streets policies or have made written commitment to do so.[69] Strong evidence indicates that policies to enhance built environments such as improving walking and cycling infrastructure, improving street connectivity, and increasing access to public transit can increase the likelihood of active travel in given populations.[70] Multilevel strategies such as infrastructure improvements (walking- and cycling-friendly environments) combined with promotional campaigns have the greatest potential to increase physical activity levels.[71-73]

This initiative sought to increase the number of residents with access to environments that provide opportunities for physical activity. Specifically, the initiative focused on increasing the number of communities across southwest Atlanta that endorsed and implemented Complete Streets policies. Specific activities implemented to promote Complete Streets included engagement and collaboration with local leaders, community-based organizations and residents; hosting community information sessions; establishing a community working group; mapping built environment impediments and priorities; review of paving and other community development plans and schedules; development of educational issue briefs for key stakeholders; and use of community health workers to support community awareness and engagement.

COMMUNITY CLINICAL LINKAGES

Results of the CHNA represent a local reality that is mirrored nationally with respect to diabetes and CVD outcomes. Educational efforts related to CVD and DMII prevention, including self-management and behavioral change activities, should be targeted to racial/ethnic minorities, who bear a significant burden of the diseases with worse outcomes.[24,74]

The iADAPT 2.0 Program is a component of the Community-Clinical Linkages Core. The goal of the program is the activation of up to 400 community health workers in underserved neighborhoods. The objective of this program is to strengthen the community health worker (CHW) infrastructure to facilitate improvement in self-management and prevention of DMII, prediabetes, CVD, and related mental health concerns; to improve linkages between community health centers and community-based interventions; and to sustain systems change for chronic disease self-management and prevention. The iADAPT 2.0 Program is designed to increase access to patient-centered medical homes and the use of nonphysician care teams incorporating CHWs in neighborhoods with greater exposure to health risks and decreased access to health services for chronic diseases.

A key component of the community–clinical linkages program is to use the services of CHWs to identify persons at risk of or diagnosed with DVM II and prediabetes. There is also strong evidence of effectiveness for interventions that engage CHWs in teams targeting blood pressure and cholesterol reduction for patients with increased CVD risk. The CHWs provide referrals to community clinics for CVD and diabetes prevention and self-management education classes and medical services. This referral program bridges a gap between neighborhoods and clinics. Referrals are tracked through CHW referral forms. An electronic medical records (EMR) system is used to track changes in health outcomes (glucose, HbA1c, blood pressure, weight, body mass index (BMI), and the total cholesterol panel. These measures are evaluated at 6- and 12-month intervals. Based on previous research, the program will reach approximately 54,000 community residents over a 3-year period.

MENTAL AND BEHAVIORAL HEALTH INTEGRATION

The rationale for integrating strategies that target mental health and substance use disorders is supported by over 80 randomized controlled studies that demonstrate the benefit of collaborative care for depression and anxiety disorders[76] and for individuals with co-morbid chronic conditions such as diabetes and cardiovascular disease.[75] These clinic-based strategies have a strong evidence base. Furthermore, emerging evidence shows that integrated approaches are promising strategies to help mitigate against the negative impact of trauma exposure[76] and eliminate disparities.[78] A review of studies examining integration of mental health with CHW strategies pointed to potential benefits of these approaches.[78] Understanding the impact of unmet needs for treatment of mental illness and substance use disorders,[79] our approach integrates mental health interventions with strategies designed to address DMII and CVD.

The Mental and Behavioral Health Core provides leadership in examining the role of selected psychosocial risk factors as comorbid conditions/factors of hypertension and DMII in the priority population. These factors include (1) depression, (2) history of trauma, (3) stress and coping strategies used, and (4) substance use. This integrative approach will look into the mental and behavioral health practices of community members, specifically as it relates to eating habits and access to nutritional foods; physical activity and environmental impact; and access to and use of primary care services for mental and behavioral health needs. Our approach combines best practices in supporting the training of CHWs to improve their ability to identify and support community-clinical linkages for individuals impacted by mental illness and substance use disorders. We also include CHW training for self-care and identification of character strengths.[80]

CENTRAL COLLABORATORS AND STAKEHOLDERS

The MSM REACH Health Intervention (REACH HI) is being implemented through a partnership led by community partners (the CCB and residents of Atlanta Georgia NPUs V, X, Y, Z, and T)[68], academic partners (the Morehouse School of Medicine PRC, Satcher Health Leadership Institute, Clinical Research Center, National Center for Primary Care, Evaluation and Institutional Assessment Unit) and agency partners (Fulton County Department of Health and Wellness, Southside Medical Center, Family Healthcare Centers of Georgia, and Morehouse School of Medicine's Family Comprehensive Health Center). Their complementary missions and goals merge to represent the expertise critical to addressing community-based health disparities through intervention approaches that are evidence-based and demonstrate a CBPR approach.

KEY EVALUATION QUESTIONS

The planned evaluation is designed to answer questions that address the project components depicted in the logic model, provide performance monitoring data for ongoing program improvement, and assess the actual impact and use of the MSM REACH HI interventions by the target population. Table 9.3 includes evaluation questions and data sources.

Table 9.3 **Evaluation Questions and Associated Data Sources**

Evaluation Questions	Pre-Post Surveys	Clinical Data	Community/ Policy Assessment	Secondary Data Analysis
1. To what extent were MSM REACH HI activities implemented as planned?				X
2. To what extent did the target population(s) demonstrate positive change toward specified behavioral and health outcomes?	X	X		X
3. To what extent were policy, system, and environmental changes in the target area initiated and maintained that were supportive of MSM REACH HI outcomes?	X		X	X

Conclusion

The comprehensive model presented, while still evolving, is built on a foundation representing demonstrable evidence on the effectiveness of CBPR approaches applied to several important health disparities. It also serves as a roadmap that connects national health disparities to the identification of local health priorities and intervention responses that resonate with communities through established and trusted community-based infrastructure. Its expansion to address clinical outcomes and the PSE that support or serve as barriers to individual behavior change has great potential to go beyond individual intervention to community research and sustainability.

Reducing the future burden of DMII and CVD depends on the success of both "top-down" national/state initiatives and "bottom-up" targeted CBPR approaches that bring together transdisciplinary teams and neighborhood residents as essential members and partners. Addressing the spectrum of prevention and risk reduction strategies also requires a coordinated PSE approach that fundamentally changes communities and environments that promote health and provide access to realistic options for physical activity and improved nutrition. To capitalize on evidence-based approaches, it is imperative that diverse stakeholders develop and evaluate promising strategies that enhance the likelihood of sustained intervention approaches centered on community strengths and assets.

References

1. Meyer, P.A., Penman-Aguilar, A., Campbell, V.A., et al. "Conclusion and Future Directions." *CDC Health Disparities and Inequalities Report—United States, 2013 Supplements* 62 (2013): 184–6.
2. Marmot, M., Friel, S., Bell, R., Houweling, T.A.J. and Taylor, S. "Closing the Gap in a Generation: Health Equity Through Action on the Social Determinants of Health." *Lancet* 372 (2008): 1661–9.
3. Global Health Observatory Data Repository. *Cardiovascular Diseases, Deaths per 100,000, Data by Country, 2015.* <http://apps.who.int/gho/data/node.main.A865CARDIOVASCULAR?lang=en>
4. Centers for Disease Control and Prevention. *Heart Disease Statistics and Maps, 2015.* <http://www.cdc.gov/heartdisease/statistics_maps.htm> (accessed February 5, 2016).
5. Centers for Disease Control and Prevention, National Center for Health Statistics. *Deaths and Mortality, 2015.* <http://www.cdc.gov/nchs/fastats/deaths.htm>
6. Centers for Disease Control and Prevention. *Heart Disease Facts.* 2015. http://www.cdc.gov/heartdisease/facts.htm Retrieved on July 9, 2015.
7. Centers for Disease Control and Prevention. *National Diabetes Statistics Report: Estimates of Diabetes and Its Burden in the United States, 2014.* Atlanta, GA: US Department of Health and Human Services.
8. Centers for Disease Control and Prevention. *National Diabetes Fact Sheet: National Estimates and General Information on Diabetes and Prediabetes in the United States, 2011.* Atlanta, GA: US Department of Health and Human Services, Centers for Disease Control and Prevention. <http://www.cdc.gov/diabetes/pubs/pdf/ndfs_2011.pdf>
9. Mozaffarian, D., Benjamin, E.J., Go, A.S., et al. "Heart Disease and Stroke Statistics—2015 Update: A Report from the American Heart Association." *Circulation* 131.4 (2015): e29–322. doi:10.1161/CIR.0000000000000152
10. American Diabetes Association. "Economic Costs of Diabetes in the U.S. in 2002." *Diabetes Care* 26 (2003): 917–32. doi: 10.2337/diacare.26.3.917
11. American Diabetes Association. "Economic Costs of Diabetes in the U.S. in 2007." *Diabetes Care* 31 (2008): 596–615. doi: 10.2337/dc08-9017
12. American Diabetes Association. "Economic Costs of Diabetes in the U.S. in 2012." *Diabetes Care* 36 (2012):1033–46. doi: 10.2337/dc12-2625
13. Centers for Disease Control and Prevention, National Center for Chronic Disease Prevention and Health Promotion, and Division of Diabetes Translation. *National Diabetes Fact Sheet, 2011.* 2011. http://www.cdc.gov/diabetes/pubs/factsheet11.htm> (accessed July 10, 2014).
14. Heidenreich, P.A., Trogdon, J.G., Khavjou, O.A., et al. "Forecasting the Future of Cardiovascular Disease in the United States: A Policy Statement from the American Heart Association." *Circulation* 123 (2011): 933–44.
15. Centers for Disease Control and Prevention. "Vital Signs: State-Specific Obesity Prevalence Among Adults—United States, 2009." *Morbidity and Mortality Weekly Report* 59.30 (2010): 951–5.
16. Centers for Disease Control and Prevention: National Diabetes Surveillance System. *Diabetes Data and Trends.* 2011. <http://www.cdc.gov/diabetes/statistics> (accessed July 31, 2012).
17. Georgia Department of Community Health. *Georgia Adult Obesity by County: Fact Sheet.* 2010. <http://health.state.ga.us/pdfs/epi/cdiee/Obese%20Adults%20in%20Georgia%20by%20County_final3.pdf> (accessed July 15, 2014).
18. US Census Bureau. *Fulton County, Ga: Quick Facts.* 2011. <http://quickfacts.census.gov/qfd/states/13/13121.html> (accessed on July 12, 2014).

19. Fryar, C.D., Chen, T. and Li, X. *Prevalence of Uncontrolled Risk Factors for Cardiovascular Disease: United States, 1999–2010*. NCHS Data Brief, No. 103. Hyattsville, MD: National Center for Health Statistics, Centers for Disease Control and Prevention, US Dept of Health and Human Services, 2012.

20. Valderrama, A.L., Loustalot, F., Gillespie, C., et al. "Million Hearts: Strategies to Reduce the Prevalence of Leading Cardiovascular Disease Risk Factors—United States, 2011." *Morbidity and Mortality Weekly Report* 60.36 (2011): 1248.

21. Centers for Disease Control and Prevention. *Heart Disease Risk Factors, 2009*. http://www.cdc.gov/mmwr/preview/mmwrhtml/su6203a26.htm. Retrieved July 20, 2015.

22. Center for Disease Control and Prevention. "Health Disparities and Inequalities Report." *Morbidity and Mortality Weekly Report Supplement* 62 (2013, November 22): 1–187.

23. Georgia Department of Public Health, Georgia Diabetes Prevention and Control Program. *2012 Georgia Diabetes Burden Report: An Overview*. 2012. <http://health.state.ga.us/programs/diabetes/index.asp>

24. Hutch, D.J., Bouye, K.E., Skillen, E., Lee, C., Whitehead, L. and Rashid, J.R. "Potential Strategies to Eliminate Built Environment Disparities for Disadvantaged and Vulnerable Communities." *American Journal of Public Health* 101.4 (2011): 587–95.

25. Varda, D.M., Chandra, A., Stern, S.A. and Lurie, N. "Core Dimensions of Connectivity in Public Health Collaboratives." *Journal of Public Health Management and Practice* 14.5 (2008): E1–7.

26. Institute of Medicine Committee on Accelerating Progress in Obesity Prevention Food and Nutrition Board. *Accelerating Progress in Obesity Prevention: Solving the Weight of the Nation*, ed. D. Glickman, L. Parker, L. Sim, H. DelValle Cook, E. Miller. Washington, DC: National Academies Press, 2012.

27. American Public Health Association and Public Health Institute. *Health in All Policies: A Guide for State and Local Governments*. 2013. <https://www.apha.org/topics-and-issues/healthy-communities/health-in-all-policies>

28. Jones, A.P., Homer, J.B., Murphy, D.L., Essien, J., Milstein, B., and Seville, D.A. "Understanding Diabetes Population Dynamics Through Simulation Modeling and Experimentation." *American Journal of Public Health* 96.3 (2006): 488–94. doi: 10.2105/AJPH.2005.063529

29. Institute for Alternative Futures. (2014). *Diabetes 2025 Forecasting Model*. <http://www.altfutures.org/diabetes2025> (accessed July 18, 2014).

30. "Moving Beyond 'Food Deserts': Reorienting United States Policies to Reduce Disparities in Diet Quality." *PLoS Medicine* 12.12 (2015): 1–9. doi:10.1371/journal.pmed.1001914

31. Walker, R.E., Keane, C.R., & Burke, J.G. "Disparities and Access to Healthy Food in the United States: A Review of Food Deserts Literature." *Health and Place* 16 (2010): 876–84. doi:10.1016/j.healthplace.2010.04.013

32. Centers for Disease Control and Prevention. *Mental Health and Chronic Diseases*. National Center for Chronic Disease Prevention and Health Promotion. Division of Population Health. Issue Brief No. 2. 2012. <http://www.cdc.gov/nationalhealthyworksite/docs/issue-brief-no-2-mental-health-and-chronic-disease-.pdf>

33. Ghitza, U.E., Wu, L., and Tai, B. "Integrating Substance Abuse Care with Community Diabetes Care: Implications for Research and Clinical Practice." *Substance Abuse and Rehabilitation* 4 (2013): 3–10.

34. Centers for Disease Control and Prevention. *Mental Health and Chronic Diseases*. National Center for Chronic Disease Prevention and Health Promotion. Division of Population Health. Issue Brief No. 2. 2012. <http://www.cdc.gov/nationalhealthyworksite/docs/issue-brief-no-2-mental-health-and-chronic-disease-.pdf>

35. Anderson, R.J., Freedland, K.E., Clouse, R.E. and Lustman, P.J. "The Prevalence of Comorbid Depression in Adults with Diabetes: A Meta-Analysis." *Diabetes Care* 24 (2001): 1069–78.

36. Rubin, R.R., Ciechanowski, P., Egede, L.E., Lin, E.H. and Lustman, P.J. "Recognizing and Treating Depression in Patients with Diabetes." *Current Diabetes Reports* 4 (2004): 119–25.

37. Ahlgren, S.S., Shultz, J.A., Massey, L.K., Hicks, B.C. and Wysham, C. "Development of a Preliminary Diabetes Dietary Satisfaction and Outcomes Measure for Patients with Type 2 Diabetes." *Quality of Life Research* 13 (2004): 819–32.
38. Liu, C., Xie, B., Chou, C.P., et al. "Perceived Stress, Depression and Food Consumption Frequency in the College Students of China Seven Cities." *Physiology and Behavior* 748–754 (2007): E51593.
39. Adams, T.B., Moore, M.T., and Dye, J. The Relationship Between Physical Activity and Mental Health in a National Sample of College Females. *Women Health* 45 (2007): 69–85.
40. Fox, K.R., Stathi, A., McKenna, J. and Davis, M.G. "Physical Activity and Mental Well-Being in Older People Participating in the Better Ageing Project." *European Journal of Applied Physiology* 100 (2007): 591–602.
41. Roshanaei-Moghaddam, B., Katon, W.J. and Russo, J. "The Longitudinal Effects of Depression on Physical Activity." *General Hospital Psychiatry* 31.4 (2009): 306–15. <http://dx.doi.org/10.1016/j.genhosppsych.2009.04.002>
42. Coughlin, S.S. "Post-traumatic Stress Disorder and Cardiovascular Disease." *The Open Cardiovasccular Medicine* 5 (2011): 164–70. <http://www.ncbi.nlm.nih.gov/pmc/articles/PMC3141329/>
43. Miller, G.E., Chen, E., and Parker, K.H. "Psychological Stress in Childhood and Susceptibility to the Chronic Diseases of Aging: Moving Towards a Model of Behavioral and Biological Mechanisms." *Psychological Bulletin* 137.6 (2011): 959–97. doi: 10.1037/a0024768 http://www.ncbi.nlm.nih.gov/pmc/articles/PMC3202072/
44. Rugulies R. "Depression as a predictor for coronary heart disease. A review and meta-analysis." *American Journal of Preventive Medicine* 23 (2002): 51–61.
45. Ma, J., Yank, V., Xiao, L., et al. "Translating the Diabetes Prevention Program Lifestyle Intervention for Weight Loss into Primary Care: A Randomized Trial." *Journal of the American Medical Association Internal Medicine* 173.2 (2013): 113–121. doi:10.1001/2013.jamainternmed.987
46. Ockene, I.S., Tellez, T.L., Rosal, M.C., et al. "Outcomes of a Latino Community-Based Intervention for the Prevention of Diabetes: The Lawrence Latino Diabetes Prevention Project." *American Journal of Public Health* 102.2 (2012): 336–42. doi:10.2105/AJPH.2011.300357
47. Reitz, J.A., Sarfaty, M., Diamond, J.J. and Salzman, B. "The Effects of a Group Visit Program on Outcomes of Diabetes Care in an Urban Family Practice." *Journal of Urban Health: Bulletin of the New York Academy of Medicine* 89.4 (2012): 709–16. doi:10.1007/s11524-012-9675-9
48. Johnson, W., Shaya, F., Khanna, N., et al. "The Baltimore Partnership to Educate and Achieve Control of Hypertension (The BPTEACH Trial): A Randomized Trial of the Effect of Education on Improving Blood Pressure Control in a Largely African American Population." *Journal of Clinical Hypertension* 13.8 (2011): 563–70. doi:10.1111/j.1751-7176.2011.00477.x
49. Albright, A.L. and Gregg, E.W. "Preventing Type 2 Diabetes in Communities Across the U.S.: The National Diabetes Prevention Program." *American Journal of Preventive Medicine* 44.4 Suppl 4 (2013): S346–51. doi:10.1016/j.amepre.2012.12.009
50. Ackermann, R.T., Finch, E.A., Brizendine, E., Zhou, H. and Marrero, D.G. "Translating the Diabetes Prevention Program into the Community. The DEPLOY Pilot Study." *American Journal of Preventive Medicine* 35.4 (2008): 357–63. doi:10.1016/j.amepre.2008.06.035
51. Katula, J., Vitolins, M., Rosenberger, E., Blackwell, C., Morgan, T., Lawlor, M., & Goff, D.J. "One-Year Results of a Community-Based Translation of the Diabetes Prevention Program: Healthy-Living Partnerships to Prevent Diabetes (HELP PD) Project." *Diabetes Care* 34.7 (2011): 1451–57. doi:10.2337/dc10-2115
52. Allen, J., Dennison-Himmelfarb, C., Szanton, S., et al. "Community Outreach and Cardiovascular Health (COACH) Trial: A Randomized, Controlled Trial of Nurse Practitioner/Community Health Worker Cardiovascular Disease Risk Reduction in Urban Community Health Centers." *Circulation: Cardiovascular Quality and Outcomes* 4.6 (2011): 595–602.

53. Harvey, I., Schulz, A., Israel, B., et al. "The Healthy Connections Project: A Community-Based Participatory Research Project Involving Women at Risk for Diabetes and Hypertension." *Progress in Community Health Partnerships: Research, Education, and Action* 3.4 (2009): 287–300. doi:10.1353/cpr.0.0088

54. Brennan, T., Spettell, C., Villagra, V., et al. "Disease Management to Promote Blood Pressure Control Among African Americans." *Population Health Management* 13.2 (2010): 65–72. doi:10.1089/pop.2009.0019

55. Proia, K.K., Thota, A.B., Njie, G.J., et al. "Team-Based Care and Improved Blood Pressure Control: A Community Guide Systematic Review." *American Journal of Preventive Medicine* 47 (2014): 86–99. doi:10.1016/j.amepre.2014.03.004

56. Suminski, R.R., Petosa, R.L. and Poston, C.W. "Neighborhoods on the Move: A Community-Based Participatory Research Approach to Promoting Physical Activity." *Progress in Community Health Partnerships: Research, Education, and Action* 3.1 (2009): 5. doi:10.1353/cpr.0.0059

57. Israel, B.A., Schulz, A.J., Parker, E.A. and Becker, A.B. "Review of Community-Based Research: Assessing Partnership Approaches to Improve Public Health." *Annual Review of Public Health* 19 (1998): 173–202.

58. Minkler, M. and Wallerstein, N., eds. *Community Based Participatory Research for Health: Process to Outcomes* (2nd ed.). San Francisco, CA: Jossey Bass, 2008.

59. Dankwa-Mullan, I., Rhee, K.B., Williams, K., et al. "The Science of Eliminating Health Disparities: Summary and Analysis of the NIH Summit Recommendations." *American Journal of Public Health* 100 Suppl 1 (2010): S12–8. doi:10.2105/AJPH.2010.191619

60. Blumenthal, D.S. "A Community Coalition Board Creates a Set of Values for Community-Based Research." *Preventing Chronic Disease* 3.1 (2006): A16.

61. Blumenthal, D.S. "How Do You Start Working with a Community?" Section 4a of "Challenges in Improving Community Engagement in Research." In *The Clinical and Translational Science Awards Community Engagement Key Function Committee Task Force on the Principles of Community Engagement* (2nd ed.). Washington, DC: Department of Health and Human Services, 2011.

62. Blumenthal, D.S. "Is Community-Based Participatory Research Possible?" *American Journal of Preventive Medicine* 40.3 (2011): 386–9. doi:10.1016/j.amepre.2010.11.011

63. Blumenthal, D.S., Smith, S.A., Majett, C.D. and Alema-Mensah, E. "A Trial of 3 Interventions to Promote Colorectal Cancer Screening in African Americans." *Cancer* 116.4 (2010): 922–9. doi:10.1002/cncr.24842

64. Henry Akintobi, T., Goodin, L., Trammel, E., Collins, D. and Blumenthal, D. "How Do You Set Up and Maintain a Community Advisory Board?" Section 4b of "Challenges in Improving Community Engagement in Research." In *The Clinical and Translational Science Awards Community Engagement Key Function Committee Task Force on the Principles of Community Engagement: Principles of Community Engagement* (2nd ed.). Washington, DC: Department of Health and Human Services, 2011.

65. Henry Akintobi, T., Goodin, L., & Hoffman, L. "Morehouse School of Medicine Prevention Research Center: Collaborating with Neighborhoods to Develop Community-Based Participatory Approaches to Address Health Disparities in Metropolitan Atlanta." *Atlanta Medicine: Journal of the Medical Association of Atlanta* 84.2 (2013): 14–17.

66. City of Atlanta. *Neighborhood Planning Unit (NPU)*. 2016. <http://www.atlantaga.gov/index.aspx?page=739>

67. City of Atlanta, Department of Planning and Community Development—Office of Planning. *2010 Census Summary Report Neighborhood Planning Unit V*. Atlanta, GA, 2010.

68. City of Atlanta Department of Planning and Community Development—Office of Planning. *2010 Census Summary Report Neighborhood Planning Unit X*. Atlanta, GA, 2010.

69. City of Atlanta Department of Planning and Community Development—Office of Planning. *2010 Census Summary Report Neighborhood Planning Unit Y*. Atlanta, GA, 2010.

70. City of Atlanta Department of Planning and Community Development—Office of Planning. *2010 Census Summary Report Neighborhood Planning Unit Z.* Atlanta, GA, 2010.

71. Lee, A., Leous, A., Botchwey, N., Guhathakurta, S. and Kennedy, J. (2012). *Quality of Life and Health in Atlanta.* Paper presented at the 2012 Georgia Planning Association Meeting, Columbus, GA.

72. The Food Trust. *Healthy Corner Store Initiative: Overview.* http://thefoodtrust.org/food-access/publications> (accessed July 16, 2014).

73. Smart Growth America. *National Complete Streets Coalitions: Policy Atlas.* 2014. http://www.smartgrowthamerica.org/complete-streets/changing-policy/complete-streets-atlas (accessed November 16, 2014).

74. Pucher, J., Buehler, R., Bassett, D.R. and Dannenberg, A.L. "Walking and Cycling to Health: A Comparative Analysis of City, State, and International Data." *American Journal of Public Health* 100.10 (2010): 1986–1992. doi:10.2105/AJPH.2009.189324

75. Ogilvie, D., Egan, M., Hamilton, V. and Petticrew, M. "Promoting Walking and Cycling as an Alternative to Using Cars: Systematic Review." *BMJ (Clinical Research ed.)* 329.7469 (2004): 763. doi:10.1136/bmj.38216.714560.55

76. De Nazelle, A., Nieuwenhuijsen, M.J., Antó, J.M., et al. "Improving Health Through Policies That Promote Active Travel: A Review of Evidence to Support Integrated Health Impact Assessment." *Environment International* 37.4 (2011): 766–77. doi:10.1016/j.envint.2011.02.003

77. Center for Disease Control and Prevention. *Health Disparities and Inequalities Report. Morbidity and Mortality Weekly Report.* 62 Suppl 3 (2013): 1–187.

78. Archer, J., Bower, P., Gilbody, S., et al. "Collaborative Care for Depression and Anxiety Problems." *Cochrane Database of Systematic Reviews* (2012)10:CD006525.

79. Coventry, P., Lovell, K., Dickens, C., et al. "Integrated Primary Care for Patients with Mental and Physical Multimorbidity: Cluster Randomized Controlled Trial of Collaborative Care for Patients with Depression Comorbid with Diabetes or Cardiovascular Disease." *British Medical Journal* 350 (2015): h638.

80. Melville, J.L., Reed, S.D., Russo, J., et al. "Improving Care for Depression in Obstetrics and Gynecology: A Randomized Controlled Trial." *Obstetrics and Gynecology* 123.6 (2014): 1237–46. http://doi.org/10.1097/AOG.0000000000000231

81. Woltmann, E., Grogan-Kaylor, A., Perron, B., Georges, H., Kilbourne, A. and Bauer, M. "Comparative Effectiveness of Collaborative Chronic Care Models for Mental Health Conditions Across Primary, Specialty, and Behavioral Health Settings: Systematic Review and Meta-Analysis." *American Journal of Psychiatry* 169 (2012): 1–15.

82. De Hert, M., Correll, C.U., Bobes, J., et al. "Physical Illness in Patients with Severe Mental Disorders: I. Prevalence, Impact of Medications and Disparities in Health Care." *World Psychiatry* 10.1 (2011): 52–77.

83. Linley, P.A., Nielsen, K.M., Gillett, R. and Biswas-Diener, R. "Using Signature Strengths in Pursuit of Goals: Effects on Goal Progress, Need Satisfaction, and Well-Being, and Implications for Coaching Psychologists." *International Coaching Psychology Review* 5.1 (2010): 6–15.

10

Community-Based Participatory
Research Addressing Infant Mortality

STEVEN S. COUGHLIN, PHD AND SELINA A. SMITH, PHD, MDIV

This chapter considers community-based participatory research (CBPR) aimed at reducing infant mortality and improving maternal and child health. The topics discussed include global disparities in infant mortality, risk factors for infant mortality, and evidence-based approaches for preventing infant mortality in low- and middle-income countries and in higher-income countries such as the United States. The role of CBPR in addressing infant mortality is highlighted, including CBPR studies conducted in the United States that addressed infant mortality and closely related maternal and newborn health topics (e.g., smoking during pregnancy) that had a randomized controlled trial, quasi-experimental, or pre/post test design. Participatory studies conducted in developing countries are also considered. Additional CBPR studies are needed that have the potential to fill in gaps in the current evidence about what intervention strategies are effective in reducing infant mortality in population subgroups that are disproportionately affected by it. This includes dissemination and implementation research and studies that translate evidence-based interventions to new populations identified by age, race, ethnicity, culture, nativity, or geographic locality. In addition, participatory action cluster randomized controlled trials of women's group interventions should be extended to additional low-resource, rural settings in sub-Saharan Africa and Latin America, as existing studies have primarily been conducted in Asia.

The infant mortality rate, an estimate of the number of infant deaths for every 1,000 live births, has long been recognized as a key indicator of the health and well-being of a nation or community. There is substantial international variation in infant mortality rates. In developed countries, infant mortality rates declined rapidly during the 1970s due to medical advances such as neonatal intensive care units for premature or seriously ill newborn infants.

About 98% of the almost 4 million deaths that occur each year among newborns during the first month of life occur in developing countries.[1] The highest neonatal mortality rates occur in sub-Saharan Africa followed by Asia and Latin America.[2]

In countries that have the highest rates, almost 10% of infants die within the first month. Globally, most deaths of infants and children under the age of 5 occur at home, without any contact with the formal health system.[3] Several factors contribute to high newborn mortality, including poverty, poor maternal reproductive health and nutrition, HIV/AIDS, infections (e.g., bacterial sepsis), low-quality delivery or antenatal care, lack of skilled attendance at birth, and lack of postnatal care.[4] In regions such as sub-Saharan Africa, most births occur at home due to the inaccessibility or absence of care.

Countries with the lowest infant mortality rates include developed countries such as Iceland, Sweden, Finland, Japan, Greece, Norway, and the Czech Republic (2.5–2.8 per 1,000 live births). In 2011, the United States had a higher infant mortality rate (6.6 per 1,000 live births) than 27 other countries. Despite the frequent provision of risk-appropriate care (i.e., level III facilities) in the United States, preterm births are a major contributor to the country's poor international ranking among developed countries. Substantial variation in infant mortality rates also occur within countries. In the United States, for example, the highest rates occur in Mississippi and Alabama.[5] More than 50% of infant deaths occur among infants with gestation of 32 weeks or less.

The most prevalent causes of infant mortality include birth defects, preterm birth (i.e., birth before 37 weeks gestation), low birth weight, maternal complications of pregnancy, infection, sudden infant death syndrome (SIDS), and unintentional injuries such as suffocation. Lack of access to appropriate healthcare is also a risk factor for infant mortality, especially during the neonatal period (< 28 days). Other risk factors for infant mortality identified in epidemiologic studies include lower socioeconomic status, lower educational attainment, and decreased access to prenatal care or underutilization of prenatal care services. Preventable causes of preterm birth and low birth weight include maternal smoking and illicit drug use. Maternal stress and racism may also contribute to poor birth outcomes.[6,7] In the United States, the infant mortality rate among African Americans is over twice the rate for Whites. The infant mortality rate is also higher among American Indians and Alaska Natives than for Whites.[8] Research conducted in developing countries has shown that intense indoor air pollution from cooking in poorly ventilated homes is associated with neonatal death.[9]

Prevention of Infant Mortality

In developed countries such as the United States, national strategies for reducing infant mortality include the use of caesarian sections and avoidance of elective deliveries at less than 39 weeks gestation, the use of regional neonatal intensive care units (e.g., Level III facilities), SIDS risk reduction, preconception and interconception care, reducing teenage pregnancy, and smoking cessation during pregnancy. It is advantageous for all women of reproductive age to adopt healthy behaviors such as maintaining a healthy diet and weight, quitting tobacco use, not drinking excessive amounts of alcohol, avoiding use of illicit drugs, and visiting a healthcare provider at recommended scheduled time periods.[10] Folic acid supplementation has a significant protective effect on neural tube defects.[11] Preventing intimate partner violence (IPV) is also relevant, as IPV against women has adverse effects on the fetus/newborn, including growth retardation, and can result in perinatal death.[12] As noted by the Centers for Disease Control and Prevention, a healthy pregnancy begins before conception and continues with appropriate prenatal care.

In developing countries, several measures for preventing infant mortality have been recommended, including the initiation of exclusive breastfeeding, hypothermia prevention and management, kangaroo mother care (skin-to-skin contact between the baby's front and the mother's chest), pneumonia management, and resuscitation.[13] For neonatal survival, a principal factor is the recognition of danger signs (e.g., a high fever) during pregnancy and the neonatal period, and the knowledge and timely decision to seek care when needed, particularly in high-mortality settings.[14] This has led to interventions aimed at improving knowledge and attitudes at the community level.

The benefits of medical interventions are greatest when there is a continuum of care through prepregnancy, pregnancy, childbirth, and the postpartum period. Maternal reproductive health and nutrition are necessary for perinatal health.[2] Care during childbirth is also essential. Antenatal care provides a means to address other healthcare needs, such as immunization against tetanus, family planning, and the prevention and treatment of HIV infection, other sexually transmitted infections, and malaria.[2] Compared to births spaced 9 to 14 months apart, children born 36 to 41 months after their next oldest sibling have a lower risk of neonatal death. There is also a lower risk of maternal death, third trimester bleeding, premature rupture of the membranes, puerperal endometritis, and anemia.[2]

The Role of CBPR in Addressing Infant Mortality

Community interventions for addressing infant mortality often involve academic–community partnerships. Community-based participatory research involves the engagement and collaboration of academic and community members on multiple aspects of research to design a more relevant and often more effective intervention. Evidence-based approaches for reducing adverse birth outcomes require developing and evaluating interventions that are culturally appropriate and tailored to the demographic and socioeconomic characteristics of the target population.

Table 10.1 summarizes CBPR studies conducted in the United States that addressed infant mortality and closely related maternal and newborn health topics (e.g., smoking during pregnancy) that had a randomized controlled trial, quasi-experimental, or pre/post test design. The studies shown were identified using PubMed with relevant search terms. Articles published in English through January 31, 2016, were identified using the following MeSH search terms and Boolean algebra commands: (((community-based participatory research) OR (action research)) AND (infant mortality)). Although the search criteria did not specify a begin date, the earliest article that met the search criteria was published in 2004. The searches were not limited to words appearing in the titles of articles. Information obtained from bibliographic searches (title and topic of article, information in abstract, geographic locality of a study, and key words) was used to determine whether to retain each article. The references in reports and review articles were also reviewed. A total of 47 citations were found. After screening the abstracts or full texts of these articles, six US CBPR studies on infant mortality or closely related maternal and newborn health topics that met the search criteria were identified (Table 10.1). The excluded citations included CBPR studies on infant mortality that involved focus groups or in-depth interviews of key informants but which did not evaluate the effectiveness of a prevention program using a randomized controlled trial, quasi-experimental, or pre/post test design.

Discussion

The studies summarized in Table 10.1 illustrate the flexibility and generality of the CBPR approach in diverse communities. A variety of study designs and intervention strategies were used by the researchers to address infant mortality or closely related health concerns in at-risk communities. The interventions included case management services for high-risk women, home visits by paraprofessional personnel, family planning, prevention of teen pregnancy (which is associated with preterm birth and other adverse reproductive outcomes), smoking cessation programs for pregnant women, and educational interventions to increase awareness of infant safety and risk behaviors and to improve adolescents' knowledge of preconception health. A common consideration in these studies was the engagement of members of the target communities to ensure that the interventions were culturally appropriate and met the concerns of community members. Several additional evaluative studies of infant mortality conducted in the United States and other countries have used qualitative methods such as focus groups and in-depth interviews of key informants.

In addition to the CBPR studies listed in Table 10.1, nine "participatory action" cluster randomized controlled trials have been conducted in developing countries in Asia and Africa to improve maternal and newborn health.[21-29] At least three more similar trials have been initiated.[4,14,30] All of the studies conducted

Table 10.1 **CBPR Studies on Infant Mortality Conducted in the United States with a Randomized Controlled Trial, Quasi-Experimental, or Pre/Post Test Design**

Citation	Study Population	Study Design	Results	Comments
Chao et al.[15]	African American residents of Antelope Valley, Los Angeles County, CA	1) Data and assessment (using 2002 vital records to identify areas with the highest rates of feto-infant mortality); 2) implementing infant mortality review and the Los Angeles Mommy and Baby (LAMB) Project (with a case-control design) to identify potential factors associated with adverse birth outcomes; and 3) developing strategic actions for targeted prevention.	In response to findings from the LAMB Project, community stakeholders gathered to develop strategic actions to address infant mortality. Resources were infused into the community, resulting in expanded case management of high-risk women, increased family-planning services, better training for nurses, and public health initiatives to increase awareness of infant safety and risk behaviors. A preconception health curriculum and brochure was developed for African American women. In addition, faith leaders incorporated health education within faith-based youth services. Between 2002 and 2003, the infant mortality rate dropped significantly, from 32.7 deaths to 16 deaths per 1,000 live births.	Perinatal periods of risk methods were used to mobilize the community
Javier et al.[16]	Filipino American parents (n = 25) and adolescents (n = 35) in San Jose, CA, who attended a culturally tailored conference on teen pregnancy	Pre/post-test comparisons of survey data collected before and after the conference	Filipino youth reported feeling uneasy in discussing their concerns about sex with parents. Both parents and youth reported that teen pregnancy was a problem in the Filipino community and that the factual content of the conference was helpful. After the conference, most of the parents who were surveyed (70%) talked with their adolescents about sex.	The conference was a partnership between the Filipino Youth Coalition, a community-based organization, and the Stanford School of Medicine Pediatric Advocacy Program

(continued)

Table 10.1 Continued

Citation	Study Population	Study Design	Results	Comments
English et al.[17]	Low-income, African American and Hispanic pregnant women in New York City and Long Island, NY	Pre/post-test evaluation of a lay health advisor-delivered perinatal tobacco cessation program	Five of the 46 clients (11%) who reported tobacco use at intake quit smoking during their enrollment in the program. Moreover, 7 additional clients reported a reduction in tobacco use by an average of 10 cigarettes per day. However, 4 clients who reported being former smokers at intake relapsed to smoking during the study period.	
Salihu et al.[18]	Residents of 8 Florida counties with high rates of infant mortality among African Americans	Pre/post-test evaluation of the Black Infant Health Community Collaborative (BIHCC) Leadership Conference in Florida	When asked how the BIHCC Leadership Conference compared with other conferences of its type, 90.6% of respondents indicated very good or better, and 100% indicated that they would recommend the conference to others. All of the respondents agreed or strongly agreed that the conference was well organized and that the sessions were appropriate and informative. All respondents reported that the conference provided them with new ideas that may be tailored to their local communities, and that they feel prepared to take action to address the problem of Black infant mortality, to analyze the problem, and to plan solutions.	CBPR was used as the guiding framework for the academic–community collaboration

| Richards & Mousseau[19] | Northern Plains American Indian female high school students ($n = 77$). | Cluster randomized controlled trial that examined the effectiveness of a culturally appropriate, 15-session, preconception health educational intervention developed by tribal community members and elders. | Postintervention scores were higher in the intervention group than the nonintervention group in overall knowledge of preconception health and obesity. | CBPR principles were followed. A tribal working group (comprising 12 individuals from the tribal health and human services committee, Indian Health Services midwifery department, tribal home visiting program, parent council, family and child education program, tribal health education, school administration, cultural instructors, tribal court, and domestic violence prevention workers) met quarterly to review all media messages, manuscripts, survey instruments, and other areas of project implementation. |

(continued)

Table 10.1 Continued

Citation	Study Population	Study Design	Results	Comments
Barlow et al.[20]	Expectant American Indian teens (n = 322, mean age 18.1 yrs) from 4 southwestern reservation communities	Randomized controlled trial of a paraprofessional-delivered home-visiting intervention consisting of 43 one-on-one structured lessons with a culturally congruent format. Each home visit lasting ≤ 1 hour occurred weekly through the third trimester of pregnancy, biweekly until 4 months postpartum, monthly between 4 and 12 months postpartum, and bimonthly between 12 and 36 months postpartum. The participants were randomized to receive either the Family Spirit Intervention plus optimized standard care or optimized standard care alone. Optimized standard care consisted of transportation to recommended prenatal and well-baby clinic visits, pamphlets about child care and community resources, and referrals to local services.	From pregnancy to 36 months, mothers in the intervention group had significantly greater parenting knowledge and parental locus of control and lower past-month use of marijuana (odds ratio [OR] = 0.65) and illegal drugs (OR = 0.67). Children in the intervention group had fewer externalizing, internalizing, and dysregulation problems.	The Family Spirit Intervention was developed over a decade through CBPR.

in low-resource settings are trials in which women from the target communities assisted with delivering the interventions.[31] The trials involved participatory action (also referred to as participatory learning and action), which shares some features with CBPR (i.e., the studies were community-placed and included the involvement of women's group members or lay health advisors).

Participatory learning and action is an approach for learning about and engaging with communities and is intended to facilitate a process of collective analysis and learning.[32] The approach can be used in identifying needs, planning projects and programs, and monitoring or evaluating them. Like CBPR, it promotes the participation of communities in issues and interventions affecting their lives. The participatory learning and action approach has been used mostly with rural communities in the developing world, where it has been found to be useful for understanding the perspectives of the rural poor, helping to discover their ideas about the nature and causes of the issues that affect them, and considering potential solutions.[32] It enables local people to share their perceptions and to identify, prioritize, and appraise issues from their knowledge of local conditions. Conventional studies by academic researchers tend to consult with communities and then take away the findings for analysis, with no assurance that they will be acted on. In contrast, participatory learning and action provides a catalyst for the community to act on what is learned.[32]

Although the trials conducted in low-resource settings do not include all of the elements of CBPR (e.g., the use of a community advisory committee or the participation of members of the target community in the design of the study, data analysis, and dissemination of the findings), the findings from these studies hold promise for reducing infant mortality and improving maternal and newborn health in low-resource settings, which warrants their discussion here.

In Nepal, Manandhar et al.[21] conducted a cluster randomized trial that showed a 30% reduction in risk of neonatal death over a 2-year period (OR = 0.70). The intervention was based on participation in women's groups, in which a facilitator encouraged the participants to identify perinatal health problems in their own environment. The participants were provided with information about childbirth and care of newborns, which led to positive changes in behaviors. Similar trials have been conducted in Bangladesh, India, Malawi, and Nigeria.[23-29] In addition, a trial in rural Sindh in southern Pakistan combined meetings with trained lay health workers and home visits by traditional birth attendants (*Dais*), who also received training.[24] A meta-analysis conducted by Prost et al.[31] included seven of the trials undertaken in rural, low-resource settings in Bangladesh, India, Malawi, and Nepal, in which the effects of women's groups practicing learning and action on neonatal and maternal mortality were assessed. The meta-analysis showed that exposure to women's groups was associated with a 23% reduction in neonatal mortality (OR = 0.77, 95% confidence interval [CI] 0.65, 0.90) and a 37% reduction in maternal mortality (OR = 0.63, 95% CI 0.32, 0.94). These results, which may not be generalizable to urban settings, compare favorably with those of other trials in which trained birth attendants provided antenatal and intrapartum home visits (relative risk = 0.70, 95% CI 0.51, 0.96).[33]

Conclusion

Additional CBPR studies are needed that have the potential to fill in gaps in the current evidence about what intervention strategies are effective in reducing infant mortality in population subgroups that are disproportionately affected by it. This includes dissemination and implementation research and studies that translate evidence-based interventions to new populations identified by age, race, ethnicity, culture, nativity, or geographic locality. Of particular interest are CBPR studies that include multicomponent intervention approaches aimed at different levels of the socioecological model. In addition, participatory action, cluster randomized controlled trials of women's group interventions should be extended to additional low-resource, rural settings in sub-Saharan Africa and Latin America, as existing studies have primarily been conducted in Asia.

References

1. Rajaratnam, J.K., Marcus, J.R., Flaxman, A.D., et al. "Neonatal, Postneonatal, Childhood, and Under-5 Mortality in 187 Countries, 1970–2010: A Systematic Analysis of Progress Towards Millennium Development Goal 4." *Lancet* 375 (2010): 1988–2008.
2. Bhutta, Z.A., Soofi, S., Cousens, S., et al. "Improvement of Perinatal and Newborn Care in Rural Pakistan Through Community-Based Strategies: A Cluster-Randomized Effectiveness Trial." *Lancet* 377 (2011): 403–12.
3. United Nations Children's Fund. *The State of the World's Children-Special Edition: Celebrating 20 Years of the Convention on the Rights of a Child.* New York: UNICEF, 2010.
4. Waiswa, P., Peterson, S.S., Namazzi, G., et al. "The Uganda Newborn Study (UNEST): An Effectiveness Study on Improving Newborn Health and Survival in Rural Uganda Through a Community-Based Intervention Linked to Health Facilities—Study Protocol for a Cluster Randomized Controlled Trial." *Trials* 13 (2012): 213. <http://www.trialsjournal.com/content/13/1/213>
5. Mathews, T.J., MacDorman, M.F. and Thoma, M.E. "Infant Mortality Statistics from the 2013 Period Linked Birth/Infant Death Data Set." *National Vital Statistics Reports* 64 (2015). <http://www.cdc.gov/nchs/data/nvsr/nvsr64/nvsr64_09.pdf>
6. Carty, D.C., Kruger, D.J., Turner, T.M., et al. "Racism, Health Status, and Birth Outcomes: Results of a Participatory Community-Based Intervention and Health Survey." *Journal of Urban Health* 88 (2011): 84–97.
7. Oyana, T.J., Matthews-Juarez, P., Cormier, S.A., et al. "Using an External Exposome Framework to Examine Pregnancy-Related Morbidities and Mortalities: Implications for Health Disparities Research." *International Journal of Environmental Research and Public Health* 13 (2016): 13. <http://www.mdpi.com/1660-4601/13/1/13>
8. MacDorman, M.F. and Mathews, T.J. *Understanding Racial and Ethnic Disparities in U.S. Infant Mortality Rates.* NCHS Data Brief no. 74. Centers for Disease Control and Prevention, National Center for Health Statistics, 2011.
9. Mavalankar, D., Trivedi, C. and Gray, R. "Levels and Risk Factors for Perinatal Mortality in Ahmedabad, India." *Bulletin of the World Health Organization* 69 (1991): 435–42.

10. Centers for Disease Control and Prevention. "Infant Mortality." <http://www.cdc.gov/repro-ductivehealth/MaternalInfantHealth/InfantMortality.htm>

11. Lumley, J., Watson, L., Watson, M., et al. "Periconceptual Supplementation with Folate and/or Multivitamins for Preventing Neural Tube Defects." *Cochrane Database of Systematic Reviews* 3 (2001): CD001056.

12. Coker, A.L., Sanderson, M. and Dong, B. "Partner Violence During Pregnancy and Risk of Adverse Pregnancy Outcomes." *Paediatric and Perinatal Epidemiology* 18 (2004): 260–9.

13. Darnstadt, G.L., Bhutta, Z.A., Cousens, S., et al. "Evidence-Based, Cost-Effective Interventions: How Many Newborn Babies Can We Save?" *Lancet* 365 (2005): 977–88.

14. Wallin, L., Malqvist, M., Nga, N.T., et al. "Implementing Knowledge into Practice for Improved Neonatal Survival: A Cluster-Randomized, Community-Based Trial in Quang Ninh Province, Vietnam." *BMC Health Services Research* 11 (2011): 239. <http://www.biomedcentral.com/1472-6963/11/239>

15. Chao, S.M., Donatoni, G., Bemis, C., et al. "Integrated Approaches to Improve Birth Outcomes: Perinatal Periods of Risk, Infant Mortality Review, and the Los Angeles Mommy and Baby Project." *Maternal and Child Health Journal* 14 (2010): 827–37.

16. Javier, J.R., Chamberlain, L.J., Rivera, K.K., et al. "Lessons Learned from a Community-Academic Partnership Addressing Adolescent Pregnancy Prevention in Filipino American Families." *Progress in Community Health Partnerships* 4 (2010): 305–13.

17. English, K.C., Merzel, C. and Moon-Howard, J. "Translating Public Health Knowledge into Practice: Development of a Lay Health Advisor Perinatal Tobacco Cessation Program." *Journal of Public Health Management and Practice* 16 (2010): E9–19.

18. Salihu, H.M., August, E.M., Alio, A.P., et al. "Community-Academic Partnerships to Reduce Black-White Disparities in Infant Mortality in Florida." *Progress in Community Health Partnerships* 5 (2011): 53–66.

19. Richards, J. and Mousseau, A. "Community-Based Participatory Research to Improve Preconception Health Among North Plains American Indian Adolescent Women." *American Indian Alaska and Native Mental Health Research* 19 (2012): 154–85.

20. Barlow, A., Mullany, B., Neault, N., et al. "Paraprofessional-Delivered Home-Visiting Intervention for American Indian Teen Mothers and Children: 3-Year Outcomes from a Randomized Controlled Trial." *American Journal of Psychiatry* 172 (2015): 154–62.

21. Manandhar, D.S., Osrin, D., Shrestha, B.P., et al. "Effect of a Participatory Intervention with Women's Groups on Birth Outcomes in Nepal: Cluster-Randomised Controlled Trial. *Lancet* 364 (2004): 970–9.

22. Azad, K., Barnett, S., Banerjee, B., et al. "Effect of Scaling Up Women's Groups on Birth Outcomes in Three Rural Districts in Bangladesh: A Cluster-Randomised Controlled Trial." *Lancet* 375 (2010): 1193–1202.

23. Tripathy, P., Nair, N., Barnett, S., et al. "Effect of a Participatory Intervention with Women's Groups on Birth Outcomes and Maternal Depression in Jharkhand and Orissa, India: A Cluster-Randomised Controlled Trial." *Lancet* 375 (2010): 1182–92.

24. Bhutta, Z.A., Lassi, Z.S., Blanc, A. and Donnay, F. "Linkages Among Reproductive Health, Maternal Health, and Perinatal Outcomes." *Seminars in Perinatology* 34 (2010): 434–45.

25. More, N.S., Bapat, U., Das, S., et al. "Community Mobilization in Mumbai Slums to Improve Perinatal Care and Outcomes: A Cluster Randomized Controlled Trial." *PLoS Medicine* 9 (2012): e1001257.

26. Lewycka, S., Mwansambo, C., Rosato, M., et al. "Effect of Women's Groups and Volunteer Peer Counselling on Rates of Mortality, Morbidity, and Health Behaviours in Mothers and Children in Rural Malawi (MaiMwana): A Factorial, Cluster-Randomised Controlled Trial." *Lancet* 381 (2013): 1721–35.

27. Findley, S.E., Uwemedimo, O.T., Doctor, H.V., et al. "Early Results of an Integrated Maternal, Newborn, and Child Health Program, Northern Nigeria, 2009 to 2011." *BMC Public Health* 13 (2013): 1034 <http://www.biomedcentral.com/1471-2458/13/1034>

28. Fottrell, E., Azad, K., Kuddus, A., et al. "The Effect of Increased Coverage of Participatory Women's Groups on Neonatal Mortality in Bangladesh: A Cluster Randomized Trial." *JAMA Pediatrics* 167 (2013): 816–25.

29. Colbourn, T., Nambiar, B., Bondo, A., et al. "Effects of Quality Improvement in Health Facilities and Community Mobilization Through Women's Groups on Maternal, Neonatal and Perinatal Mortality in Three Districts of Malawi: MaiKhanda, a Cluster Randomized Controlled Effectiveness Trial." *International Health* 5 (2013): 180–95.

30. Shrestha, B., Bhandari, B., Manandhar, D.S., et al. "Community Interventions to Reduce Child Mortality in Dhanusha, Nepal: Study Protocol for a Cluster Randomized Controlled Trial." *Trials* 12 (2011): 136. <http://www.trialsjournal.com/content/12/1/136>

31. Prost, A., Colbourn, T., Seward, N., et al. "Women's Groups Practising Participatory Learning and Action to Improve Maternal and Newborn Health in Low-Resource Settings: A Systematic Review and Meta-Analysis." *Lancet* 381 (2013): 1736–46.

32. Thomas, S. "What Is Participatory Learning and Action (PLA): An Introduction." University of Wolverhampton, Centre for International Development and Training. <http://idp-key-resources.org/documents/0000/d04267/000.pdf>

33. Lassi, Z.S., Haider, B.A. and Bhutta, Z.A. "Community-Based Intervention Packages for Reducing Maternal and Neonatal Morbidity and Mortality and Improving Neonatal Outcomes." *Cochrane Database of Systematic Reviews* 11 (2010): CD007754.

11

Colorectal Cancer Disparities and Community-Based Participatory Research

SELINA A. SMITH, PHD, MDIV, BENJAMIN E. ANSA, MD, MSCR,

AND DANIEL S. BLUMENTHAL, MD, MPH

Introduction

Colorectal cancer is the second-leading cause of cancer-related death in the United States and is responsible for approximately 50,000 deaths every year. Yet the majority of these deaths are preventable. Colorectal cancer incidence can be reduced through dietary modification, and screening with colonoscopy can reduce mortality by over 50%.[1] However, unhealthy dietary practices and widespread lack of screening persist. Improved community-based approaches are needed to alter these facts.

Cancer of the Colon and Rectum

The colon, or large intestine, is typically about 150 centimeters (60 inches) long in an adult; its terminal segment is the rectum. Its course through the abdomen is shown in Figure 11.1.

Its primary function is to absorb water from the digested food that passes through it. Cancer most commonly develops from adenomatous polyps that arise from the glands in the colon's lining, the mucosa (Figure 11.2). These cancers are known as adenocarcinomas. Their prognosis depends on the stage at which they are diagnosed. A cancer that is limited to the mucosa is classified as Stage 0. If it has penetrated the submucosa it is Stage I; if it has penetrated the muscle layer it is Stage II. Once the cancer has penetrated the serosa—the outer surface of the colon—it is classified as Stage III. At this stage, it may be found in lymph nodes that lie near the colon. Cancers that have spread (metastasized) to distant organs are classified as Stage IV.

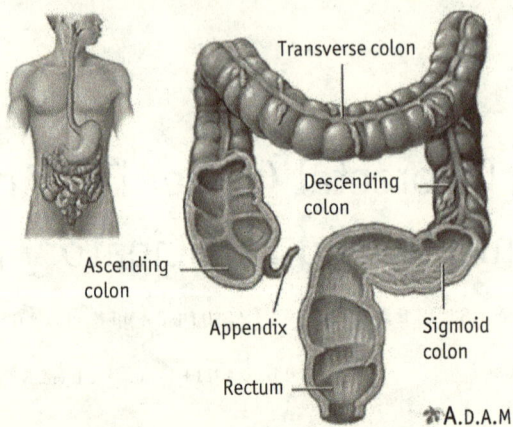

Figure 11.1 Diagram of the colon and rectum.

Common symptoms of colorectal cancer include bloody stools, gross blood passed through the anus, abdominal pain, weight loss, diarrhea, or constipation. Stage IV cancers may present with symptoms related to the organ to which the cancer has metastasized—for instance, a patient may present with jaundice if the cancer has spread to the liver.

Treatment of a Stage 0 cancer may consist of excision through a colonoscope and no other therapy may be needed. For Stage I and higher cancers, abdominal surgery is indicated, and this may be followed by chemotherapy, particularly for stage IV cancers. The 5-year survival rate for colorectal cancers diagnosed at Stage 0–II is over 90%; for Stage III, over 70%; but for Stage IV, only about 13%.[2]

Colorectal cancer mortality rates may be reduced through primary prevention (reducing or eliminating risk factors or susceptibility) or secondary prevention

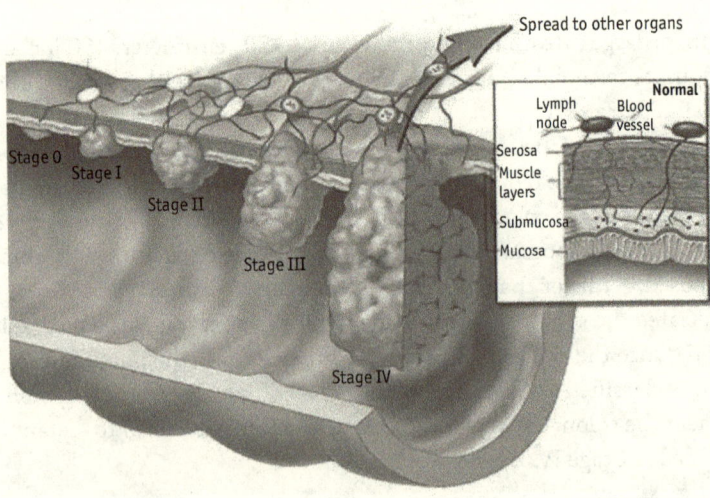

Figure 11.2 Adenomatous polyps.

Box 11.1 **Colorectal Cancer Screening Schedule
(American Cancer Society)**

TESTS THAT FIND POLYPS AND CANCER

- Flexible sigmoidoscopy every 5 years*
- Colonoscopy every 10 years
- Double-contrast barium enema every 5 years*
- CT colonography (virtual colonoscopy) every 5 years*

TESTS THAT MAINLY FIND CANCER

- Guaiac-based fecal occult blood test (gFOBT) every year*,**
- Fecal immunochemical test (FIT) every year*,**
- Stool DNA test (sDNA) every 3 years*

---

* If the test is positive, a colonoscopy should be done.

** The multiple stool take-home test should be used. One test done in the office is not enough. A colonoscopy should be done if the test is positive.

(screening—that is, early detection of presymptomatic cancer). Primary prevention of colorectal cancer can be achieved by improving diet (see risk factors, below), increasing physical activity, controlling weight, eliminating tobacco use, and moderating alcohol consumption. Screening modalities include fecal occult blood testing, fecal immunochemical testing, fecal DNA testing, or endoscopy (sigmoidoscopy or colonoscopy). Endoscopy can also achieve primary prevention by identifying and removing adenomatous polyps before they become cancerous; in fact, the majority of lesions found and removed during endoscopy are polyps rather than cancers. The screening schedules generally recommended are shown in Box 11.1.

EPIDEMIOLOGY

About 9% of cancers in both men and women are cancers of the colon or rectum. Colorectal cancer represents about 8% of cancer-related deaths in men (ranking third, behind lung and prostate cancer) and 9% of cancer-related deaths in women (ranking third, behind lung and breast cancer). Since prostate cancer does not occur in women and breast cancer is rare in men, colorectal cancer is overall the second-leading cause of cancer-related death.

Risk factors for colorectal cancer[3] include:

- Age: Approximately 90% of colorectal cancers occur in individuals over the age of 50.
- Inflammatory bowel disease: The relative risk of contracting colorectal cancer in persons with Crohn's disease or ulcerative colitis is between 4- and 20-fold.

- Family history of colorectal cancer: Persons with one first-degree relative with a history of the disease have about double the relative risk of contracting colorectal cancer; for persons with more than one such relative, the relative risk is about four-fold. This increased risk may be due to genetic factors, environmental factors, or some combination of these.
- Specific genetic conditions: hereditary conditions for which specific genes have been identified include familial adenomatous polyposis (FAP) and hereditary nonpolyposis colorectal cancer (HNPCC), also called Lynch syndrome. The colorectal cancer risk for persons with these conditions may approach 80%.
- Adenomatous polyps identified during screening endoscopy.
- Tobacco: about 12% of colorectal cancers are thought to be due to smoking.
- Alcohol: this is particularly a risk factor associated with the development of colorectal cancer at a younger age.
- Diet: diets high in red meat, processed meat, and animal fat and low in fiber are thought to be at least partially responsible for up to 70% of colorectal cancers.
- Lack of physical activity and obesity: these interrelated factors may be at least partially responsible for a third to a fourth of colorectal cancers.

In the United States, the age-adjusted incidence rate for colorectal cancer in men is about 54/100,000; the mortality rate is about 20/100,000. For women, the incidence rate is about 40/100,000 and the mortality rate is about 14/100,000. Both the incidence rates and mortality rates for colorectal cancer have been declining (Figure 11.3); for women, the decrease actually started in the 1940s. At least some of the decrease is likely due to screening. With most cancers, increased screening (secondary prevention) would be expected to lead to an increase in incidence and, in fact, a transient increase in colorectal cancer incidence can be seen in the mid-1990s; but, as noted earlier, endoscopy leads to primary prevention when adenomatous polyps are removed, and more polyps than cancers are found on endoscopy.

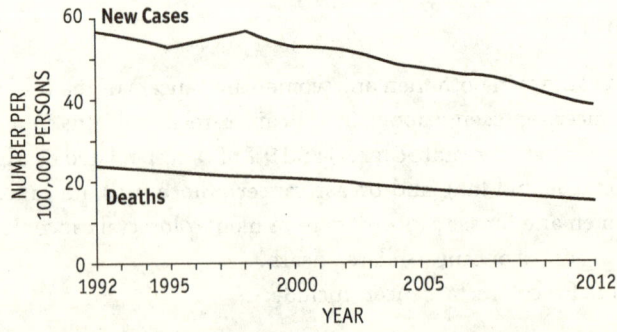

Figure 11.3 Colorectal incidence and mortality rates in the United States. National Cancer Institute. <http://seer.cancer.gov/statfacts/html/colorect.html>

Table 11.1 **Colorectal Cancer Incidence Rates: New Cases/100,00 Population, Age-Adjusted, by Race and Ethnic Group. SEER, 2008–2012**

Race/Ethnicity	Male	Female
All Races	48.9	37.1
White	47.8	36.3
Black	61.2	46.0
Asian	42.2	31.3
Native American	46.3	35.7
Hispanic	43.3	30.0
Non-Hispanic	49.7	38.1

Like most other cancers (and most other major causes of death), colorectal cancer exhibits a significant racial disparity, with African Americans bearing the heaviest burden of disease. This is exhibited in Tables 11.1 and 11.2.[2]

Historically, Black-White disparities have not always been present. As seen in Figure 11.4, until the 1980s, colorectal cancer incidence and mortality rates were similar in Blacks and Whites (incidence and mortality rates for Asians, Native Americans, and Hispanics were not routinely collected until the 1990s; generally, they were previously lumped together as "other"). For the last 30 or so years, incidence and mortality disparities between African Americans and other population groups have been widening.[4]

Additional evidence regarding the causes of racial/ethnic disparities in colorectal cancer incidence can be gathered by examining international rates of the disease.[5] The highest rates are found in Australia, New Zealand, and Western Europe, while the lowest rates are found in sub-Saharan Africa—the opposite of what one would expect if the Black-White disparities in the United States were based on genetic inheritance.

Table 11.2 **Colorectal Cancer Mortality Rates: Deaths/100,00 Population, Age-Adjusted, by Race and Ethnic Group. SEER, 2008–2012**

Race/Ethnicity	Male	Female
All Races	18.6	13.1
White	18.0	12.7
Black	26.9	17.8
Asian	13.0	9.4
Native American	18.8	15.6
Hispanic	15.6	9.6
Non-Hispanic	18.9	13.4

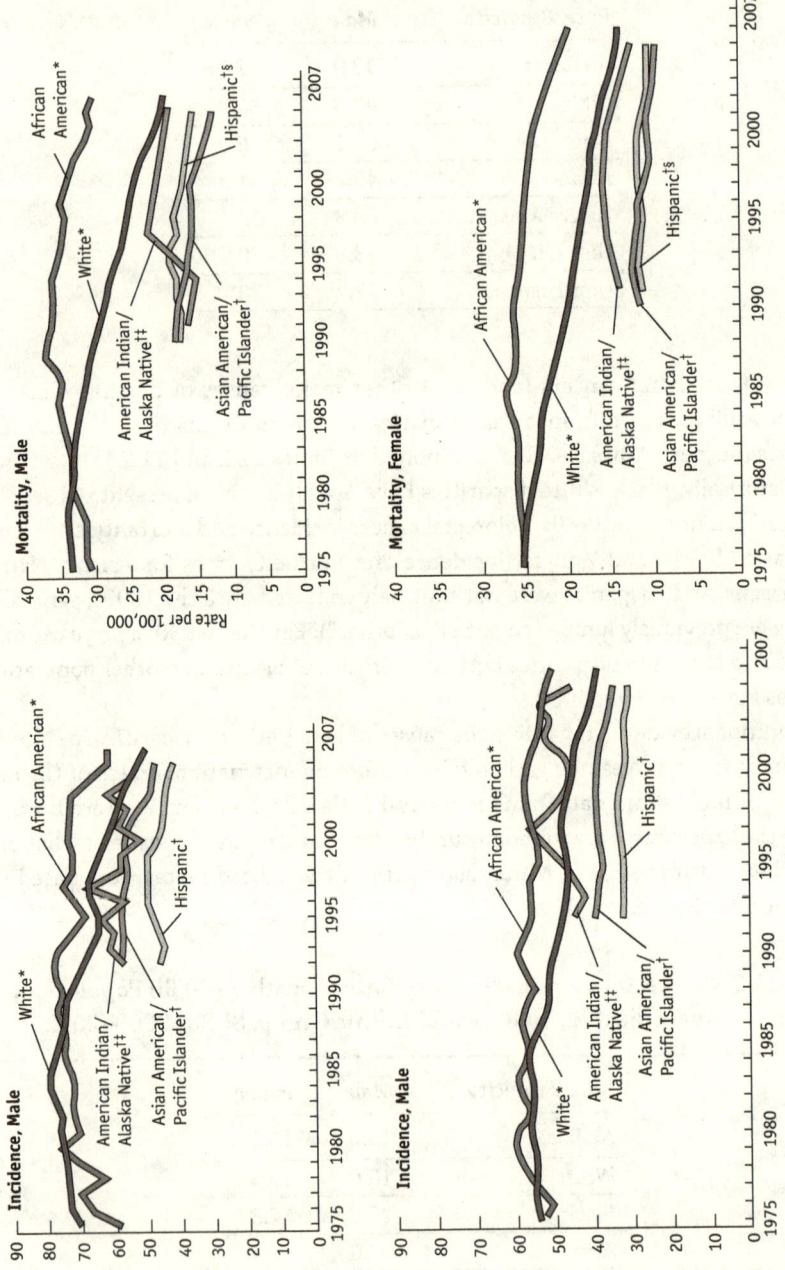

Figure 11.4 Colorectal cancer disparities.

Table 11.3 **Educational Attainment and Colorectal Cancer Incidence**

	# of Participants (Colorectal Cancer Cases)	Incidence/10,000 Person-Years
Postgraduate	103,164 (1305)	13.2
College degree	98,292 (1408)	15.0
Some college	120,507 (1815)	15.9
Posthigh school	51,612 (857)	17.6
High school	101,580 (1681)	17.5
<12 years	31,333 (610)	21.2

To what cause or causes, then, can we attribute the disparities? The possibilities include:

Lifestyle behaviors: African American diets have been found in some studies to be associated with a higher risk of colorectal cancer compared with Africans[6] as well as with White Americans.[7] Physical activity is associated with reduced risk of colorectal cancer and sedentary behavior with increased risk.[8]

Screening: The CDC's Behavioral Risk Factor Surveillance System (BRFSS) indicates that African Americans are more likely than Whites to be screened by the less-sensitive and less-specific fecal occult blood test, while Whites are more likely to be screened by endoscopy. According to BRFSS figures, only about two-thirds of age-eligible individuals of either race have been screened, and the percentage who have been screened according to recommended schedules is probably lower, since the BRFSS survey asks about fecal occult blood test in the last 2 years (rather than 1 year, as recommended) and asks only about whether the respondent has ever had endoscopy screening.[9]

Diagnosis and treatment: numerous studies have documented that African Americans are less likely than Whites to receive timely, state-of-the-art diagnostic studies and treatment for many diseases, colorectal cancer among them.[10]

Social determinants: Factors such as income, education, housing, and social class are the most powerful predictors of health status. As an example, colorectal cancer incidence is inversely related to educational attainment (Table 11.3).[11]

Community-Based Participation

Community-engaged approaches hold promise for addressing racial/ethnic disparities in colorectal cancer screening, incidence, and mortality.[12–14] As described elsewhere in this book, community-based participatory research (CBPR), a partnership approach equitably involving community members, organizational representatives, and investigators in the research process,[15] promotes ownership of colorectal cancer disparities by the community, which in turn influence solutions to this problem. Unlike traditional research, CBPR elicits participation of community members in each research component, including identifying the health concern, designing the study, seeking funding, recruiting and retaining study participants, developing data collection instruments, designing and implementing interventions, and disseminating results (Figure 11.5).

Prior to engaging a community in a CBPR approach to colorectal cancer disparities, investigators must learn the structure, demography, and interactions within segments of a community (community ecology); establish an alliance for combined action (community coalition); and undergo a systematic process for determining difference between current conditions and desired outcomes (needs assessment).

LEARNING THE COMMUNITY ECOLOGY

Communities comprise various populations and organizations interacting on multiple planes. In an ecological framework, individuals are connected at intrapersonal (micro), interpersonal (meso), and institutional (macro) levels. In assessing a community's ecology, the focus is on the context of individual and interpersonal health behavior related to social and psychological influences that consider community and organizational influences. In this framework,[16] environmental influences on health behavior (e.g., dietary intake, physical activity, and screening) related to colorectal cancer incidence, screening, and mortality disparities are addressed on multiple levels:

1. *Individual* identifies personal (e.g., age, education, and income) and behavioral factors that may affect attitudes, beliefs, and behaviors. In the context of colorectal cancer, this refers to dietary preferences and habits, other lifestyle practices, beliefs about cancer, and attitudes toward screening and toward the healthcare system more generally.
2. *Interpersonal* examines closest personal relationships—family members, coworkers, peers, church members—to determine influences on and contributors to behaviors. These personal relationships are likely to have a major impact on lifestyle practices, beliefs about cancer, and attitudes toward screening and the healthcare system.
3. *Organizational* includes settings such as schools, workplaces, and neighborhoods in which relationships occur and identifies characteristics of these settings that may influence behaviors.
4. *Community* considers relationships among organizations, institutions, and informational networks. Locations in the community, built environment, businesses, which may influence norms, including health, economics, and education,

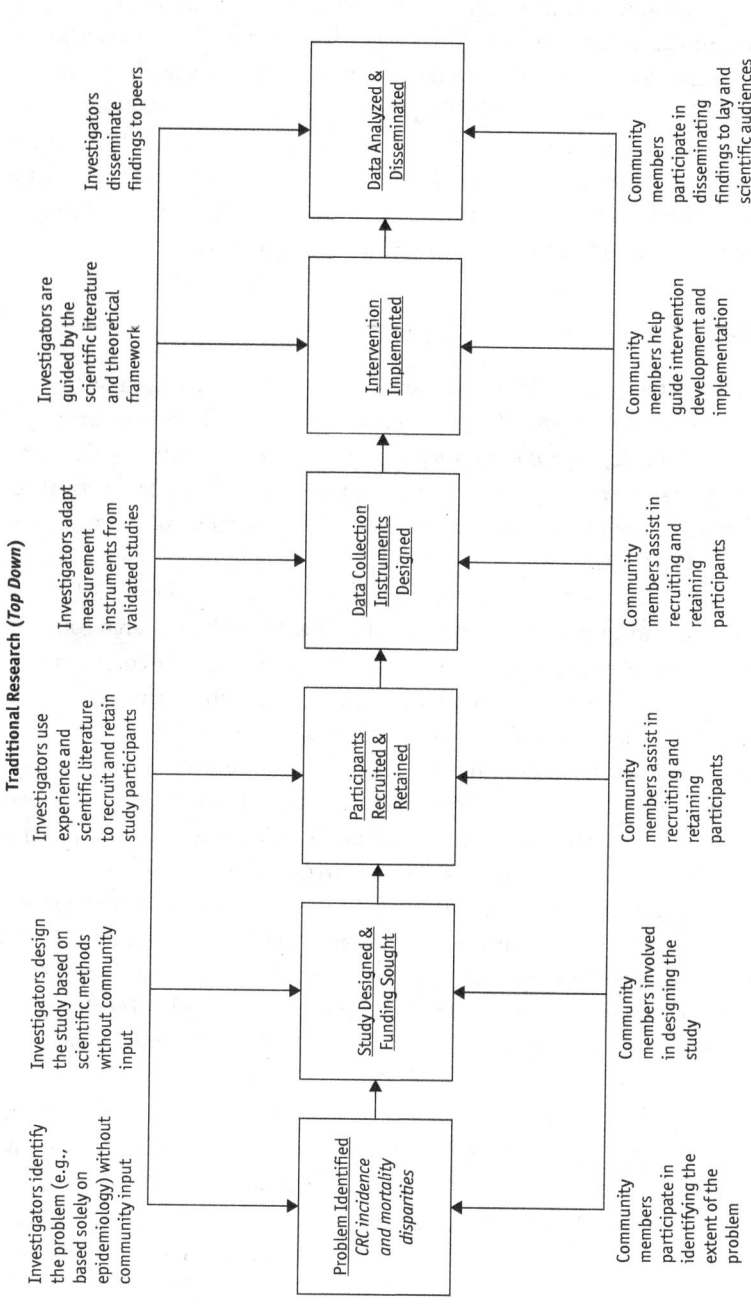

Figure 11.5 Traditional versus community-based approach to CRC disparity research.

are included. It is, in fact, these relationships to which the term "community ecology" usually refers. For instance, many low-income minority communities are located in "food deserts" (areas in which there is an absence of stores that sell healthful foods) and this, more than food preferences or attitudes, may determine diet. Similarly, the presence or absence of healthcare services may be the most important determinant of screening. As noted earlier, social determinants are the most important factors affecting the health status of populations.

5. *Policy* determines community infrastructure and how resources at local, state, and national levels are allocated. For instance, the Centers for Disease Control provides funding to some states (and not others) to establish programs to promote and facilitate colorectal cancer prevention and screening.[17]

ESTABLISHING A COMMUNITY COALITION

This section addresses the challenge of building a community coalition to conduct CBPR on colorectal cancer. The community coalition will be organized by a researcher, an advocate, or a community organizer who understands the community ecology, has earned the trust of the community, and can bring together leaders from the churches, schools, hospitals, public agencies, urban planning committees, and so forth.[18]

But in a sense, this exercise is a contradiction in terms: in a pure CBPR initiative, it is the community, not the researcher, that identifies the research topic. In a low-income African American community, the topic chosen by the community is likely to be a health problem with proximate social roots, such as drug abuse, violence, or sexually transmitted infections. If a chronic disease is chosen, it is likely to be one with a higher incidence rate than colorectal cancer—for instance, high blood pressure or diabetes. But the researcher may have funding from a cancer-oriented agency such as the National Cancer Institute or may be working for a cancer-oriented organization such as the American Cancer Society.

In such a case, a compromise may be called for[19]: The coalition's first project may be one focused on the community's first choice—for instance, an educational initiative to remind people to get their blood pressure checked. The second project may be focused on colorectal cancer; if there is money available for that project, the community coalition will recognize the practical value of moving it up in the queue.

In another model, rather than building a coalition of community leaders from a broad assortment of sectors, the coalition can be built around cancer generally, or colorectal cancer specifically. In this model, the organizer will seek out cancer survivors, friends and relatives of cancer victims, representatives of cancer-focused agencies, and others who are moved for personal reasons to become cancer advocates.

In either case, the needs assessment process becomes one of determining needs around colorectal cancer, rather than health needs generally. Needs assessments are usually conducted by a combination of subjective data and objective data.[20] The former include key informant interviews, focus groups, and surveys. The latter include demographic data (e.g., Census data) and morbidity and mortality data (typically from the Centers for Disease Control, state and local health departments, and cancer registries).

Subjective data will include (at a minimum) information on dietary practices, physical activity, knowledge, attitudes and beliefs about colorectal and other cancers, and attitudes toward screening. Objective data will include colorectal cancer incidence and mortality rates as well as demographic data about the community in which the research is to be conducted.

PLANNING THE PROJECT

The researcher or research team may be challenged to adhere to the CBPR model. The type of project to be conducted may have been dictated by the funding agency, or the researcher may wish to develop a project that is consistent with a particular health promotion theory. But if the health problem to be researched is dictated by noncommunity forces, and the project plan is as well, the project is no longer CBPR.

More appropriately, the research protocol can be developed jointly with the community coalition. Will the focus be primary prevention (e.g., diet, physical activity, colonoscopy) or secondary prevention (e.g., screening by fecal tests and/ or endoscopy)? What type of intervention should be tested (e.g., participant education, provider reminders, reduced out-of-pocket expense)? How will recruitment be conducted? These are the sorts of broad parameters that can be identified by the community coalition, while the details that determine scientific validity can be worked out by the research team. Table 11.4 lists types of interventions to increase colorectal cancer screening that have been reviewed by the Community Preventive Services Task Force, an expert committee supported by the Centers for Disease Control. The Task Force has recommended types of interventions for which there is evidence of effectiveness and has also identified types of interventions for which evidence regarding effectiveness is lacking and for which, therefore, additional research is needed.

If the community coalition favors testing an intervention that is not consistent with the researcher's favorite health promotion theory, (s)he should identify a theory that fits the intervention, rather than insist on an alternative intervention that fits the favored theory.

CONDUCTING THE PROJECT

The participation of community leadership in conducting the project is essential, but cannot be expected unless the community leadership has been treated as an equal partner to this point. Community commitment to the success of the

Table 11.4 **Interventions to Increase Colorectal Cancer Screening**

Client-Oriented Interventions	*Recommendation*
Client Reminders	Recommended July 2010
Client Incentives	Insufficient Evidence July 2010
Small Media	Recommended December 2005
Mass Media	Insufficient Evidence October 2009
Group Education	Insufficient Evidence October 2009
One-on-One Education	Recommended March 2010
Reducing Structural Barriers	Recommended March 2010
Reducing Client Out-of-Pocket Costs	Insufficient Evidence October 2009
Provider-Oriented Interventions	
Provider Assessment and Feedback	Recommended October 2009
Provider Incentives	Insufficient Evidence October 2009
Provider Reminder and Recall Systems	Recommended February 2006

research project is particularly essential in a colorectal cancer project because it is likely that the project will otherwise likely have difficulty recruiting, followed by an excessive rate of attrition. Finding ways to promote colorectal cancer prevention is challenging, and people who are part of a study that aims to do so frequently drop out. Motivating research participants to alter their dietary habits is difficult under the best of circumstances, and more so when they live in a food desert. Equally difficult for participants is increasing leisure-time physical activity when they live in a "fitness center desert." Neither of the options for colorectal cancer screening—undergoing endoscopy or providing fecal smears—is appealing. Hence, unless they are members of a supportive community, people may be reluctant to participate and if they do participate initially, they may soon change their minds.

ANALYZING AND DISSEMINATING THE RESULTS

Community members cannot be expected to conduct or understand sophisticated statistical analyses of results, but they can help explain them. Why, for instance, might one intervention have been successful while others have not?

Similarly, community members may have little interest in having their names as authors on publications in the scientific literature (sometimes they do) but they may have substantial interest in communicating to their friends and neighbors the results of the project in which they have participated. If members of the community coalition are representatives of agencies, neighborhood organizations, churches, or other community institutions, these will be ideal outlets for information about the outcomes of the CBPR project.

FOLLOW-UP

No matter the outcome of the research project, it may be deemed a failure if it results only in a publication in a journal that then sits on shelves. It may be viewed as a success, however, if it results in one of the following:

- Dissemination of a successful intervention: If the project tested an intervention that resulted in lifestyle changes or increased colorectal cancer screening in participants, it deserves to be implemented on a larger scale. This may happen through health departments, community clinics, nonprofit organizations, or other outlets.
- Policy change: If the project identified a barrier such as (for instance) an absence of access to fresh fruits and vegetables, policy makers may be convinced to establish programs to remove the barrier. In this example, it might be in the form of a city- or county-supported weekly farmers' market.

An Illustrative Project

A recent CBPR project conducted to test three interventions intended to increase colorectal cancer screening in African Americans illustrates many of the points discussed in this chapter.[21] Initiatied in 1998, the project is ongoing at least through 2017.

The project began with the organization of two community coalitions: The first, the Metropolitan Atlanta Coalition on Cancer Awareness (MACCA), comprised cancer advocates and survivors as well as businesspeople with a civic commitment to fight cancer. It was the Atlanta representative of the National Black Leadership Initiative on Cancer, a movement that eventually generated over 30 coalitions in locales across the country. The second, the Community Coalition Board of the CDC-funded Morehouse School of Medicine Prevention Research Center (PRC), was organized around health problems more generally in one predominantly low-income African American section of southeast Atlanta. Hence, one of the coalitions was able to "waive" the health needs assessment component of the CBPR process, since the coalition was established with a cancer focus. The other went through a needs assessment process both at the board (coalition) level and, later, through a community survey. It established HIV/AIDS and other STIs as its lead interest.

In 2005, Morehouse investigators obtained a grant from the CDC to support a community intervention trial of three interventions to increase colorectal cancer screening among African Americans aged 50–75 years. The grant proposal was developed with input from the MACCA, but the grant was awarded to the Morehouse Prevention Research Center, which was also funded by CDC. By this time, the Center was doing well with grant funding supporting research on its first priority—HIV/AIDS/STI prevention—so the Community Coalition Board was quite amenable to accepting additional funding to support research on cancer prevention, even though this was a lower priority.

The three interventions to be tested were developed in consultation with the MACCA. Participants were randomized into four cohorts, three of which were to receive an experimental intervention, with the fourth serving as a control. The interventions were:

- One-on-one education: Each participant was to meet individually with a health educator in three weekly sessions to learn about colorectal cancer and its prevention and treatment
- Group education: Participants were to meet in groups of 8–15 with a health educator in four weekly sessions.
- Reduced out-of-pocket expense: Participants did not attend any educational sessions but were to be reimbursed for any personal expenses associated with screening, up to 500 dollars.

The control or comparison cohort was to receive no special intervention. All four cohorts received some literature that had been produced by the National Cancer Institute. The project was approved by the Morehouse Institutional Review Board as well as by the PRC Community Coalition Board.

Community health workers were hired to recruit participants, and the PRC Community Coalition Board provided some assistance. Recruitment was done in churches, senior centers, and clinics. In all, 369 participants were enrolled in the project, but as the project progressed, there was a high attrition rate. This was likely due to lack of leadership in the MACCA; the coalition eventually collapsed, and the PRC Community Coalition Board was involved in multiple projects. At follow-up 6 months after the conclusion of the interventions, there were 259 participants who had completed the intervention and could be located to determine whether they had been screened. Table 11.5 illustrates the results.

Table 11.5 **Outcomes of the Colorectal Cancer Screening Intervention Trial**

Cohort	# Contacted	#Screened	%Screened	p Value Intervention vs. Control
Control	63	11	17.5	–
Reduced Out-of-Pocket Expense	63	14	22.2	ns
One-on-One Education	68	17	25.0	ns
Group Education	65	22	33.9	0.0341
Total	259	64	24.7	

Of the three interventions, only the group education intervention made a statistically significant difference in the screening rate compared with the control group. This came as a surprise to some, who had predicted that the reduced-out-of-pocket-expense intervention would be the most efficacious. Hence, the result was not consistent with the hypothesis that finances are the most important barrier to screening among African Americans; it was, however, consistent with social learning theory.[22] This project was dutifully written up and reported in a journal;[21] but that was not the end. The PRC and the research team next entered into a partnership with the local health department and demonstrated that the intervention was as effective in a practice setting as it was efficacious in a research environment.[23] With funding from the state Department of Public Health, it was offered in several locations in Georgia. Directions for implementing the intervention were submitted to the National Cancer Institute (NCI) and published on NCI's *Research-Tested Intervention Programs (RTIPs)* website[24] so that other organizations and health departments can use it. Finally, through 2017, it is being tested by 17 NBLIC community coalitions to determine the best sites and conditions for implementation.[25]

This project, then, illustrates several points that are important to consider when a CBPR approach is used to discover ways in which to reduce the disparity in colorectal cancer incidence and mortality rates in African Americans as compared with Whites and other racial and ethnic groups.

- A typical community coalition in an African American community may not rank cancer generally, or colorectal cancer specifically, high on its list of priority issues. To conduct colorectal cancer CBPR, therefore, it will be necessary to strike a compromise with the coalition; or, alternatively, organize a cancer-focused community coalition of cancer survivors and advocates.
- Prevention research often suffers from a high rate of participant attrition.[26] Substantial community involvement is needed to prevent this.
- Research that is guided by the community should not be shaped to fit a health promotion theory favored by a university investigator. It is more appropriate to identify a theory post hoc that is consistent with the research design and its outcomes.
- If any research project is to lead to a program that will reduce disparities, it cannot be a one-off that is published in a journal and then never heard of again. It must lead to widespread implementation of an intervention, policy change, or both.

Racial disparities in colorectal cancer (and other conditions) have persisted for decades, so discovering approaches to reducing and eliminating them will be challenging. Success is more likely if the research is guided by the community in a CBPR approach.

References

1. Zauber, A.G., Winawer, S.J., O'Brien, M.J., et al. "Colonoscopic Polypectomy and Long-Term Prevention of Colorectal Cancer Deaths." *New England Journal of Medicine* 366 (2012): 687–96.

2. National Cancer Institute. *SEER Fact Sheets: Colon and Rectum Cancer.* <http://seer.cancer.gov/statfacts/html/colorect.html> (accessed January 15, 2016).

3. Haggar, F.A. and Boushey, R.P. "Colorectal Cancer Epidemiology: Incidence, Mortality, Survival, and Risk Factors." *Clinics in Colon and Rectal Surgery* 22 (2009): 191–7.

4. American Cancer Society. *Colorectal Cancer Facts and Figures 2011–2013.* Atlanta: American Cancer Society, 2011.

5. International Agency for Research on Cancer. *GLOBOCAN 2012: Estimated Cancer Incidence, Mortality and Prevalence Worldwide in 2012.* <http://globocan.iarc.fr/Pages/fact_sheets_cancer.aspx> (accessed January 15, 2016).

6. O'Keefe, J.D., Chung, D., Nahmoud, N., et al. "Why Do African Americans Get More Colon Cancer Than Native Africans?" *Journal of Nutrition* 137 Suppl 1 (2007): 175S–182S.

7. Satia, J.A., Tseng, M., Galanko, J.A., Martin, C. and Sandler, R.S. "Dietary Patterns and Colon Cancer Risk in Whites and African Americans in the North Carolina Colon Cancer Study." *Nutrition and Cancer* 61 (2009): 179–93.

8. Howard, R.A., Freedman, D.M., Park, Y., Hollenbeck, A., Schatzkin, A., and Leitzmann, M.F. "Physical Activity, Sedentary Behavior, and the Risk of Colon and Rectal Cancer in the NIH-AARP Diet and Health Study." *Cancer Causes and Control* 19 (2008): 939–53.

9. Joseph, D.A., King, J.B., Miller, J.W. and Richardson, L.C.; Centers for Disease Control and Prevention (CDC). "Prevalence of Colorectal Cancer Screening Among Adults—Behavioral Risk Factor Surveillance System, United States, 2010." *Morbidity and Mortality Weekly Report Supplement.* 61.2 (2012): 51–6.

10. Shavers, V.L. and Brown, M.L. "Racial and Ethnic Disparities in the Receipt of Cancer Treatment." *JNCI J Natl Cancer Inst.* 94(2002): 334–57.

11. Mouw, T., Koster, A., Wright, M.E., et al. "Education and Risk of Cancer in a Large Cohort of Men and Women in the United States." *PLoS One* 3.11 (2008): e3639.

12. Thompson, V.L., Drake, B., James, A.S., et al. "A Community Coalition to Address Cancer Disparities: Transitions, Successes and Challenges." *Journal of Cancer Education* 30.4 (2015): 616–22.

13. Gwede, C.K., Jean-Francois, E., Quinn, G.P., et al. "Tampa Bay Community Cancer Network Partners: Perceptions of Colorectal Cancer Among Three Ethnic Subgroups of US Blacks: A Qualitative Study." *Journal of the National Medical Association* 103.8 (2011): 669–80.

14. Gwede, C.K., William, C.M., Thomas, K.B., et al. "Exploring Disparities and Variability in Perceptions and Self-Reported Colorectal Cancer Screening Among Three Ethnic Subgroups of U.S. Blacks." *Oncology Nursing Forum* 37.5 (2010): 581–91.

15. Smith, S.A., Whitehead, M.S., Sheats, J.Q., Ansa, B.E., Coughlin, S.S., Blumenthal, D.S. "Community-Based Participatory Research Principles for the African American Community." *Journal of the Georgia Public Health Association* 5.1 (2015): 52–56.

16. Stokols, D. "Translating Social Ecology Theory into Guidelines for Community Health Promotion." *American Journal of Health Promotion* 10 (1996): 282–98.

17. Centers for Disease Control and Prevention: Colorectal cancer control program. https://www.cdc.gov/cancer/crccp/ Accessed June 1, 2016.

18. Braithwaite R.L., Murphy F., Lythcott N., Blumenthal D.S. Community organization and development for health promotion within an urban black community: a conceptual model. *Health Educ.* (1989) Dec;20(5):56–60.

19. Blumenthal D.S. Is community-based participatory research possible? *Am J Prev Med.* (2011) Mar;40(3):386–9.

20. Blumenthal D.S. Clinical community health: revisiting "the community as patient". *Educ Health* (Abingdon). (2009) Aug;22(2):234.

21. Blumenthal D.S., Smith S.A., Majett C.D., Alema-Mensah E. A trial of 3 interventions to promote colorectal cancer screening in African Americans. *Cancer.* (2010) Feb 15;116(4):922–9.

22. Bandura A: Social Learning Theory. General Learning Press, New York NY, (1971).

23. Smith S, Johnson L, Wesley D, Turner KB, McCray G, Sheats J, Blumenthal D. Translation to practice of an intervention to promote colorectal cancer screening among African Americans. *Clin Transl Sci.* (2012) Oct;5(5):412–5.

24. National Cancer Institute: Research Tested Intervention Programs (RTIPs): http://rtips.cancer.gov/rtips/programDetails.do?programId=1124686 Accessed 3 June 2016.

25. Smith, S.A. and Blumenthal, D.S. Efficacy to effectiveness transition of an Educational Program to Increase Colorectal Cancer Screening (EPICS): study protocol of a cluster randomized controlled trial. *Implement Sci.* 8.1 (2013): 86.

26. Blumenthal, D.S., Sung, J., Williams, J., Liff, J., and Coates, R. Recruitment and Retention of Subjects for a Longitudinal Cancer Prevention Study in an Inner-city Black Community. *Health Services Research* (1995) 30:197–205.

12

Community-Based Participatory Research Studies on Breast and Cervical Cancer Screening

STEVEN S. COUGHLIN, PHD, EMILY YOUNGBLOM, MPH,

AND DEBORAH J. BOWEN, PHD

In this chapter, we provide an overview of the public health significance of breast and cervical cancer and briefly discuss (1) disparities in incidence and mortality rates according to race, ethnicity, urban versus rural residence, and geographic locality; (2) the primary prevention of breast cancer; (3) the primary prevention of cervical cancer; (4) breast cancer screening through screening mammography, and (5) cervical cancer screening. We then highlight the important role of community-based participatory research (CBPR) studies in addressing breast cancer and cervical cancer in diverse communities including faith-based interventions. Finally, we discuss lessons learned from CBPR studies on breast and cervical cancer screening and provide recommendations for further research.

The Public Health Importance of Breast Cancer and Cervical Cancer

In the United States, breast cancer accounts for more cancer deaths in women than any site other than lung cancer. An estimated 40,450 deaths from breast cancer will occur in 2016.[1] Breast cancer is the most commonly diagnosed invasive cancer in the United States for women of all racial and ethnic groups, with an estimated 246,660 new cases diagnosed in 2016.[1] Worldwide, about 521,907 deaths from breast cancer occur each year.[2]

Because of widespread screening in developed countries, there are fewer deaths from cervical cancer than breast cancer. In 2016, about 4,120 deaths from cervical cancer will occur and about 12,990 new cases of cervical cancer will be diagnosed in the United States.[1] Worldwide, about 265,672 deaths from cervical cancer occur each year.[2] About 85% of cervical cancer deaths occur in developing countries.

Disparities in Breast and Cervical Cancer in the United States

Age-standardized breast cancer incidence rates in the United States are higher among non-Hispanic White women than non-Hispanic Black women, Asian and Pacific Islander, American Indian and Alaska Native, or Hispanic women, although Black women have a higher breast cancer mortality rate than women from other racial groups.[1] Black-White differences in survival persist even after accounting for disease stage and tumor characteristics.[3,4] Since 1975, the 5-year relative survival rate for breast cancer has increased for both African American and White women.[1] However, there remains a substantial racial difference. In the most recent time period, the 5-year relative survival rate was 79% for African American women and 92% for White women.[1] This disparity in breast cancer survival is due to both later stage at diagnosis and poorer stage-specific survival among African American women.[1] Both routine screening and access to treatment are important to address breast cancer disparities. In the United States, Black race and Hispanic ethnicity have been associated with later stage at breast cancer diagnosis. Studies have shown that African American women are less likely than White women to receive timely follow-up after an abnormal or inconclusive screening mammogram.[5,6] Compared with White women in the United States, African American women tend to have more aggressive breast cancers that present more frequently as estrogen receptor negative tumors.[7] Among premenopausal women, tumors that are estrogen receptor negative, progesterone receptor negative, and HER2 negative ("triple negative" tumors) are more common among Black women than among White women.[8]

For cervical cancer, age-standardized incidence rates are higher among non Hispanic Black women and Hispanic women than among non-Hispanic White women.[1] American Indian and Alaska Native women also have higher cervical cancer incidence rates than non-Hispanic women. Although cervical cancer incidence rates in the United States are lower among Asian and Pacific Islander women than other racial groups, Laotian and Cambodian women have very high rates of cervical cancer. Cervical cancer mortality rates are higher among non-Hispanic black, American Indian and Alaska Native, and Hispanic women than among non-Hispanic White women.[1] Geographic disparities in cervical cancer incidence and mortality exist in the United States. For example, rates are relatively high in Appalachia and in the US-Mexico border region.

Primary Prevention of Breast Cancer

A variety of risk factors for breast cancer have been well established by epidemiologic studies including race, ethnicity, family history of cancer, and genetic traits, as well as modifiable exposures such as increased alcohol consumption, physical inactivity, obesity, exogenous hormones, and certain female reproductive factors.[1,7] Efforts to prevent breast cancer and other chronic illnesses have focused on promoting physical activity, healthy diet and nutrition, and avoidance of excessive alcohol consumption. It is likely that, in addition to biological and genetic factors, social and environmental factors (for example, severe stress due to living in poverty) have an adverse impact on access to timely screening and treatment and may also influence how breast cancer is expressed.[3,4,9] Recent advances in understanding the molecular biology of breast cancer have prompted efforts to better understand approaches for preventing the disease among higher-risk women who are genetically predisposed to developing the disease.

Primary Prevention of Cervical Cancer

Oncogenic human papillomavirus (HPV) types (mainly types 16 and 18) cause almost all cervical cancers.[10] An HPV infection is commonly transmitted sexually.[11] About 43% of US females ages 14–59 years have a current genital HPV infection.[12] Most infections will clear within 1 year without intervention[13-16] but females with persistent infections can develop serious disease if left untreated. The HPV vaccines available in the United States include a bivalent vaccine that prevents infection with HPV types 16 and 18; a quadrivalent vaccine that prevents infection with HPV types 6, 11, 16, and 18; and a 9-valent vaccine that prevents infection with HPV types 6, 11, 16, 18, 31, 33, 45, 52, and 58. Both the bivalent and quadrivalent vaccines offer protection against HPV types 16 and 18, which account for 66% of all cervical cancers, and the 9-valent vaccine protects against five additional types accounting for an additional 15% of cervical cancers. Both the quadrivalent and 9-valent vaccines protect against HPV types causing 90% of genital warts.[16] Guidelines currently recommend that all 11- to 12-year-old females receive two doses of either HPV vaccine, with catch-up vaccination for 13- to 26-year-old females.[16] In addition to HPV infection, factors that increase a woman's risk of cervical cancer include human immunodeficiency virus (HIV) infection, a compromised immune system, and cigarette smoking.

Early Detection of Breast Cancer Through Screening Mammography

The US Preventive Services Task Force (USPSTF) recommends screening mammography every 2 years as there is convincing evidence from randomized controlled trials that screening mammography reduces breast cancer mortality, with a greater absolute reduction for women aged 50 to 74 years than for younger women.[17] For women who are aged 40 to 49 years (who are not at increased risk by virtue of a known genetic mutation) the USPSTF concludes that the decision to start regular, biennial screening mammography before the age of 50 years should be an individual one and take patient context into account, including the patient's values regarding specific benefits and harms. The American Cancer Society has also provided recommendations for breast cancer screening.[18]

Early Detection of Cervical Cancer

Screening aims to identify high-grade precancerous cervical lesions to prevent development of cervical cancer and early-stage asymptomatic invasive cervical cancer. The USPSTF recommends cervical screening for women ages 21 to 65 years every 3 years with cytology (Papanicolaou test).[19] The USPSTF concludes that HPV testing combined with cytology (cotesting) every 5 years in women ages 30 to 65 years offers a comparable balance of benefits and harms, and is therefore a reasonable alternative for women in this age group who would prefer to extend the screening interval. The American Cancer Society and the World Health Organization have also provided recommendations for routine cervical screening.[18,20]

Role of CBPR in Addressing Breast Cancer and Cervical Cancer in Diverse Communities

We believe that the use of CBPR methods has improved the design, implementation, and evaluation of interventions to prevent breast and cervical cancer by targeting these risk factors in population samples. As discussed by Coughlin et al. in chapter 1, CBPR involves the engagement and collaboration of academic and community members on multiple aspects of research to design a more relevant and hopefully more effective intervention. Here we have selected a few projects that have used CBPR differently in their interventions to reduce the burden of breast and cervical cancer. We selected these studies because to us they provided strong examples of the use of CBPR methods in the design and evaluation of interventions to promote screening. The studies were not pilot projects with a small "n" or only formative research. We also tried to select studies that dealt with diverse populations to illustrate the strength of CBPR in engaging these multiple groups.

CBPR IN ACTION TO PREVENT CANCER

In recent decades, a rich literature has developed on CBPR intervention studies on breast and cervical cancer screening among African American women, Hispanic women, women in the Appalachian region of the United States, and other racial, ethnic, and cultural groups.[21-44] Some studies have been conducted in collaboration with churches or other faith communities. The church is the most important social institution in many communities.[27,38] In view of its important cultural role, service orientation, and multitude of contributions through social networks and organizational structures, the church is an ideal setting in which to offer health promotion activities for African Americans, Hispanics, and other minorities. This is particularly true of vulnerable groups such as the poor, elderly, medically underserved, and people who have been harmed by a history of neglect, oppression, or discrimination.[27,38] Several notable studies are summarized below.

The goal of the Forsyth County Cancer Screening Project in North Carolina was to improve the use of breast and cervical cancer screening among low-income, predominately African American women aged 40 and older. The multicomponent intervention strategies included chart reminders, examination room prompts, in-service meetings, and patient-directed literature in clinic settings, and community outreach strategies including educational sessions, distribution of literature, community events, media, and church programs.[21] The proportion of women reporting regular use of mammography increased 31%–56% ($p < .001$) in the intervention city.

In the Witness Project in Arkansas, Erwin et al. studied the effectiveness of a culturally competent breast cancer education program in which cancer survivors were trained to promote early detection and increased breast self-examination and mammography among rural, underserved African American women.[22,28] The setting for the intensive educational program was African American churches in two intervention counties and two control counties in the Mississippi River Delta region of Arkansas. Breast self-examination and mammography significantly increased in the intervention counties ($p < .005$).

In the Los Angeles mammography Promotion in Churches Program (LAMP), a church-based telephone mammography counseling intervention was implemented with the assistance of Latino, African American, and White peer counselors.[23,30,38] Thirty churches were randomized to telephone counseling and control conditions. Telephone interviews were conducted to assess intervention effects on mammography adherence. Over a 1-year follow-up period, the telephone peer counseling intervention reduced the nonadherence rate from 23% to 16% and maintained mammography adherence among participants who were adherent at baseline.[38]

A faith-based breast and cervical cancer screening intervention for African American women living in urban communities was conducted as part of the Centers for Disease Control and Prevention (CDC) Racial and Ethnic Approaches to Community Health (REACH) program.[35] A formative evaluation of the program was conducted involving focus groups of women in each of the nine participating churches. Key findings included the acceptability of receiving cancer education within the context of a faith community, the importance of pastoral input, the effectiveness of personal testimonies and lay health advocates, the saliency of biblical scripture in reinforcing health messages, and the effectiveness of multimodal learning aids.[35]

Studts et al.[39] conducted a community-based randomized trial of a faith-placed intervention to reduce cervical cancer burden in Appalachia. The study was conducted in four Kentucky counties to assess the effectiveness of a faith-placed lay health advisor intervention to increase Pap test use among middle-aged and older women. Women aged 40–64 years and overdue for screening were recruited from churches and individually randomized to an intervention group (n = 176) or a wait-list control group (n = 169). The intervention provided lay health advisor home visits and newsletters addressing barriers to screening. The main outcome was self-reported receipt of a Pap test. Treatment group participants (17.6% screened) had over twice the odds of wait-list controls (11.2% screened) of reporting Pap test receipt post intervention (odds ratio = 2.56, 95% CI: 1.03–6.38, p = .04).

Mishra et al.[40] examined the effectiveness of a theory-guided, culturally tailored cervical cancer education program designed to increase Pap smear use among Samoan women residing in the US Territory of American Samoa. A two-group, pre/post test design was used. Principles of CBPR were followed. The sample included 398 Samoan women age 20 and older recruited from Samoan churches. Women in the intervention group received a culturally tailored cervical cancer education program in three weekly sessions. The primary outcome was self-reported receipt of a Pap smear. Women in the intervention group were twice as likely to self-report Pap smear use at the post-test (adjusted odds ratio = 2.0, 95% confidence interval: 1.3–3.2, p < .01).

A randomized controlled trial in Texas tested an intervention to promote breast cancer prevention activities among low-socioeconomic-status urban adults.[41] Through advisory board involvement and focus groups, the investigators designed an educational program to help adults consider methods of preventing breast cancer, with significant changes in several breast cancer prevention behaviors.

Several studies have used promotoras to support women in increasing screening.[42-44] In all of these studies, the idea for using promotoras came from engaged discussions with community members about what would help them to increase their use of screening services. Each of these studies was able to show positive results using promotoras, ranging from increased community awareness to actual behavior change in participants.

SUMMARY

These are just illustrative examples of the many CBPR studies that have been conducted to examine the effectiveness of intervention strategies to promote breast and cervical cancer screening among diverse groups of women. The intervention approaches examined in these studies extend across many of the intervention approaches highlighted in Guide to Community Preventive Services systematic reviews including small media, one-on-one education, small group education, client reminders, reducing structural barriers, and provider reminders.[45]

One of the commonalities identified in Table 12.1 is the use of community advisory boards found in most of the studies portrayed in this table. Advisory

Table 12.1 **CBPR Studies of Breast and Cervical Cancer Screening, Illustrating How CBPR Influenced the Study Activities**

Name of Study	Citation	Study Design	Study Population	CBPR Activities	How CBPR Influenced the Study Activities
FoCaS (Forsyth County Cancer Screening) Project	Pasket et al.[21]	4 phases in 2 cities over 4 years: 1) Surveys 2) in-reach and outreach interventions (Winston-Salem only) 3) follow-up survey 4) transfer of interventions to comparison city (Greensboro)	Women age > 40 years living in low income housing communities in Winston-Salem and Greensboro, NC. (populations were primarily African American and > 60 years old)	**Interventions implemented in the housing communities included:** (a) "Women's Fest," a free party held in the community that included food, educational classes, cholesterol, blood pressure and diabetes screening, prizes, and information booths (b) a church program that included a ministers' luncheon and a lay health educator program, "Taking Care of Our Sisters", for female church members (c) educational brochures especially designed to address identified barriers such as "Where to Get a Mammogram" (d) mass media techniques (public bus ads, newspaper and radio ads on African-American media) (e) monthly classes in each housing community conducted by a lay health educator (f) birthday cards with the FoCaS logo (g) targeted mailings and door knob hangers with invitations to events (h) one-on-one educational sessions in women's homes.	Face to face interviews and focus groups were used to gather information on barriers, attitudes, current breast and ovarian cancer screening practices, and optimum intervention strategies. A community-based advisory board was involved throughout the intervention. Ongoing feedback on intervention activities was sought from community advisers.

(continued)

Table 12.1 Continued

Name of Study	Citation	Study Design	Study Population	CBPR Activities	How CBPR Influenced the Study Activities
				Clinic-focused interventions implemented included: (a) in-service and primary care conference training for providers on issues including clinical breast exam proficiency, cultural sensitivity, and techniques to integrate prevention in primary care (b) visual prompts in the exam rooms, e.g., "Have you screened today? (c) educational games, e.g., "Find the Lump Game" to teach clinical breast exam techniques (d) an abnormal test protocol that included alert stickers, a referral process for managing the care of women with abnormal test results, and a tracking system (e) poster and literature distribution in the waiting rooms (f) one-on-one counseling sessions and personalized letters for follow-up testing for women who had abnormal test results.	
Witness Project	Erwin et al.[22]	In this study, a quasi-experimental pretest and post-test design was used to measure the effectiveness of	African American women living in 4 counties in Arkansas: (Phillips and Monroe were	Members of a Witness Project team, which was composed of 7 local African American women who had survived breast or cervical cancer, spoke in groups at local churches and community meetings. Cancer survivors	Members of the community who had survived breast or cervical cancer were available to answer any questions that the study participants had.

		the Witness Project in increasing the practice of breast self-examination and mammography by rural African American women in two counties. Program participants were compared with a control population of African American women from two other counties who did not participate in the intervention.	intervention counties, Chicot and Desha were control). Primarily low income, low education. Recruited through local church or community groups.	(Witness role models) spoke about their experiences, highlighting the importance of early detection and treatment for survivorship, and the need to take responsibility for their own health (empowerment and assertiveness). They stressed the need to spread these messages throughout the African American community. These programs began with a hymn and prayer, and included biblical quotations and statements of faith by the Witness models. Breast self-examination (BSE) was taught and resources for free and reduced-cost mammograms were discussed.	The intervention talks were designed to be community-based and culturally sensitive, and incorporated spirituality and faith.
LAMP (Los Angeles Mammography Promotion in Churches Program) telephone Counseling	Derose et al.[23]	Church-based telephone mammography counseling intervention utilizing female church members as peer counselors	African American, Latina, or Anglo (white) women (50-80 years old) involved in a local Los Angeles church group.	26 local women from 12 of the 15 intervention churches were hired and trained as counselors. Three telephone centers at two churches were organized. Culturally specific and small group interactions were most effective for training.	Members of the community were invited to participate in focus groups to help adapt the intervention to the site. Focus groups specific to mammography were conducted, and this was used to develop a counseling script in both English and Spanish. Bilingual consultants that were familiar with the target population were hired to review the scripts and make recommendations.

(continued)

Table 12.1 Continued

Name of Study	Citation	Study Design	Study Population	CBPR Activities	How CBPR Influenced the Study Activities
LAMP (Los Angeles Mammography Promotion in Churches Program) telephone Counseling	Duan et al.[30]	30 churches were randomized to telephone counseling and control conditions; data were used in assessing intervention effects on mammography adherence. Separate analyses were conducted for maintaining adherence and conversion to adherence	African American, Latina, or Anglo (white) women (50–80 years old) involved in a local Los Angeles church group.	1 session of telephone counseling was conducted annually for 2 years. Part-time peer counselors from participating churches called participants from those churches to provide mammography counseling by phone. The counseling was individualized to address barriers. Women were informed about their risk status and about breast cancer prevalence rates. They were also encouraged to ask their physicians for a referral and information about convenient screening facilities. Primary outcome measure was annual mammography screening adherence status (undergoing at least 1 mammogram during the previous 12 months). During annual telephone surveys, status was self-reported by participants.	Members of the community were hired to serve as peer telephone counselors, ensuring that the target population had someone of similar religious and ethnic background to talk to and ask questions of.
Racial and Ethnic Approaches to Community Health (REACH)	Matthews et al.[35]	Faith based breast and cervical cancer early detection and prevention intervention for African American women in urban communities	Members of churches in communities with high proportion of African Americans, members living at or below the poverty level, and rates of breast cancer.	Women were exposed to 6 months of education and outreach activities focused on increasing cancer knowledge and early detection. "Standard" components were delivered to all participating churches, and "variable" interventions were initiated and delivered at each individual church. The standard educational curriculum was based on a "train the trainer" model, which required that each church identify one to two church	Focus groups with 30–40 participants were run by a female congregation member in order to solicit feedback on program development. After the intervention, focus groups were held as a means of soliciting in-depth program evaluation.

		members to receive training to become lay health educators. The educators then delivered both the standard and variable educational activities at their churches, taught from a culturally specific, faith-oriented education curriculum developed by team. The curriculum also included demonstrations of breast self-examinations and information about local resources for mammograms and Pap smears. These events were publicized by the educators and reinforced by an announcement from the pastor.		
Faith Moves Mountains (FMM)	Studts et al.[39]	Faith-placed lay health advisor (LHA) intervention to increase Pap test use among middle-aged and older women in Appalachian Kentucky. Single-blind, 2-armed, 4-year community-based randomized controlled trial to reduce invasive cervical cancer (ICC).	29 local churches were recruited. Female congregants were invited to participate, and were eligible if 40–64 years old, spoke English, and had not had regular cervical cancer screening.	Participants were randomized into treatment or control conditions. The treatment group received intervention. 10 LHAs were selected with similar demographics as study population, and were trained as health advisors. They did tailored home visits (2 hours) with participants and sent out a newsletter on cervical cancer screening information. After the intervention, a follow up was done with all participants (control and intervention group) to reassess cervical cancer screening status. FMM depended upon the efforts of local residents, often requiring a delicate balance of community needs and scientific procedures. Project staff consisted of local community members. Project staff members were the only ones delivering cervical cancer screening and prevention information, in the form of educational lunches held at the church. These lunches ensured that the target population had a basic understanding of the importance of screening before the intervention took place.

(continued)

Table 12.1 Continued

Name of Study	Citation	Study Design	Study Population	CBPR Activities	How CBPR Influenced the Study Activities
Cervical Cancer Education Program	Mishra et al.[40]	2-group (intervention and control). Women were randomized to the control or intervention group. Pretests and posttests were designed to assess efficacy of the intervention.	Women age > 20 years recruited from Samoan churches. All women were of Samoan ancestry and had no history of a Pap-smear within two years, cervical cancer, or a hysterectomy.	The education program consisted of 3 parts: English and Samoan language cervical cancer education booklets (with Samoan women as models), skill building and behavioral exercises, and interactive group discussion sessions. Samoan female health educators delivered the education programs in Samoan while respecting cultural and religious norms. This was done over 3 consecutive weeks in 20 groups of 8-14 women per group. Pre- and posttest surveys were conducted in person. Interviewers received about 10 hours of training in the conduct of interviews. Both control and intervention groups were given the pre- and post-test surveys. Post-test survey was done about 6 months after the pre-test survey (and after intervention). Women in the control group only received the booklets after the post-test surveys.	The study included extensive open-dialogue, active participation, and group involvement, allowing learners to become more personally involved in the subject of interest. The intervention was designed to address factors such as knowledge, doctor-patient communication, perceptions of disease susceptibility and severity, cultural beliefs, and self-efficacy.
Dallas Cancer Disparities Research Coalition pilot study	Cardarelli et al.[41]	Participants were divided into 2 groups: one receiving the intervention (n=59) and one serving as a control group (n=60).	Age > 40 years, living in South Dallas (intervention) or West Dallas (control). Both geographical areas are low income. No history of cancer, English speaking.	An 8-week breast cancer education curriculum was developed, using both the Health Belief Model and social cognitive theory. Each session was 1.5 hours long and held once a week at a local elementary school. Education content focused on prevention of breast cancer, and included cooking demonstrations. Participants also received written educational materials.	Research staff built a strong relationship with local universities and the South Dallas community. Community members serve on the advisory board, which completed a series of focus groups in the community to identify perceptions of cancer

				Educational sessions were delivered by both local peers and health professionals. A baseline (before intervention) and follow up (after intervention) survey was administered to both populations to determine efficacy.	disparities and community strengths and assets to promote cancer prevention.
AMIGAS: Ayundando a las Mujeres con Informacion, Guia, y Amor para su Salud (helping women with information, guidance, and love for their health)	Byrd et al.[44]	Participants were randomized into 4 study arms: full AMIGAS program with video and flipchart, AMIGAS without video, AMIGAS without flipchart, and control	Mexican origin > 21 years with no previous history of cancer, no hysterectomy, no cervical cancer screening within the past 3 years. Living in El Paso, Houston, or Yakima Valley, TX.	Programs were developed using theory-based and evidence-based health promotion interventions. The program intervention consisted of a video novella using role models to discuss barriers to facilitators for cervical cancer screening; a flip chart reviewing the information in the video; games and activities, including cards to help participants understand a woman's stage of change, a contract sheet titled "mi promesa" (my promise) for women to write promises to themselves to get screened or think about screening, and a training manual. Women in the control group received no education from the promotoras.	Local promotoras (lay health workers) were hired to recruit women into the study and deliver the program materials. A community advisory board was solicited to participate throughout the program development and testing. Initial testing of the educational material was done through 2 half-day workshops with bilingual promotoras who worked with the target population. Further pretesting was done over 3 pilot sessions.
Cultivando la Salud (Cultivating Health)	Fernandez et al.[43]	2 groups were chosen: intervention (Merced, CA and Eagle Pass, TX) or control (Anthony, NM and Watsonville, CA)	Low income, low literacy, Hispanic, female farmworkers age > 50 years who were nonadherent to mammography or Pap test screening guidelines	Women in the intervention group were contacted by lay health workers to set up a 1-on-1 session in their home. Each session lasted 1–2 hours, and consisted of a presentation and discussion using Cultivando la Salud materials. Information on local breast and cervical cancer screening were also provided. 2 weeks after the intervention, participants were recontacted by lay health workers to follow up and see if any other assistance was needed.	The baseline surveys were piloted with 200 low-income Hispanic women, and were refined. Focus groups were also held to determine what items should be included in the survey. The intervention was occasionally observed by a project supervisor to offer feedback on program delivery.

(continued)

Table 12.1 Continued

Name of Study	Citation	Study Design	Study Population	CBPR Activities	How CBPR Influenced the Study Activities
A CBPR Approach to Cervical Cancer in the Apsáalooke population	Christopher et al.[42]	Longitudinal social network intervention	Apsáalooke women of Montana	A three-step community-based approach was used to determine suitable community members for the role of cervical cancer prevention lay health advisor (LHA). To ascertain the qualities an Apsáalooke woman would look for in an LHA, this question was asked on a survey. Next, open community meetings were held to determine women that had the identified attributes. The project advisor (from the community) determined the identified women's ability to carry out the tasks. Finally, the women were invited to be Messengers (LHAs). Assessments were done to make sure they understood the information they were being asked to teach.	The principal investigator promised work in partnership with the community in all phases of the project by holding community meetings, having all project meetings open to the public, sharing all data, coanalyzing data with community members, and collaborating with local entities. Community members offered feedback regarding the effectiveness and need for Messengers for Health.

Project staff provided the Messengers with information about cervical health and outreach, and they were given an opportunity to receive information, comprehend it, and share it in one-on-one, role-playing with another community member. During the intervention, Messengers provided cervical cancer education and general health education directly to women and indirectly to men (e.g., via family members). These were done in participants' homes or in community locations. The Messengers received education from project staff and guest lecturers during monthly meetings and yearly retreats. Pre and posttest surveys were administered to determine efficacy of the intervention.

boards allow for advice and discussion about detailed issues, often needing trust and honesty that comes with exposure to the ideas of research and of community issues that comes with increased contact time. The thoughts shared in advisory boards can be compared to qualitative data collection through interviews and focus groups. These methods do not require as much trust, but provide input from a broader and potentially more diverse group of community members, making them a valuable method for CBPR as well. Both focus groups and interviews can be repeated during the study, continuing the efforts to gather feedback and ideas throughout the project.

Discussion

Additional CBPR studies are needed to address breast and cervical cancer screening in population subgroups where screening rates are relatively low. This includes many low-income, uninsured, and underinsured women, which contributes to higher mortality rates among these population subgroups.[1,3] Racial and ethnic differences in health insurance coverage and access to healthcare services are likely to play a role as women who have a regular healthcare provider are more likely to receive a provider recommendation to get a cancer screening test.[46-48] Many CBPR studies on breast cancer, cervical cancer, or both have provided health education through small media, small group sessions, mass media, or other intervention strategies. Studies have found that some women have misconceptions about the etiology of breast or cervical cancer, misconceptions about their risk of the disease, and barriers to receiving screening and timely treatment (for example, fear of the disease and mistrust of the healthcare system due to historical injustices).[3,49] For example, at-risk African American women are less likely than White women to be informed about current guidelines and recommendations related to breast cancer prevention and early detection.[50] In conducting CBPR studies in diverse communities, there is a need for culturally appropriate, targeted health messages for women to increase their knowledge and awareness of health behaviors for the early detection of breast and cervical cancer.[9] Health promotion messages that are culturally targeted for a group address the unique needs of individuals, increase their motivation, tend to be perceived as more personally relevant, and lead to a greater likelihood of behavior change. The targeting of health promotion messages to a cultural group such as Hispanic, Vietnamese, Native Hawaiian, or African American women increases the relevance of the messages to members of the target audience.[51] Culturally appropriate interventions address the cultural values of the group, reflect the attitudes and norms of the group, and reflect the behavioral preferences and expectations of the group's members.

Of particular interest are CBPR studies that have the potential to fill in gaps in the current evidence about what intervention strategies are effective in increasing screening in population subgroups that are disproportionately affected by breast or cervical cancer. This includes dissemination and implementation research and studies that translate evidence-based interventions to new populations identified by race, ethnicity, culture, nativity, or geographic locality. Of particular interest are CBPR studies that include multicomponent intervention approaches aimed at different levels of the socioecological model. Studies conducted in collaboration with recent immigrants and socioeconomically disadvantaged populations should also be a priority.

References

1. American Cancer Society. *Cancer Facts and Figures 2016.* Atlanta, GA: American Cancer Society, 2016.
2. International Agency for Cancer Research. *Globocan.* <http://globocan.iarc.fr/Pages/fact_sheets_population.aspx>
3. Gerend, M.A. and Pai, M. "Social Determinants of Black-White Disparities in Breast Cancer Mortality: A Review." *Cancer Epidemiology, Biomarkers and Prevention* 17 (2008): 2913–23.
4. Coughlin, S.S. "Intervention Approaches for Addressing Breast Cancer Disparities Among African American Women." *Annals of Translational Medicine and Epidemiology* 1 (2014). pii: 1001.
5. McCarthy, B.D., Yood, M.U., Boohaker, E.A., Ward, R.E., Rebner, M. and Johnson, C.C. "Inadequate Follow-up of Abnormal Mammograms." *American Journal of Preventive Medicine* 12 (1996): 282–8.
6. Hunter, C.P. "Epidemiology, Stage at Diagnosis, and Tumor Biology of Breast Carcinoma in Multiracial and Multiethnic Populations." *Cancer* 88 (2000): 1193–202.
7. Coughlin, S.S. and Cypel, Y. "Epidemiology of Breast Cancer in Women." In *Breast Cancer Metastasis and Drug Resistance: Challenges and Progress,* ed. A. Ahmad. New York: Springer, 2013.
8. Wheeler, S.B., Reeder-Hayes, K.E. and Carey, L.A. "Disparities in Breast Cancer Treatment and Outcomes: Biological, Social, and Health System Determinants and Opportunities for Research." *Oncologist* 18 (2013): 986–93.
9. Leeks, K.D., Hall, I.J., Johnson-Turbes, C.A., et al. "Formative Development of a Culturally Appropriate Mammography Screening Campaign for Low-Income African American Women." *Journal of Health Disparities Research and Practice* 5 (2012): 42–61.
10. Gillison, M.L., Chaturvedi, A.K. and Lowy, D.R. "HPV Prophylactic Vaccines and the Potential Prevention of Noncervical Cancers in Both Men and Women." *Cancer* 113 Suppl 10 (2008): 3036–46.
11. Reiter, P.L., Katz, M.L. and Paskett, E.D. "HPV Vaccination Among Adolescent Females from Appalachia: Implications for Cervical Cancer Disparities." *Cancer Epidemiology Biomarkers and Prevention* 21 (2012): 2220–30.
12. Weinstock, H., Berman, S. and Cates, W., Jr. "Sexually Transmitted Diseases Among American Youth: Incidence and Prevalence Estimates, 2000." *Perspectives on Sexual and Reproductive Health* 36 (2004): 6–10.
13. Hariri, S., Unger, E.R., Sternberg, M., et al. "Prevalence of Genital Human Papillomavirus Among Females in the United States, the National Health and Nutrition Examination Survey, 2003–2006." *Journal of Infectious Diseases* 204 (2011): 566–73.
14. Moscicki, A.B., Shiboski, S., Broering, J., et al. "The Natural History of Human Papillomavirus Infection as Measured by Repeated DNA Testing in Adolescent and Young Women." *Journal of Pediatrics* 132 (1998): 277–84.

15. Franco, E.L., Villa, L.L., Sobrinho, J.P., et al. "Epidemiology of Acquisition and Clearance of Cervical Human Papillomavirus Infection in Women from a High-Risk Area for Cervical Cancer." *Journal of Infect Diseases* 180 (1999): 1415–23.

16. Petrosky, E., Bocchini, J., Hariri, S., et al. "Use of 9-Valent Human Papillomavirus (HPV) Vaccine: Updated HPV Vaccination Recommendations of the Advisory Committee on Immunization Practices." *Morbidity and Mortality Weekly Report* 64 (2015): 300–4.

17 US Preventive Services Task Force. *Final Recommendation Statement Breast Cancer Screening.* November 2016. <http://www.uspreventiveservicestaskforce.org/Page/Document/UpdateSummaryFinal/breast-cancer-screening>

18 Smith, R.A., Manassaram-Baptiste, D., Durado Brooks, D., et al. "Cancer Screening in the United States, 2015: A Review of Current American Cancer Society Guidelines and Current Issues in Cancer Screening." *CA: A Cancer Journal for Clinicians* 65 (2015): 30–45.

19 US Preventive Services Task Force. *Final Recommendation Statement Cervical Cancer Screening.* <http://www.uspreventiveservicestaskforce.org/>

20 *Comprehensive Cervical Cancer Control: A Guide to Essential Practice* (2nd ed.). Geneva: World Health Organization, 2014.

21 Paskett, E.D., Tatum, C.M., D'Agostino, R., Jr., et al. "Community-Based Interventions to Improve Breast and Cervical Cancer Screening: Results of the Forsyth County Cancer Screening (FoCaS) Project." *Cancer Epidemiology Biomarkers and Prevention* 8 (1999): 453–9.

22 Erwin, D.O., Spatz, T.S., Stotts, R.C. and Hollenberg, J.A. "Increasing Mammography Practice by African American Women." *Cancer Practice* 7 (1999): 78–85.

23 Derose, K.P., Fox, S.A., Reigadas, E., and Hawes-Dawson J. "Church-Based Telephone Mammography Counseling with Peer Counselors." *Journal of Health Communication* 5 (2000): 175–88.

24 Mann, B.D., Sherman, L., Clayton, C., et al. "Screening to the Converted: An Educational Intervention in African American Churches." *Journal of Cancer Education* 15 (2000): 46–50.

25 Husaini, B.A., Sherkat, D.E., Bragg, R., et al. "Predictors of Breast Cancer Screening in a Panel Study of African American Women." *Women's Health* 34 (2001): 35–51.

26 Husaini, B.A., Sherkat, D.E., Levine, R., et al. "The Effect of a Church-Based Breast Cancer Screening Education Program on Mammography Rates Among African-American Women." *Journal of the National Medical Association* 94 (2002): 100–6.

27 Markens, S., Fox, S.A., Taub, B. and Gilbert M.L. "Role of Black Churches in Health Promotion Programs: Lessons from the Los Angeles Mammography Promotion in Churches Program." *American Journal of Public Health* 92 (2002): 805–10.

28 Erwin, D.O. "Cancer Education Takes on a Spiritual Focus for the African American Faith Community." *Journal of Cancer Education* 17 (2002): 46–9.

29 Holt, C.L., Kyles, A., Wiehagen, T. and Casey, C. "Development of a Spiritually Based Breast Cancer Educational Booklet for African American Women." *Cancer Control* 10 (2003): 37–44.

30 Duan, N., Fox, S., Derose, K.P., Carson, S. and Stockdale, S. "Identifying Churches for Community-Based Mammography Promotion: Lessons from the LAMP Study." *Health Education and Behavior* 32 (2005): 536–48.

31 Holt, C.L. and Klem, P.R. "As You Go, Spread the Word: Spiritually Based Breast Cancer Education for African American Women." *Gynecologic Oncology* 99 (2005): S141–2.

32 Husaini, B.A., Emerson, J.S., Hull, P.C., et al. "Rural-Urban Differences in Breast Cancer Screening Among African American Women." *Journal of Health Care for the Poor and Underserved* 16 (2005): 1–10.

33 Powell, M.E., Carter, V., Bonsi, E., et al. "Increasing Mammography Screening Among African American Women in Rural Areas." *Journal of Health Care for the Poor and Underserved* 16 (2005): 1–10.

34 Darnell, J.S., Chang, C.H. and Calhoun, E.A. "Knowledge About Breast Cancer and Participation in a Faith-Based Breast Cancer Program and Other Predictors of Mammography Screening Among African American Women and Latinas." *Health Promotion and Practice* 7 (2006): 201S–12S.

35 Matthews, A.K., Berrios, N., Darnell, J.S. and Calhoun, E. "A Qualitative Evaluation of a Faith-Based Breast and Cervical Cancer Screening Intervention for African American Women." *Health Education and Behavior* 33 (2006): 643–63.

36 Holt, C.L., Lee, C. and Wright, K. "A Spiritually Based Approach to Breast Cancer Awareness: Cognitive Response Analysis of Communication Effectiveness." *Health Communication* 23 (2008): 13–22.

37 Katz, M.L., Kauffman, R.M., Tatum, C.M., et al. "Influence of Church Attendance and Spirituality in a Randomized Controlled Trial to Increase Mammography Use Among a Low-Income, Tri-Racial, Rural Community." *Journal of Religion and Health* 47 (2008): 227–36.

38 Duran, N., Fox, S.A., Pitkin Derose, K. and Carson, S. "Maintaining Mammography Adherence Through Telephone Counseling in a Church-Based Trial." *American Journal of Public Health* 90 (2000): 1468–71.

39 Studts, C.R., Tarasenko, Y.N., Schoenberg, N.E., et al. "A Community-Based Randomized Trial of a Faith-Placed Intervention to Reduce Cervical Cancer Burden in Appalachia." *Preventive Medicine* 54 (2012): 408–14.

40 Mishra, S.I., Luce, P.H. and Baquet, C.R. "Increasing Pap Smear Utilization Among Samoan Women: Results from a Community Based Participatory Randomized Trial." *Journal of Health Care for the Poor and Underserved* 20 Suppl 2 (2009): 85–101.

41 Cardarelli, K., Jackson, R., Martin, M., et al. "Community-Based Participatory Approach to Reduce Breast Cancer Disparities in South Dallas." *Progress in Community Health Partnerships* 5 (2011): 375–85.

42 Christopher, S., Gidley, A.L., Letiecq, B., et al. "A Cervical Cancer Community-Based Participatory Research Project in a Native American Community." *Health Education and Behavior* 35 (2008): 821–34.

43 Fernandez, M.E., Gonzales, A., Tortolero-Luna, G., et al. "Effectiveness of Cultivando la Salud: A Breast and Cervical Cancer Screening Promotion Program for Low-Income Hispanic Women." *American Journal of Public Health* 99 (2009): 936–43.

44 Byrd, T.L., Wilson, K.M., Smith, J.L., et al. "AMIGAS: A Multicity, Multicomponent Cervical Cancer Prevention Trial Among Mexican American Women." *Cancer* 119 (2013): 1365–72.

45 Sabatino, S.A., Lawrence, B., Elder, R., et al. "Effectiveness of Interventions to Increase Screening for Breast, Cervical, and Colorectal Cancers. Nine Updated Systematic Reviews for the Guide to Community Preventive Services." *American Journal of Preventive Medicine* 43 (2012): 97–118.

46 Rimer, B.K., Trock, B., Engstrom, P.F., Lerman, C. and King, E. "Why Do Some Women Get Regular Mammograms?" *American Journal of Preventive Medicine* 7 (1991): 69–74.

47 Lerman, C., Rimer, B., Trock, B., Balshem, A. and Engstrom P.F. "Factors Associated with Repeat Adherence to Breast Cancer Screening." *Preventive Medicine* 19 (1990): 279–90.

48 Zapka, J.G., Stoddard, A., Maul, L. and Costanza, M.E. "Interval Adherence to Mammography Screening Guidelines." *Medical Care* 29 (1991): 697–707.

49 Phillips, J.M., Cohen, M.Z. and Moses, G. "Breast Cancer Screening and African American Women: Fear, Fatalism, and Silence." *Oncology Nursing Forum* 26 (1999): 561–71.

50 Wolff, M., Bates, T., Beck, B., et al. "Cancer Prevention in Underserved African American Communities: Barriers and Effective Strategies—A Review of the Literature." *Western Journal of Medicine* 102 (2003): 36–40.

51 Skinner, C.S., Strecher, V.J. and Hospers, H. "Physicians' Recommendations for Mammography: Do Tailored Messages Make a Difference?" *American Journal of Public Health* 84 (1994): 43–49.

13

Overview of Community-Based Participatory Research in Environmental Health

STEPHANI S. KIM, MPH AND ERIN N. HAYNES, DRPH, MS

Community-based participatory research (CBPR) incorporates the community to collaborate in the research process. Community members and groups are involved in the design and implementation of the study, as well as interpreting results and disseminating information back to the whole community. Environmental health is an ideal field to use CBPR approaches, since often communities raise health and environmental concerns over various contaminants and environmental issues. This chapter highlights five environmental health studies that used CPBR practices in the United States and China. The studies span various environmental pollutants, such as hog waste, air pollution, heavy metals, and organic pollutants, and human health outcomes, including but not limited to asthma, cancer, and cognitive development. Each case study highlights the formation of academic-community partnerships, the role of the community partners, and actions that resulted from the partnership.

Introduction

Community-based participatory research (CBPR) has been defined as "a methodology that promotes active community involvement in the processes that shape research and intervention strategies, as well as in the conduct of research studies."[1] The CBPR approach incorporates community into the research paradigm from inception of research question, study design, dissemination of results, to development of interventions or policy recommendations to effect change. The environmental health research community was one of the early adopters of this academic–community partnership strategy. The field of environmental health lends itself to community-engaged research, as it is the community residents who are grappling with issues of exposure, noise, smell, and possible health consequences and are often the ones initiating the research agenda.

In the United States, the National Institute of Environmental Health Sciences (NIEHS) has taken a leading role in promoting CBPR in research. The NIEHS implemented the Partnerships in Environmental Public Health (PEPH) umbrella program to fund community/stakeholder participation in research[2] and has endorsed the following six principles for effective CBPR in environmental health research, outlined in Box 13.1.

Briefly, principle one, "*Defines community as a unit of identity*," is often one of the largest challenges faced by CBPR researchers. Community can refer to residents of a particular geographic area, an ethnic population, workers from a defined industry, or individuals connected by social networks. Ultimately, the community is those who are most affected by the environmental health issue and who are most likely to be affected by the research.

Principle two, "*Promotes active collaboration and participation at every stage of research*," establishes the community partner as a member of the scientific team and includes the community partner(s) in every step of the research process. Research teams are typically composed of scientists with expertise in their respective field; and the scientific community has long recognized the importance of cross-disciplinary or interdisciplinary teams as the most effective in addressing challenging research questions. Researchers working in CBPR expanded the research team to include community stakeholders. These stakeholders may be representatives from the public health community, such as local physicians, public officials, and decision-makers who can address or implement the research findings, and concerned community residents, such as residents experiencing the environmental problems or who have concern about their health or the health of their children potentially exposed to environmental chemicals or other toxicants. The inclusion of these community experts enhances the conduct of the research study. Community partner team members have increased the capacity of the research team by increasing capacity of data collection, analysis, and

---

Box 13.1 **NIEHS Endorsed Principles for Effective Community-Based Participatory Research in Environmental Health**

1. Defines community as a unity of identity.
2. Promotes active collaboration and participation at every stage of the research process.
3. Fosters colearning of all team members.
4. Ensures that research projects are community-driven.
5. Disseminates research results in useful terms.
6. Ensures research and intervention strategies are culturally appropriate.

interpretation; reduction of iatrogenic effects of research; enhancing the relevance of research for community; and maximizing the data disclosure process or the return of research results, thereby leading to improved policy and practice.[3–8]

Principle three, *"Fosters colearning of all research team members,"* acknowledges the expertise of community partners. Environmental health scientists, although expert in their respective field, do not have expertise about the particular community, that is the issues faced by residents, how the community "works," trusted leaders, and so forth. The expertise of the community partner is essential for the conduct of the research study. Both partners, academic and community, need to rely on and appreciate the expertise that the other brings to the research team. Within environmental health research, principle four, *"Ensures projects are community-driven,"* places the guiding force of the study in the concerns or issues raised by community members. The scientific team members rely on the issues identified by the community as the basis for the research. Principle five, *"Disseminates research results in useful terms,"* is critical for building and maintaining trust among all research partners. Involvement of community partners in the development of data disclosure strategies ensures that the approach is culturally appropriate, understandable to the target audience, respectful of the target community, and useful for next steps taken by the community. Principle six requires that the conduct of CBPR in environmental health research *"Ensures that research and intervention strategies are culturally appropriate."* Research that includes active participation from the target community has a strong likelihood of developing research and data disclosure strategies that are based in the cultural context of the community, thereby increasing community participation in the research.

This chapter illustrates how these principles have been applied in five community–academic environmental health research studies. These examples include US residents who are predominantly underrepresented communities and have struggled to understand their exposure from oil and metal refineries, hog farms, and port traffic, and a community in China balancing economic development with a healthy environment for human health. Within each case study, we describe the environmental health issue of concern, how the partnership began, the role of the partners (academic and community), and what we know from the literature about how the issue resolved. We begin with one of the earliest examples of CBPR in environmental health: the academic–community partnership formed between concerned residents of communities surrounded by large hog farms and an epidemiologist from North Carolina University, Dr. Steve Wing.

Case Study 1: North Carolina Hog Farms

North Carolina is the second largest pork producing state in the United States, with farms concentrated in the eastern part of the state.[9] Over a span of 20 years, the number of hog farms in the United States dropped by 70% to fewer than

56,000 farms in 2012, but productivity in the pork industry increased.[10] Prior to 1992, only a small fraction of hogs were raised on farms of more than 2,000 animals, but by 2012, 97% of hogs were being raised on farms with over 2,000 animals.[11] The majority of the hog farms are located in low-income counties. These counties also have a higher proportion of African Americans. Many of the large hog farms were built around predominantly black neighborhoods, surrounding black churches and schools.[12,13]

In the early 1990s, the pork industry announced that it would build 17 new hog production facilities in Halifax County in northeastern North Carolina. There was the promise of economic development in a predominantly low-income, minority population.[12,14] The residents were soon concerned about the potential noxious odors, air pollution, and ground water contamination from the CAFOs. However, since there was so scientific evidence to back up claims, the residents did not have power against the pork industry's development. Residents grew frustrated when they took their concerns about health and pollution to government officials, where they were told that it was anecdotal with no clear patterns. They began keeping diaries and taking photographs to document health problems, waste spills, and hog carcasses. In 1996, a grassroots organization, Concerned Citizens of Tillery, collaborated on a CBPR project with the University of North Carolina School of Public Health funded by NIEHS's Environmental Justice: Partnership for Communication program.[12]

Community partners identified study populations and sources of data, chose and defined variables, and interpreted the results alongside the researchers.[12] They also served as community consultants, who traveled with trained interviewers from UNC to homes of study participants to administer the health survey.[12] These consultants played a critical role in building trust between the UNC investigators and the study population. The study found an increased frequency of runny nose, headache, sore throat, coughing, diarrhea, and eye irritation in residents living in hog farm communities than in a cattle-farming community that was used as a comparison group.[15]

Prior to submitting the reports to the North Carolina State Department of Health and Human Services, UNC researchers held meetings with the three communities to discuss the preliminary findings. The community members and partners decided they did not wish to release the names of the communities in the report. The UNC researchers removed information that characterized the communities to keep them from being identified.[12] The same day the results were announced in a press release, Dr. Wing received a request to release the names of study participants, location of their homes, responses from the questionnaire, and all documents related to the study from lawyers for the North Carolina Pork Council.[16] Although UNC Chapel Hill counseled Dr. Wing to provide the requested information, he hired a lawyer and was able to redact documents to protect the identities of communities and participants.[16]

In 1997, the North Carolina General Assembly placed a moratorium on building hog farms with the traditional waste pits and spraying methods. In 2007, the moratorium became a law, with the state and the pork production industry funding studies to find improved methods of waste management. Although residents continue to suffer from the odors years after the study, there has been progress to control the environmental quality for nearby communities.[13,17]

Case Study 2: Northern California Household Exposure Study

Richmond, California, is home to one of the largest oil refineries in the United States. The refinery, owned by Chevron, processes over 240,000 barrels of crude oil each day over a space of 2,900 acres. Crude oil is necessary to make diesel fuel, jet fuel, gasoline, and lubricants. Richmond residents were found to have an increased risk incidence of breast cancer, which was higher than the state rate.[18] Residents of the city also have an increased risk of respiratory diseases that have been linked to industrial emissions, and the county has one of the state's highest asthma prevalence rates (15%).[18]

Individuals can be exposed to crude oil if they live near an oil refinery or if there is a spill or leak. Humans can also be exposed through contaminated seafood.[19] When crude oil is burned it contains chemicals that are toxic to humans, including lead, carbon dioxide, carbon monoxide, polycyclic aromatic hydrocarbons (PAHs), particulate matter (PM), sulfur dioxide, and volatile organic compounds (VOCs).[19] These chemicals are associated with adverse health effects, such as neurodevelopmental problems, respiratory disease, cardiovascular disease, and cancer.

A community primarily composed of low-income and minority residents noticed that many people in their community were being diagnosed with cancer, particularly breast cancer, along with asthma and problems with child development. The residents of Liberty Village and Atchison Village in Richmond, Contra Costa County, California, were concerned that the Chevron oil refinery, along with a truck, rail, and shipping corridor, might be related to their health issues. The 2000 Census revealed that the population of the two villages were 61% Latino, 18% African American, and 3% Asian American; 26% of residents were below the federal poverty level. This raised environmental justice concerns.

The Northern California Household Exposure Study (HES) was a collaborative research project by Silent Spring Institute, Brown University, the University of California, Berkeley, and Communities for a Better Environment (CBE), an environmental justice organization that focuses on organizing the community and changing policies and legislation (http://www.cbecal.org/). Silent Spring Institute focuses on environment and women's health, particularly breast cancer (http://www.silentspring.org/).

In the HES, community members collaborated in all aspects of the study, and the research partners communicated regularly through conference calls, in-person meetings, and training sessions.[20] Members of CBE were trained to collect environmental samples from homes and conduct interviews. They were the ones to approach residents in Atchison Village and Liberty Village.[18] The study included advisory councils, which comprised leaders from four community-based organizations: Breast Cancer Action, Breast Cancer Fund, Commonweal, and West County Toxics Coalition. The advisory board also included two residents from Richmond, one environmental health scientist, and one state public health official.[20] The council met annually and made suggestions for the study, including adding a comparison group in a rural area.

The research team conducted an exposure study in Richmond from 2004 to 2009 to characterize pollutants from indoor and outdoor sources.[18] A rural neighborhood in Bolinas was used as a comparison community. The team identified 80 compounds in the outdoor air and 104 compounds indoors in Richmond compared to 60 compounds in the outdoor air and 69 in the indoor air in Bolinas.[18] Of the 56 compounds that the two communities had in common, 33 were detected at significantly higher levels in the outdoor Richmond air versus one compound that was significantly higher in Bolinas. Compounds at higher levels in Richmond included sulfates, nickel, and vanadium, which are related to refineries, and fine particulate matter ($PM_{2.5}$), elemental carbon, and PAHs, which are related to transportation and combustion.[18] They also found that nearly half of the homes in Richmond were above California's annual ambient air quality standard for $PM_{2.5}$ and that levels were higher indoors than outdoors in both communities.[18] Correlation analysis showed that some of the chemicals were seeping into the homes from the outdoors, in particular sulfates, nickel, and vanadium, which are more harmful components found in $PM_{2.5}$.[18]

While this project was being conducted, changes in permits for refineries were proposed that would have increased the release of pollutants into the environment. The research group and CBE testified before the Richmond Planning Commission. Participants in the study testified using their own data, environmental measurements, and stories to paint a powerful picture of the health effects on the community.[18] The planning commission attempted to restrict high-sulfur refining of crude oil but, in July 2008, the original Chevron proposal was approved after increasing gas prices allowed the company to offer the city of Richmond $60 million in mitigation benefits.[18] In November 2008, newly elected council members and Richmond residents supported and passed a ballot that required Chevron to pay an annual business license fee of $26.5 million.[18] Later, a court decision required that Chevron prepare a cumulative impact assessment prior to approval of refinery expansion. A recent agreement between Chevron and the city has yielded a large corporate contribution for social benefits, though there is dispute about who will control that process.

In December 2015, the San Francisco Bay Area Air Resources Board planned to vote on "the strictest controls in the nation" to reduce pollution from the five largest oil refineries in the Bay Area by cutting 16% of overall emissions a year.[21] This came after a fire at the Chevron Richmond refinery sent over 10,000 people to the hospital with sore throats, noses, and eye irritation.[21] Chevron and the other refineries, including Shell, Phillips 66, Tesoro, and Valero claim that the controls are too strict without enough evidence that it will benefit public health, whereas CBE and other environmental justice groups contend that the controls are not sufficient.[21]

Communities for a Better Environment gained important benefits from the project, including exposure reduction, recognition for political acumen, an opportunity to engage and educate community residents, and scientific training for members. They used the HES as a jumping-off point to seek a survey of Richmond's health status, for which Silent Spring negotiated a research grant, and the Berkeley partners collaborated with CBE on conducting a survey that showed high asthma rates and other indicators of poor health.

Case Study 3: Southern California Goods Movement, THE (Trade, Health, Environment) Impact Project

"Goods movement," or the transport of imported goods (mostly from Asia) into the United States, is essential for economic growth and trade; however, with the mass movement of goods, particularly through the ports/rail yards/and on roadways, there are related adverse health effects. Two of the largest ports in the United States are located in Southern California, at the Los Angeles and Long Beach Ports. At the time of the study, the two ports received up to 40% of all US imports.[22]

The combined emissions from the ships, trains, and trucks, along with the cranes and other yard equipment, create an environment heavy with diesel particulate matter. In 2012, the International Agency for Research on Cancer (IARC) declared diesel engine exhaust as a Group 1 carcinogen, or "carcinogenic to humans based on sufficient evidence that exposure is associated with increased risk for lung cancer."[23] Rail yards, highways, and shipping ports also emit particulate matter (PM), metals, sulfur dioxide, and PAHs, which are known to cause a variety of diseases in humans, particularly in children, who are more vulnerable to air pollution.[24,25]

At the time the Union Pacific Intermodal Container Transfer Facility (ICTF) was built in the 1980s, demographic data indicated that the communities surrounding the site were predominately working poor people of color.[26] The Final Environmental Impact Report (EIR) from 1986 stated, "Air quality impacts of the ICTF on adjacent residential areas are anticipated to be insignificant" despite the air pollution concerns of residents at a nearby mobile park.[26] Since then residents have raised concerns about the chemical pollution and noise from the goods movement ports.[26,27]

In 2006 THE (Trade, Health, Environment) Impact Project was launched to address adverse health effects related to diesel exposure. THE Impact Project was a CBPR collaboration between a local university and college and four advocacy groups that were concerned about the goods movement's impact on human health, including the Community Outreach and Engagement Program (COEP) at the Environmental Health Sciences Center at the University of Southern California (USC), the Urban and Environmental Policy Institute at Occidental College (http://www.oxy.edu/urban-environmental-policy-institute), East Yard Communities for Environmental Justice (EYCEJ) in Los Angeles (http://eycej.org/), Center for Community Action and Environmental Justice (CCAEJ) in Riverside (http://www.ccaej.org/), Coalition for a Safe Environment (CFASE), and the Long Beach Alliance for Children with Asthma (LBACA, http://lbaca.org/).[27] From its formation, the goal of THE Impact Project was "to shift the policy debate and make the goods movement industry accountable for its decision-making by taking under consideration the health and environmental impacts from multiple sources of air pollution."[27]

Prior to the formalized collaboration of THE Impact Project, there were informal relationships between USC's COEP and various community-based organizations with funding from NIEHS. With increasing success of research and community outreach from the informal collaborations, and funding from a foundation, the California Endowment, in 2005 allowed the groups to create a formal partnership.[27] The community partners recruited residents from Riverside, Wilmington, Long Beach, and Commerce who were then trained by USC staff on diesel particulate matter and goods movement. These residents made up the Neighborhood Assessment Teams, also called "A" teams, which functioned as citizen scientists in their respective communities. They measured air pollution and counted traffic in the neighborhood. Researchers analyzed data collected by the "A" teams and the results were disseminated to the communities and government agencies. The "A" teams were also able to collect data on new issues for which USC researchers previously had little or no information, so that scientists were also informed of community knowledge.[27] This academic–community partnership provided data and resources that were not being collected or could not be collected by any single entity, including the industries, the government, or academic researchers. Because of the relationships that the residents have with the community, the team was also able to collect information that researchers might not have been able to.[27]

In 2006, the project and its six partners were major players in the passage of the Ports of Los Angeles and Long Beach Clean Air Action Plan (CAAP), which created a 5-year plan to decrease pollution from the ports by 45%. Members of

THE Impact Project were also invited to sit on the CAAP implementation task force formed by the mayor of Los Angeles, which allowed for a delayed implementation of a 2010 update that would have been weaker than the 2006 version.[27] Members of the project have continued to be active in testifying at public hearings about new construction of rail yards and roadways. They have been effective in asking for environmental impact reports that include potential threats to human health. The CBPR approach used by Hricko and her collaborators empowered residents to continue the battle to a cleaner environment in and around their neighborhoods.

Case Study 4: Rural Eastern Ohio Ferromanganese Refinery, Marietta Community Actively Researching Exposure Study (CARES)

Manganese (Mn) is an essential nutrient for normal physiologic function, yet at high levels of exposure, Mn can be neurotoxic.[28] When Mn is ingested, it is subject to homeostatic control and it travels through the digestive system;[29] however, when Mn is inhaled it can enter directly into the circulatory system, bypassing the liver and accumulating in the brain.[30] In occupational studies, Mn has been shown to affect the central nervous system, causing symptoms similar to Parkinson's disease, and to have adverse effects in the lung, cardiac, and reproductive systems.[31]

Marietta, Ohio, is home to the largest ferromanganese refinery in North America and is the world's largest producer of Mn alloys and Mn-based products.[32] Concerned about their exposure to Mn, the community organized themselves as Neighbors for Clean Air (NCA). The community had experienced "bitter metallic taste, headaches, burning eyes, fatigue, muscle aches, tremors, and nose bleeds."[33] Caroline Beidler, a resident of Marietta and concerned citizen, organized NCA to capture their experiences of this "toxic mist."[33] The community logged their experiences in the form of a "stink diary." The NCA mobilized to collect "swipe" samples for metals analysis and petitioned their state representative to help them identify their exposure and potential health effects. The NCA also reached out to a larger environmental organization, Ohio Citizen Action (OCA). The OCA worked with the NCA to develop an environmental audit of the industry and sought out academic expertise. The OCA invited Dr. Erin Haynes (a coauthor of this chapter) to provide expertise on the health effects of manganese. The development of this partnership and subsequent pilot studies that led to a larger epidemiologic study is detailed elsewhere.[33] Briefly, during the initial meeting, the community outlined their numerous research questions related to their exposure. "Does Mn affect cognitive development of children?" was their leading concern. During the meeting, a community advisory board (CAB) was formed to help guide the research. A few community partners on the CAB served as advisors for the research and as part of the academic–community research team. The community–academic team jointly conducted qualitative and quantitative pilot studies before preparing and submitting a CBPR research proposal to NIEHS. The funded study, Marietta Community Actively Researching Exposure Study (CARES), or Marietta CARES, was conducted using a CBPR approach from inception of the research idea to dissemination of research results.

In the pilot studies, both qualitative and quantitative data were collected. The community partners were involved in writing the qualitative research questions to determine the level of concern about Mn in the larger community, perception of risk, barriers to improving air quality, and whether the larger community would participate in a research study and allow their children to participate. The CAB reviewed and approved final drafts of the survey before submission to the University of Cincinnati (UC) institutional review board (IRB). Community partners also provided expertise on survey participant recruitment. Data were entered into REDCAp by academic team members, and shared with community partners for interpretation and preparation of the manuscript.[33] In the quantitative component of the pilot studies, the community identified possible locations for the study, reviewed the protocol for the cultural appropriateness of the recruitment and consent language, reviewed summary data, and assisted with preparation of manuscripts for publication.[34]

In the conduct of the full-scale epidemiologic study, Marietta CARES, community expertise was key to identification of study location, recruitment strategies, data collection, data entry, data interpretation, development of data disclosure strategies, and manuscript development. Community expertise was also enhanced as colearning equipped them to have an active role in the conduct of the study, as they were employed by UC in roles of research assistants, environmental sampling team members, co-investigators, and coprincipal investigator. Beilder was the coprincipal investigator of the research study and was hired to lead the environmental sampling team (EST). She coordinated the collection of all participant home environmental sampling. Community members were recruited to be part of the EST and provided with training using HUD-approved training modules for home dust, water, and soil collection.

Community partners were also trained to collect personal and stationary air samples,[34] postural balance assessment,[35] collection of biological samples, and parent and child neurodevelopmental assessments.[36] To ensure data integrity, these research study components required extensive training, data monitoring, and oversight from environmental health experts at UC. Prior to building the online child educational pages for the CARES website, the team evaluated the website using feedback from children to enhance its usefulness for the children in Marietta.[37] Similarly, the community–academic team evaluated the online journalist training related to "air particles and health."[38]

The CBPR approach to this research empowered the community residents to take action as they become immersed in the conduct of the epidemiologic research study. The CAB continued to provide study guidance throughout the research. Once the study was funded, the ferromanganese industry that had previously rejected the community's repeated requests to meet with them, invited NCA to meet with their leadership, thereby providing dialogue between the community and the industry. Moreover, the data collected within CARES has been useful to the community as they had peer-reviewed literature to cite in their responses to the Environmental Protection Agency's ruling for emissions from ferromanganese industries.[39]

Case Study 5: The China Jintan Child Cohort Study

China's population reached one billion in the early 1980s.[40] India, the next country to reach a population of one billion, would not reach this point until 2001, nearly 20 years after China. In 2015, China, with a population of 1.3 billion, was named the second largest economy in the world by the World Bank.[41] China has experienced rapid economic and social development since the late 1970s; however, it has come at a great cost to the environment and the health of its people.

China faces a wide range of environmental problems from outdoor and indoor air pollution, water contamination from fecal waste and chemicals from various industries, deforestation, and issues with sustainability.[42] The Chinese central government acknowledges these problems and has made improving environmental policies a priority.[42] In addition, though rare, "grassroots" efforts to combat environmental issues are beginning to form. The following case study highlights efforts to use CBPR methods in a cohort study in Jintan.

The China Jintan Child Cohort Study (CJCCS) was established in 2004 as a partnership between governmental health and medical agencies (Jintan Department of Health, Jintan Hospital, and Jintan Maternal and Child Health Center), parents and teachers from community schools, and researchers from four universities (University of Pennsylvania, China Southeastern University, Shanghai Jiaotong University, and Hong Kong University).[43] The study was initiated to address concerns of lead exposure, other environmental exposures, nutrition, and health outcomes in children.

Jintan is located between Shanghai and Nanjing in Jiangsu Province. As of June 1, 2015, Jintan City became Jintan District of Changzhou City. Jintan District has many rivers, canals, and lakes, with water occupying one-fifth of its surface area. It was traditionally a farming community, but industry has expanded and now accounts for over 80% of the city's GDP.[44] The city houses a variety of smelters and factories that have led to environmental pollution.[43] Parents of young children raised concerns of lead exposure and nutritional factors and adverse health effects to local public health workers.

Previous studies had shown elevated levels of lead in children from hair samples, but because of limited capabilities, the public health workers reached out to an investigator from the University of Pennsylvania (UPenn), who was originally from the region and had maintained contact with academics and professionals in China. Local public health leaders formalized an invitation to the investigator to form a collaboration, which then expanded to include the Shanghai Key Laboratory for Children's Environmental Health as an academic partner with a children's environmental component, as it was the only lab in China with a focus on children's environmental health. Also, CJCCS includes three additional academic partners, including China Southeastern University, which focuses on nutrition; Nanjing Brain Hospital, which focuses on child cognitive development; and Hong Kong University's Psychology Department, which focuses on assessing child behavioral outcomes.[43]

The Jintan public health workers were interested in determining major sources of lead exposure, if current levels were adversely affecting neurobehavior and cognitive development in children, and approaches to reduce exposure and reduce adverse health outcomes.[43] The PI, local health staff, and community members began designing a study protocol. A working group of the health department, JMCHC, Jintan Hospital, and a local school board determined appropriate communities and community partnerships.[43]

The team of academic researchers and public health workers identified communities by establishing a working group of government, hospital, and school board members. This working group identified four preschools (Jianshe, Huacheng, Xuebu, and Huashan) that covered urban, suburban, and rural populations within Jintan.[43] Once the schools were identified, a steering committee of parent representatives was formed to add to the list of community partners, which already included the hospital, schools, and local health department. These community partners were active in all parts of the study from developing to research protocol to completing fieldwork to disseminating the findings.[43]

When conducting a study in another country where English is not the primary language, translating validated instruments and documents correctly can be difficult. In addition, in other cultures childrearing might be different from childrearing in the United States; for example, in China there is more involvement of grandparents than there is in the United States. Also, behavior assessment often has a cultural context. The steering committee evaluated the questionnaires, which were then revised based on their suggestions while considering cross-cultural applications.[45]

Research staff was hired from within the community partner groups. The nurses and teachers were able to bridge the gap between study participants and the research team. The use of locals as research staff played a vital role in recruitment and follow-up, with 88% participating in the first follow-up.[43]

Preliminary analysis of data from recruitment showed a median blood lead level (BLL) of 6.2 µg/dL, and 7.8% of the children had elevated BLL (≥10 µg/dL).[43] In 2012, the US Centers for Disease Control and Prevention lowered the level of concern for BLL from 10 µg/dL to 5 µg/dL.[46] Lead is known to be associated with a number of adverse health effects even at low levels, therefore the CDC aims to keep BLLs for 95% of the US population under 5 µg/dL.[46] The team also found that higher BLLs had certain predictors, including being female, older, having siblings, living in a crowded neighborhood or in a rural area, smoking in the home, and eating breakfast less than five times a week.[43] The academic team reported its preliminary findings in 2008 to the city council and community. This led to other actions by the community partners to look at other routes of exposures.[43] As of 2015, the children from the kindergarten cohort were in high school and the research teams continued to follow the children with plans to collect additional data in coming years with the help of the community partners.[47]

Though China faces overwhelming obstacles associated with a variety of environmental pollution, it is not too late to change lifestyles and policies to protect public health of its people. There is a tendency to distrust government and even academics when it comes to environmental pollution and its effects on human health, but CBPR is an ideal method to build relationships between all stakeholders and improve the environment and public health.

Future of CBPR in Environmental Health

Through these examples of highly impactful community-engaged environmental health research, it is clear that the CBPR approach allows for "trust between researchers and community, increased relevance of research question, increased quantity and quality of data collection, increased use and relevance of data, increased dissemination, translates research into policy, emergence of new research questions, extend research and intervention beyond specific project, and builds infrastructure and sustainability."[8]

Also, CBPR lends itself well to the growing movement of citizen science. Citizen science was popularized by the National Audubon Society, employing bird watchers to track and monitor bird migrations. There is an increasing number of citizen science opportunities.[48–50] Research studies are using community members to collect data for their research. The largest research areas to use citizen science are biology, conservation, and ecology.[51] Citizen science extends beyond the CBPR approach; however, CBPR can be strengthened using the tools provided by citizen science.

Studies using CBPR can also be enhanced using novel technology for real-time environmental and biological sampling. These new technologies are combining GPS with air monitoring and health outcome data, equipping community residents with tools to engage with researchers and collect their own data. Dr. Kim

Anderson and her team at Oregon State University have developed a wristband that passively samples chemicals not only in air and water but also from the skin.[52] The wristband is being used in several studies, including Dr. Haynes and the CARES partnership. There is an increasing number of small-scale and hand-held particle counters to measure various types of exposures in and around homes. Participating community members can be trained to use and maintain these tools for use in research studies.

In addition, online resources are becoming accessible to the public. The Environmental Protection Agency (EPA) uses the EJSCREEN: Environmental Justice Screening and Mapping Tool, which allows users to select a location in the United States to look for possible nearby environmental quality issues along with demographic and socioeconomic information. The EJSCREEN can be used by both research and community members to identify potential risk factors for a

Table 13.1 **Best Practices from CBPR in Environmental Health**

Study	Best Practices
North Carolina Hog Farms (NC, USA)	• Community meetings • Community partners involved in planning of study, collecting data, interpreting results, and disseminating information
Northern California HES (CA, USA)	• Regular communication between all partners • Annual meeting • Used community members to collect data
THE Impact Project (CA, USA)	• Created formal partnership between academic institutions and community groups • Residents completed the neighborhood assessments • Residents were able to collect "new" information previously unknown to researchers
Marietta CARES (OH, USA)	• Community meetings • Research question came from the community • Community leader was a coinvestigator for the study • Community partners involved in each step of study
Jintan Child Cohort Study (Jintan, China)	• Partnership of academic institutions, local government, hospitals, schools, and the community • Steering committee also included parents of children from the schools • Research questions addressed community concerns • Research staff hired from the local community (teachers, nurses) • Used locals to translate study materials

particular community. The EPA noted that "this screening information may be of interest to community residents or other stakeholders as they search for environmental or demographic information and can also support a wide range of research and policy goals."[53]

In 2009 the EPA followed NIEHS's example and released a request for research applications (RFA) that specifically had a community engagement component. The funded studies focused on developing methods for cumulative risk assessment on mixtures of nonchemical and chemical stressors since human health is determined by a combination of factors. In addition to NIEHS, the W.K. Kellogg Foundation founded the Community Health Scholars Program to train postdoctoral fellows in CBPR practices in hopes "to increase the number of new faculty members committed to CBPR and the development of successful academic/community partnerships."[54] Although the program ended in 2012, alumni from the program established an alumni network to continue collaborating on "attaining health equity and equality" in the United States.[55]

The remarkable history of CBPR in environmental health research provides strong examples of academic–community partnerships. Table 13.1 summarizes examples of best practices used in the five case studies. Combined with the new technologies, online resources, and tools offered by citizen science, the future of CBPR in environmental health is bright. Environmental health community–academic partnerships have demonstrated the power of engaging community in research.

Acknowledgments

The authors recognize the significant contribution of Dr. Steve Wing, Dr. Phil Brown, Dr. Julia Brody, Dr. Andrea Hricko, and Dr. Jianghong Liu, who provided valuable insight and editorial comments on their case studies.

References

1. O'Fallon, L.R., Tyson, F.L. and Dearry, A., eds. *Successful Models of Community-Based Participatory Research: Final Report.* Research Triangle Park, NC: National Institute of Environmental Health Sciences, 2000.
2. Birnbaum, L.S. "NIEHS Supports Partnerships in Environmental Public Health." *Prog Community Health Partnership* 3 (2009):195–196.
3. Israel, B.A., Schulz, A.J., Parker, E.A. and Becker, A.B. "Review of Community-Based Research: Assessing Partnership Approaches to Improve Public Health." *Annual Review of Public Health* 19 (1998): 173–202.
4. Israel, B.A., Schulz, A.J., Parker, E.A. and Becker, A.B. "Community-Based Participatory Research: Policy Recommendations for Promoting a Partnership Approach in Health Research." *Edu for Health* 14 (2001): 182–97.
5. Israel, B. A., Eng, E., Schulz, A. J., and Parker, E. A. *Methods in Community-Based Participatory Research for Health.* San Francisco: Jossey-Bass, 2005.

6. Macaulay, A.C, Commanda, L.E., Freeman, W.L., et al. "Participatory Research Maximizes Community and Lay Involvement." *British Medical Journal* 319 (1999): 774–8.

7. Minkler, M. and Wallerstein, N., eds. *Community-Based Participatory Research for Health: From Process to Outcomes* (2nd ed.). San Francisco: Jossey-Bass, 2008.

8. O'Fallon, L.R. and Dearry, A. "Community-Based Participatory Research as a Tool to Advance Environmental Health Sciences." *Environmental Health Perspectives* 110 (2002):155–9.

9. NCGE (North Carolina in the Global Economy). "Hog Farming." Duke University, 2015. (accessed August 19, 2015).

10. Food & Water Watch. "Factory Farm Nation." 2015. (accessed August 19, 2015).

11. Food & Water Watch. "Fact Sheet: Pork Processing Highly Concentrated, Hog Production Vertically Integrated." 2011. (accessed August 19, 2015).

12. Wing, S. "Social Responsibility and Research Ethics in Community-Driven Studies of Industrialized Hog Production" *Environmental Health Perspectives* 110 (2002): 437–44.

13. Hardy, S. "The Price of Pork." *Endeavors*, 2012, January 4. (accessed August 19, 2015).

14. Wing, S., Cole D. and Grant G. "Environmental Injustice in North Carolina's Hog Industry." *Environmental Health Perspectives* 108 (2000): 225–31.

15. Wing, S. and Wolf, S. "Intensive Livestock Operations, Health, and Quality of Life Among Eastern North Carolina Residents." *Environmental Health Perspectives* 108 (2000): 233–38.

16. Wing, S. "Environmental Injustice Connects Local Food Environments with Global Food Production." In *Local Food Environments: Food Access in America*, ed. K. B. Morland. Boca Raton, FL: CRC Press, 2015.

17. Henderson, B. "NC Hog Farm Neighbors Seek Court Help to Stop the Stink." *News Observer*. 2015, January 1. (accessed August 19, 2015).

18. Brody, J.G., Morello-Frosch, R., Zota, A., et al. "Linking Exposure Assessment Science with Policy Objectives for Environmental Justice and Breast Cancer Advocacy: The Northern California Household Exposure Study." *American Journal of Public Health* Suppl 3 (2009): S600–9.

19. NIH (National Institute of Health). "Tox Town: Crude Oil." 2015. (accessed 20 November 20, 2015).

20. Brown, P., Brody, J.G., Morello-Frosch, R., et al. "Measuring the Success of Community Science: The Northern California Household Exposure Study." *Environmental Health Perspective* 120 (2012): 326–31.

21. Cuff, D. "Plan to Curb Bay Area Oil Refinery Emissions Touted as Toughest in Nation." *Inside Bay Area News*. 2015, November 27. (accessed December 3, 2015).

22. Air Resources Board. *Emission Reduction Plan for Ports and Goods Movement in California, Final*. California EPA. 2006, April 20. (accessed November 24, 2015).

23. IARC (International Agency for Research on Cancer). "IARC: Diesel Engine Exhaust Carcinogenic." WHO press release 213. 2012. (accessed November 24, 2015).

24. EPA (Environmental Protection Agency). "Diesel Exhaust and Your Health." 2015. (accessed November 24, 2015).

25. EPA (Environmental Protection Agency). "Diesel Particulate Matter." (2015). (accessed November 24, 2015).

26. Hricko, A., Rowland, G., Eckel, S., et al. "Global Trade, Local Impacts: Lessons from California on Health Impacts and Environmental Justice Concerns for Residents Living Near Freight Rail Yards." *International Journal of Environmental Research and Public Health* 11 (2014): 1914–41.

27. Garcia, A.P., Wallerstein, N., Hricko, A., et al. "THE (Trade, Health, Environment) Impact Project: A Community-Based Participatory Research Environmental Justice Case Study." *Environmental Justice* 6 (2013): 17–26.

28. ATSDR (Agency for Toxic Substances and Disease Registry). "Toxicological Profile for Manganese." CDC CAS# 7439-96-5 (2012). (accessed November 19, 2015).

29. Papavasiliou, P.S., Miller, S.T. and Cotzias, G.C. "Role of Liver in Regulating Distribution and Excretion of Manganese." *American Journal of Physiology* 211 (1966): 211–6.

30. Elder, A., Gelein, R., Silva, V., et al. "Translocation of Inhaled Ultrafine Manganese Oxide Particles to the Central Nervous System." *Environ Health Perspect* 114 (2006): 1172–8.
31. Crossgrove, J. and Zheng, W. "Manganese Toxicity Upon Overexposure." *NMR Biomed* 17 (2004): 544–53.
32. Eramet Marietta, Inc. "Company History." 2016. (accessed January 20, 2016).
33. Haynes, E., Beidler, C., Wittberg, R., et al. "Developing a Bidirectional Academic-Community Partnership with an Appalachian-American Community for Environmental Health Research and Risk Communication." *Environ Health Perspect* 119 (2011): 1364–72.
34. Haynes, E., Heckel, P., Ryan, P., et al. "Environmental Manganese Exposure in Residents Living Near a Ferromanganese Refinery in Southeast Ohio: A Pilot Study." *NeuroToxicology* 31 (2010): 468–74.
35. Rugless, F., Bhattacharya, A., Succop, P., et al. "Childhood Exposure to Manganese and Postural Instability in Children Living Near a Ferromanganese Refinery in Southeastern Ohio." *Neurotoxicology and Teratology* 41 (2014): 71–9.
36. Haynes, E., Sucharew, H., Kuhnell, P., et al. "Manganese Exposure and Neurocognitive Outcomes in Rural School-Age Children: The Communities Actively Research Exposures Study (Ohio, USA)." *Environmental Health Perspectives* 123 (2015): 1066–71.
37. Meloncon, L., Haynes, E., Varelmann, M. and Groh, L. "Building a Playground: General Guidelines for Creating Educational Web Sites for Children." *Tech Commun* 57 (2010): 398–416.
38. Parin, M., Yancey, E., Beidler, C. and Haynes, E. "Efficacy of Environmental Health e-Training for Journalists." *Stud Media Commun* 2 (2014): 71–80.
39. EPA (Environmental Protection Agency). "Rule and Implementation Information for Ferromanganese and Silicomanganese Production." Docket ID EPA-HQ-OAR-2010-0895. 2015, September 10. (accessed January 19, 2016).
40. United Nations Population Division. "India Becomes a Billionaire: World's Largest Democracy to Reach One Billion Persons on Independence Day." United Nations (2001). (accessed March 18, 2016).
41. The World Bank. "China." September 8, 2015. (accessed March 18, 2016).
42. Ali, R., Olden, K. and Xu, S. "Community-Based Participatory Research: A Vehicle to Promote Engagement for Environmental Health in China." *Environmental Health Perspectives* 116.10 (2008): 1281–4.
43. Liu, J., McCauley, L., Leung, P., et al. "Community-Based Participatory Research (CBPR) Approach to Study Children's Health in China: Experiences and Reflections." *International Journal of Nursing Studies* 48 (2011): 904–13.
44. Jiangsu. "Jintan." Jiangsu.net (2014). (accessed March 18, 2016).
45. Liu, J., Leung, P., Sun R., Li, H., and Liu, J. "Cross-Sectional Application of Achenbach System of Empirically Based Assessment (ASEBA): Process of Instrument Translation in Chinese Challenges and Future Directions." *World Journal of Pediatrics* 8 (2012): 5–10.
46. Centers for Disease Control and Prevention (CDC). "Lead." 2016, January 29. (accessed March 18, 2016).
47. Liu, J., Cao, S., Chen, Z., et al. "Cohort Profile Update: The China Jintan Child Cohort Study." *International Journal of Epidemiology* 44.5 (2015): 1548–48l.
48. Chillrud, S. and Jack, D. "NYC Cyclist Air Quality Study." *Scientific American*. June 16, 2015. (accessed January 19, 2016).
49. Chichewica, R. "Citizen Science Soil Collection Program." *Scientific American*. April 7, 2015. (accessed January 19, 2016).
50. Malaspina, D. "The Smell Experience Project." *Scientific American*. 2016. (accessed January 19, 2016).
51. Kullenberg, C. and Kasperowski, D. "What Is Citizen Science?—A Scientometric Meta-Analysis." *PLOS One* 11 (2016): e0147152.
52. O'Connell, S.G., Kincl, L.D. and Anderson, K.A. "Silicone Wristbands as Personal Passive Samplers." *Environmental Science and Technology* 18 (2014): 3327–35.

53. EPA (Environmental Protection Agency). "Purposes and Uses of EJSCREEN" 2015. (accessed January 11, 2016).

54. W.K. Kellogg Foundation Community Health Scholars Program. *Stories of Impact* [brochure]. Ann Arbor: University of Michigan, School of Public Health, Community Health Scholars Program, National Program Office, 2001.

55. W.K. Kellogg Foundation. "Announcements." Kellogg Health Scholars. 2016. (accessed April 19, 2016).

14

Community-Based Participatory Research Studies on Interpersonal Violence

Ending the Cycle of Poverty and Violence

STEVEN S. COUGHLIN, PHD

This chapter provides an overview of the population health significance of inter-personal violence, its causes, and the prevention of interpersonal violence and intimate partner violence through evidence-based interventions. The roles of poverty and lack of economic opportunity in fueling youth violence, violence against women, and other forms of interpersonal violence are highlighted, as is the important role of CBPR studies in addressing interpersonal violence in diverse communities. Finally, lessons learned from CBPR studies on interpersonal violence are discussed and recommendations offered for further research including studies that examine the combined effectiveness of programs for violence prevention and creating economic opportunities.

The Population Health Importance of Interpersonal Violence

Each year, violence causes more than 1.6 million deaths worldwide.[1,2] More than 90% of these deaths occur in low- and middle-income countries.[3] Worldwide, an estimated 200,000 youth aged 10 to 29 years are murdered each year; about 83% of these deaths occur in males. Homicide is the fourth leading cause of death in young people. In addition to age and gender, disparities in homicide mortality have been identified according to race, ethnicity, socioeconomic status, and geographic locality.[4] Homicide rates also vary widely between countries. For example, in some countries in Latin America and Africa, youth homicide rates are ≥ 100 times higher than rates for countries in Western Europe and the Western Pacific.[1,3]

Youth violence includes bullying, slapping, hitting, and more serious acts such as robbery and assault that can result in injury or death. Young people can be a victim, an offender, or a witness to the violence.[5] People exposed to violence can develop mental health conditions such as posttraumatic stress disorder, major depression, and alcohol or drug abuse, and they are at increased risk of suicide.[3,6] The relation between exposure to violence-related trauma and posttraumatic stress disorder is one of dual causality. People suffering from posttraumatic stress disorder may attempt to self-medicate with alcohol or illicit drugs, which increases their risk of interpersonal violence, disrupted family relationships, unsafe sex, and becoming homeless or a victim of sexual violence.[6]

Other important categories of interpersonal violence include child abuse (physical, sexual, or emotional abuse), intimate partner violence (physical, sexual, or psychological harm by a current or former partner or spouse), and elder abuse.[5] In 2013, there were 678,932 victims of child abuse and neglect reported to Child Protective Services in the United States.[5] About 1,520 children died from abuse and neglect in 2013. Intimate partner violence is also frequent. About one in three women in the United States report ever having experienced physical violence, rape, or stalking by an intimate partner.[7] Important disparities in intimate partner violence and other forms of domestic violence have been identified. For example, male-to-female domestic violence is over two times more frequent among Hispanics and African Americans than among non-Hispanic Whites.[8]

Because behavior is influenced by events and exposures during earlier stages in life and early child development, a life-course approach can contribute to understanding the causes of interpersonal violence.[3] Maltreated children are at increased risk of either perpetrating or becoming the victim of interpersonal violence later in life. Many factors account for youth violence including individual characteristics (e.g., a history of involvement in crime, aggressive behavior, psychological conditions such as conduct disorder or substance abuse); family factors (e.g., poor parental supervision or parental involvement in crime); relationships with peers; and community characteristics such as poverty, income inequality, unemployment, neighborhood crime, gangs, and ease of access to guns and illicit drugs.[3]

The Linkages of Poverty and Violence

An estimated one in every four persons who live in developing countries, or about 1.2 billion people, live in conditions of extreme poverty.[9] Vulnerable populations living in poverty suffer from a wide range of adverse health outcomes including interpersonal violence.[10] Poverty is the main underlying cause of ill health in many rural and urban communities in Africa, Asia, Oceania, and Latin America. In many societies, gender-based violence reinforces gender inequities, negatively affects women's economic productivity, disrupts educational attainment, and perpetuates the cycle of poverty among women.[11,12] This includes gender-based violence against refugees and internally displaced persons.[13] Violence and poverty, particularly the combination of the two, contribute to an array of public health problems including HIV/AIDS, sexually transmitted diseases, and mental health conditions such as substance abuse and depression.[14-16] For example, in a CBPR study conducted in an impoverished community in Cape Town, South Africa, Mosavel et al.[16] found that many of the women who participated in focus groups were concerned about daily hardships, lack of employment and money, the complexity and fears of raising children with limited financial resources, hunger, poor and unsafe housing, overcrowded conditions, and the pervasiveness of violence and crime, and how these structural conditions contribute to children's risk behaviors.

Poverty also contributes to interpersonal violence in developed countries. In the United States, for example, youth who reside in socioeconomically deprived counties have an eightfold increased risk of homicide mortality than their counterparts who reside in the most affluent counties.[4] The relation between poverty and interpersonal violence is bidirectional, as high crime rates can depress neighborhood housing values and deter businesses and potential employers from moving into distressed communities. There are likely to be cyclical relationships between increased interpersonal violence, drugs, gangs, and other forms of criminal activity and the lack of economic opportunities for youth and other community members.

Prevention of Interpersonal Violence

An increasing number of studies have examined the effectiveness of community-engaged approaches for preventing youth violence and other forms of interpersonal violence.[3] However, relatively few studies have been conducted in low- and middle-income countries. Prevention efforts aim to reduce factors that place youth at risk for perpetrating violence, and promote factors that protect at-risk youth. Informational resources on prevention programs and strategies that have been research-tested and found to be effective at preventing violence among youth are summarized in Box 14.1.

The Guide to Community Preventive Services recommends school-based programs to reduce violence along with individual or group cognitive-behavioral therapy. The World Health Organization Violence Prevention Unit identified several promising violence prevention strategies including parenting programs; early childhood development programs; school-based academic and social skills development strategies (e.g., bullying prevention); strategies for youth at higher risk of, or already involved in, violence; and community- and society-level strategies (e.g., reducing access to alcohol, drug control programs, reducing access to and misuse of firearms and alleviating concentrated poverty).[3] For many programs for preventing youth violence (e.g., structured leisure time activities, vocational training, mentoring, and gang and street violence prevention programs), there is insufficient evidence to assess their effectiveness.[3]

Box 14.1 **Sources of Information About Evidence-Based Prevention Programs and Strategies for Violence Prevention in Communities**

The Community Guide for Violence Prevention
http://www.thecommunityguide.org/violence/index.html

Preventing Youth Violence: An Overview of the Evidence
http://apps.who.int/iris/bitstream/10665/181008/1/9789241509251_eng.pdf?ua=1&ua=1&ua=1

Striving To Reduce Youth Violence Everywhere (STRYVE) Strategies Selector Tool
http://vetoviolence.cdc.gov/apps/stryvestrategy/strategyselector/

The National Registry of Evidence-Based Programs and Practices (NREPP)
http://www.nrepp.samhsa.gov/

Crimesolutons.gov www.crimesolutions.gov

Blueprints for Healthy Youth Development
http://www.colorado.edu/cspv/blueprints

Violence Prevention Evidence Base http://www.preventviolence.info/evidence_base.aspx

---

In addition to societal safeguards such as child protection services, law enforcement, and the criminal justice system, prevention strategies for child abuse and other forms of child maltreatment focus on influencing individual behaviors, family relationships, and societal culture.[17-19] The US Department of Health and Human Service's Child Welfare Information Gateway provides resources for building community support, conducting a community needs assessment, developing a child abuse and neglect prevention program, and evaluating its effectiveness.[20]

Efforts to prevent intimate partner violence focus on promoting healthy, respectful, nonviolent relationships, and screening by healthcare providers.[21,22] Such efforts can aim for more than one level of the socioecological model, for example, individual, interpersonal (relationship), organizational (healthcare), and community. Resources for preventing intimate partner violence include CDC's *Dating Matters: Strategies to Promote Healthy Teen Relationships*, and *Preventing Intimate Partner and Sexual Violence: Program Activities Guide*.[5]

The Role of CBPR in Addressing Interpersonal Violence in Diverse Communities

The CBPR approach lends itself to addressing interpersonal violence in diverse communities through raising awareness about prevention, developing partnerships across different sectors, enhancing community capacity to evaluate prevention programs, and helping to establish a policy framework.[3] Community interventions for violence prevention often involve several stakeholders and coalitions of community partners (e.g., educational institutions such as schools, health institutions, law enforcement, criminal justice, child protection agencies, nonprofit organizations, and the business sector). Evidence-based approaches for preventing youth violence require developing and evaluating interventions that are culturally appropriate and tailored to the demographic and socioeconomic characteristics of the target population. Community-based participatory research involves the engagement and collaboration of academic and community members on multiple aspects of research to design a more relevant, and often more effective, intervention.

Community-based participatory research studies on violence prevention that had a randomized controlled trial or pre/post design are summarized in Table 14.1. The studies were identified using PubMed with relevant search terms. Articles published in English through January 31, 2016, were identified using the following MeSH search terms and Boolean algebra commands: (((community-based participatory research) OR (action research)) AND (violence OR assault)). Although the search criteria did not specify a begin date, the earliest article that met the search criteria was published in 2007. The searches were not limited to words appearing in the titles of articles. Information obtained from bibliographic searches (title and topic of article, information in abstract, and key words) was used to determine whether to retain each article. The references in reports and review articles were also reviewed. A total of 153 citations were found. After screening the abstracts or full texts of these articles, 7 CBPR studies on violence were identified that met the search criteria, of which six were conducted in the United States and one in South Africa.[23–29] The excluded citations included CBPR studies on violence that involved focus groups or in-depth interviews of key informants but that did not evaluate the effectiveness of a violence prevention program using a randomized controlled trial or pre/post design.

These examples illustrate CBPR studies on the effectiveness of intervention strategies to prevent interpersonal violence among diverse groups of people. The intervention approaches examined in these studies extend across many of the intervention approaches highlighted in Guide to Community Preventive Services systematic reviews and WHO reports including school-based programs and cognitive-behavioral therapy. Many additional evaluative studies of violence prevention programs have used qualitative methods such as focus groups, in-depth interviews of key informants, and concept mapping.

One of the commonalities identified in Table 14.1 is the frequent use of natural leaders, teachers, or peer educators to deliver programs aimed at violence prevention, that is, a "train the trainer approach." Another commonality is the use of community advisory boards, found in most of the studies portrayed in this table. Advisory boards allow for advice and discussion about detailed issues, often needing trust and honesty that comes with exposure to the ideas of research and

Table 14.1 CBPR Studies on Violence Prevention with a Randomized Controlled Trial or Pre/Post Design

Citation	Study population	Study design	Results	Comments
Kim et al.[23]	Poor women in eight villages in Limpopo province, South Africa	Cluster-randomized trial of a microfinance intervention combined with training on HIV infection, gender norms, domestic violence, and sexuality. Outcome measures included intimate partner violence (IPV) in the past year and nine indicators of empowerment	The risk of IPV in the past year was reduced by more than half (adjusted risk ratio = 0.45, 95% confidence interval (CI) = 0.23, 0.91). Improvement in all indicators of empowerment was observed.	To foster solidarity and collective action, the participatory learning program encouraged wider community mobilization to engage both youth and men. Women deemed "natural leaders" by their peers underwent one additional week of training and then worked to address HIV infection and IPV.
Kelly et al.[24]	Predominately Mexican American third-, fourth-, and fifth-grade students (n = 312) at 14 elementary schools in South Texas	Cluster randomized controlled trial of a 10-session *El Joven Noble* violence prevention program	No significant differences were observed between intervention and control group students on the four outcome variables. However, high-risk students in the intervention group showed significant changes in their scores on nonviolence efficacy (p < .05).	Academic researchers and community members worked together to design, implement, and evaluate the intervention. The community and school district members had previously joined together after suffering the deaths of children from a wave of violence that was affecting their local community. Community members were concerned about the growing influence of violent gangs in their neighborhoods.

Kataoka et al.[25]	Predominately low-income, Mexican American sixth-grade students ($n = 123$) from two middle schools in Los Angeles. Students were eligible if they endorsed substantial violence exposure and posttraumatic stress symptoms in the clinical range.	Randomized controlled trial of a 10-session cognitive-behavioral intervention for trauma in schools	Compared with students in the delayed intervention group, students in the early intervention group had a significantly higher Spring Semester mean grade in math (2.0 vs. 1.6) but not language arts (2.2 vs. 1.9)	A community-research partnership developed, implemented, and evaluated the intervention program to improve the well-being of students traumatized by violence.
Enriquez et al.[26]	Low-income, predominately first-generation Hispanic American freshmen ($n = 26$) and sophomore students ($n = 25$) from one high school in Kansas City, Missouri	Pre/post test design with no control group, of the *Familias En Nuestra Escuela* teen violence prevention intervention	A significant increase was observed in ethnic pride ($p < .05$). Nonsignificant changes were observed in the desired direction on measures of self-efficacy for self-control, couple violence, and gender attitudes. Physical fighting decreased over the course of the academic year ($p < .05$).	The small-group intervention was facilitated by teachers. The study was limited by the lack of a control group and the small sample size.

(continued)

Table 14.1 Continued

Citation	Study population	Study design	Results	Comments
Wahab et al.[27]	59 African American survivors of IPV	Pre/post test of a 6-month motivational interviewing intervention for depression, which was led by a peer IPV advocate. The topics discussed focused on depression and IPV (safety planning, experiences with recent violence, intimate partner relationship, effects of violence on children, and parenting within violent relationships).	Significant improvements in depression severity were observed, with a reduction in PHQ-9 scores from 13.9 to 7.9 ($p < .001$). Improvements were also observed related to views about depression, depression self-efficacy, and depression self-management behaviors ($p < .001$ in each instance).	Parenting, finances, education, employment, and self-care were also explored; the study participants chose what they wanted to focus on during the individual sessions.
Clark et al.[28]	17 adult female survivors of domestic violence (70.6% white)	Nonrandomized feasibility study of a 12-week, trauma-sensitive yoga intervention delivered once a week for 30–40 minutes at the end of group psychotherapy sessions. The primary outcomes were anxiety, depression, and PTSD symptoms.	At baseline, 60.0% of the women had clinically significant levels of depressive symptoms (PHQ-9 score ≥ 10); nearly all (86.7%) had clinically significant levels of anxiety; and 50% had PCL-C scores (≥44) consistent with PTSD.	The study followed CBPR approach in its conceptualization and design and involved academic researchers and a community agency that provides advocacy and psychotherapy for men, women, and children affected by domestic violence. The study was limited by the small sample size, nonrandomized design, and losses to follow-up (30%).

| Ritchwood et al.[29] | Rural African American youth ($n = 331$) aged 10–14 years from five counties in rural eastern North Carolina. About 60% of the youth had a caregiver income of < $20,000 per year, and 29% had a caregiver income of < $5,000 per year. | Quasi-experimental community-based trial of the Teach One Reach One (TORO) intervention to reduce teen dating violence | Youth Ambassadors reported significant reductions in acceptance of couple violence between baseline and follow-up ($p < .001$). Youth in the comparison group reported higher levels of family conflict ($p = .02$) and lower levels of family cohesion ($p = .01$) at follow-up. | All of the participants reported that the study was personally meaningful and that the results would be useful to others. | The educational sessions were delivered by lay health advisors. CBPR principles were followed. |

of community issues that comes with increased contact time. Almost all of the studies targeted socioeconomically disadvantaged or marginalized populations.

Discussion

Several CBPR studies on interpersonal violence have examined the effectiveness of small group educational sessions, school-based programs, cognitive-behavioral therapy, trauma-sensitive yoga, and other intervention strategies. In conducting CBPR studies in diverse communities, there is a need for culturally appropriate, tailored health and safety messages. Health promotion messages that are culturally tailored for a group address the unique needs of individuals, increase their motivation, tend to be perceived as more personally relevant, and lead to a greater likelihood of behavior change. Culturally appropriate interventions address the cultural values of the group, reflect the attitudes and norms of the group, and reflect the behavioral preferences and expectations of the group's members.

Although the CBPR approach and action research are directly applicable to addressing unemployment and lack of economic prosperity in distressed communities, only a handful of CBPR studies have combined health interventions with interventions aimed at helping people to go back to school, get a job, or start a small business.[16,23,30] In view of the many linkages between interpersonal violence and poverty, and their cyclical relationship, there is a need for innovative CBPR studies aimed both at preventing interpersonal violence and alleviating unemployment, lack of education, and economic development.

Additional CBPR studies are needed that have the potential to fill in gaps in the current evidence about what intervention strategies are effective in reducing interpersonal violence in population subgroups that are disproportionately affected by it. This includes dissemination and implementation research and studies that translate evidence-based interventions to new populations identified by gender, age, race, ethnicity, culture, nativity, or geographic locality. Of particular interest are CBPR studies that include multicomponent intervention approaches aimed at different levels of the socioecological model. Studies conducted in collaboration with higher risk, marginalized, and socioeconomically disadvantaged populations should also be a priority.

References

1. Krug, E.G., et al., eds. *World Report on Violence and Health*. Geneva: World Health Organization, 2002.
2. *Injuries and Violence: The Facts*. Geneva: World Health Organization, 2010.
3. *Preventing Youth Violence: An Overview of the Evidence*. Geneva: World Health Organization, 2015.

4. Singh, G.K., Azuine, R.E., Siahpush, M. and Kogan, M.D. "All-Cause and Cause-Specific Mortality Among US Youth: Socioeconomic and Rural-Urban Disparities and International Patterns." *Journal of Urban Health* 90 (2013): 388–405.

5. US Centers for Disease Control and Prevention Division of Violence Prevention. "Youth Violence." <www.cdc.gov/violenceprevention/youthviolence>

6. Coughlin, S.S., ed. *Post-Traumatic Stress Disorder and Chronic Health Conditions.* Washington, DC: American Public Health Association, 2012.

7. Black, M.C., Basile, K.C., Breiding, M.J., et al. *National Intimate Partner and Sexual Violence Survey: 2010 Summary Report.* Atlanta, GA: National Center for Injury Prevention and Control and the Centers for Disease Control and Prevention, 2011.

8. Caetano, R., Field, C.A., Ramisetty-Mikler, S. and McGrath, C. "The 5-Year Course of Intimate Partner Violence Among White, Black, and Hispanic Couples in the United States. *Journal of Interpersonal Violence* 20 (2005): 1039–57.

9. UNICEF. *The State of the World's Children 2007: Women and Children—The Double Dividend of Gender Equality.* New York: United Nations Children Fund, 2006.

10. Casapia, M., Joseph, S.A. and Gyorkos, T.W. "Multidisciplinary and Participatory Workshops with Stakeholders in a Community of Extreme Poverty in the Peruvian Amazon: Development of Priority Concerns and Potential Health, Nutrition, and Education Interventions." *International Journal for Equity in Health* 6 (2007): 6.

11. Krantz, G. "Violence Against Women: A Global Public Health Issue." *Journal of Epidemiology and Community Health* 56 (2002): 242–3.

12. Gurman, T.A., Trappler, R.M., Acosta, A., et al. "By Seeing with Our Own Eyes, It Can Remain in Our Mind: Qualitative Evaluation Findings Suggest the Ability of Participatory Video to Reduce Gender-Based Violence in Conflict-Affected Settings." *Health Education Research* 29 (2004): 690–701.

13. United Nations High Commissioner for Refugees. *Sexual and Gender-Based Violence Against Refugees, Returnees and Internally Displaced Persons. Guidelines for Prevention and Response.* 2003. <http://www.unhcr.org/en-us/protection/women/3f696bcc4/sexual-gender-based-violence-against-refugees-returnees-internally-displaced.html>

14. Farmer, P. *Pathologies of Power: Health, Human Rights, and the New War on the Poor.* Berkeley: University of California Press, 2003.

15. O'Hara-Murdock, P., Garbharran, H., Edwards, M.J., et al. "Peer Led HIV/AIDS Prevention for Women in South African Informal Settlements." *Health Care for Women International* 24 (2003): 502–12.

16. Mosavel, M., Simon, C., van Stade, D. and Buchbinder, M. "Community-Based Participatory Research (CBPR) in South Africa: Engaging Multiple Constituents to Shape the Research Question." *Social Sciences and Medicine* 61 (2005): 2577–87.

17. Reynolds, A.J. and Robertson, D.L. "School-Based Early Intervention and Later Child Maltreatment in the Chicago Longitudinal Study." *Child Development* 74 (2003): 3–26.

18. Chaffin, M., Silovsky, J.F., Funderburk, B., et al. "Parent-Child Interaction Therapy with Physically Abusive Parents: Efficacy for Reducing Future Abuse Reports." *Journal of Consulting and Clinical Psychology* 72 (2004): 500–10.

19. Prinz, R.J., Sanders, M.R., Shapiro, C.J., Whitaker, D.J. and Lutzker, J.R. "Population-Based Prevention of Child Maltreatment: The U.S. Triple P System Population Trial. *Prevention Science* 10 (2009): 1–12.

20. US Department of Health and Human Services. *The Child Welfare Information Gateway* <https://www.childwelfare.gov/>

21. Schewe, P.A., ed. *Preventing Violence in Relationships: Interventions Across the Life Span.* Washington, DC: American Psychological Association, 2002.

22. Nelson, H.D., Bougatsos, C. and Blazina, I. *Screening Women for Intimate Partner Violence and Elderly and Vulnerable Adults for Abuse. Systematic Review to Update the 2004 U.S. Preventive Services Task Force Recommendation.* Evidence syntheses. Rockville, MD: Agency for Healthcare Research and Quality, 2012. Report no. 12-05167-EF-1.

23. Kim, J.C., Watts, C.H., Hargreaves, J.R., et al. "Understanding the Impact of a Microfinance-Based Intervention on Women's Empowerment and the Reduction of Intimate Partner Violence in South Africa." *American Journal of Public Health* 97 (2007): 1794–802.

24. Kelly, P.J., Lesser, J., Cheng, A.L., et al. "A Prospective Randomized Controlled Trial of an Interpersonal Violence Prevention Program with a Mexican American Community." *Family and Community Health* 33 (2010): 207–15.

25. Kataoka, S., Jaycox, L.H., Wong, M., et al. "Effects on School Outcomes in Low-Income Minority Youth: Preliminary Findings from a Community-Partnered Study of a School Trauma Intervention." *Ethnicity and Disease* 21 (2011): S1-71-7.

26. Enriquez, M., Kelly, P.J., Cheng, A.L. and Hunter, J. "An Intervention to Address Interpersonal Violence Among Low-income Midwestern Hispanic-American Teens. *Journal of Immigrant and Minority Health* 14 (2012): 292–99.

27. Wahab, S., Trimble, J., Mejia, A., et al. "Motivational Interviewing at the Intersections of Depression and Intimate Partner Violence Among African American Women." *Journal of Evidence Based Social Work* 11 (2014): 291–303.

28. Clark, C.J., Lewis-Dmello, A., Anders, D., et al. "Trauma-Sensitive Yoga as an Adjunct Mental Health Treatment in Group Therapy for Survivors of Domestic Violence: A Feasibility Study." *Complementary Therapies in Clinical Practice* 20 (2014): 152–58.

29. Ritchwood, T.D., Albritton, T., Akers, A.Y., et al. "The Effect of Teach One Reach One (TORO) on Youth Acceptance of Couple Violence." *Journal of Child and Family Studies* 24 (2015): 3805–15.

30. Benedict, S., Campbell, M., Doolen, A., et al. "Seeds of HOPE: A Model for Addressing Social and Economic Determinants of Health in a Women's Obesity Prevention Project in Two Rural Communities." *Journal of Womens Health (Larchmt)* 16 (2007): 1117–24.

15

Using Community-Based Participatory Research Approaches in HIV

Three Case Studies

MARA BIRD, PHD, BRITT RIOS-ELLIS, PHD, JASON GLOBERMAN,

MSC, DAVID GOGOLISHVILI, MPH, ALICE WELBOURN, PHD,

ULRIKE BRIZAY, PHD, LINA GOLOB, MSC, SHIRIN HEIDARI, PHD,

AND SEAN B. ROURKE, PHD, FCAHS

Communities have consistently played critical roles in responding to the human immunodeficiency virus (HIV) epidemic, and community-academic partnerships have gained increasing prominence in HIV research. The number of studies that included community participation in the field of HIV research increased substantially between 1991 and 2012, and the terms used to describe these activities have changed, moving away from "action research" (AR) to "participatory action research" (PAR), "community-based research" (CBR), and "community-based participatory research" (CBPR), with the latter being the most commonly used term, based on English-language articles indexed in PubMed.[1]

The terms CBR and CBPR are often used interchangeably, with early work of Israel et al. providing a working template and definition for the core dimensions of community-based research:

> CBR in public health is a collaborative approach to research that equitably involves all partners (for example, community members, organizational representatives, and researchers) in all aspects of the research process. The partners contribute unique strengths and shared responsibilities to enhance understanding of a given phenomenon and the social and cultural dynamics of the community, and integrate the knowledge gained with action to improve the health and well-being of community members.[2, p. 177]

The results of a literature review assessing community–academic partnerships in HIV research conducted by Brizay et al. found a variety of approaches to community participation with differences in theory and practice. Some articles discussed the involvement of community in all phases of the research process as central, while others emphasized community involvement in specific research tasks such as recruitment, data collection, intervention development, and/or interpretation of results. Furthermore, although historically researchers have largely been external to their respective communities of focus, an increasingly diverse research workforce is beginning to generate researchers who are part of and present within their communities of focus. In practice, research that involves community in all phases of the research still remains the exception. Based on the various descriptions of community participation identified through this literature review, the authors examined key phases in the research process that could act as building blocks when engaging in community–academic partnerships (Figure 15.1).

Three case studies highlighting effective community–academic research partnerships in HIV are presented here. These examples demonstrate the impact that community–academic partnerships can have specific to the three phases of research highlighted below. While CBPR often focuses on the local level, it is also useful to the broader contexts in which we live and relate. Three cases were

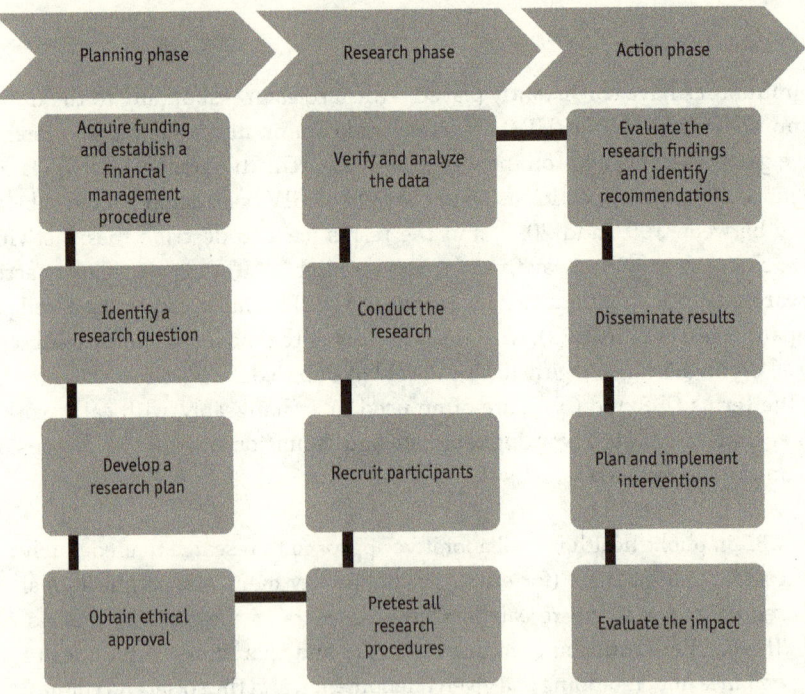

Figure 15.1 Phases of community–academic partnerships. Adapted from Brizay, U., Golob, L., Globerman, J., et al. "Community-Academic Partnerships in HIV-Related Research: A Systematic Literature Review of Theory and Practice." *Journal of the International AIDS Society* 18.1 (2015).

selected to illustrate the heterogeneity that exists in CBPR, including differing levels of analysis from local to provincial to international activities. The first study focuses on the province of Ontario, Canada; the second highlights the southwest US-Mexico border region; and the third shows how CBPR was implemented at an international level. Each case study describes the contexts of the research including community visions and need, the process by which the community was engaged in the research, and the value added through community-academic partnerships.

Positive Spaces Healthy Places (Ontario, Canada)

THE COMMUNITY NEED

In the early 2000s, frontline acquired immune deficiency syndrome (AIDS) service organizations in Ontario reported a marked increase in the number of clients living with HIV who were experiencing housing instability. Although frontline workers already knew firsthand that lack of access to stable housing was having a serious negative impact on the health of people living with HIV, Ontario and Canada lacked systematic data on the depth and breadth of their housing needs.

Started in 2005, Positive Spaces Healthy Places was the first longitudinal community-based research initiative in Canada to examine the relationship between housing stability and health for people living with HIV. Its goals were to (1) identify the range of housing options available in Ontario; (2) determine how housing and homelessness experiences vary; (3) investigate the relationship between housing quality/security and physical/ mental health, and access to healthcare, treatment, and social services; (4) examine how housing changes for people living with HIV over time; (5) increase understanding and awareness about housing needs and experiences; and (6) identify the characteristics of healthy housing.

With support from provincial and federal funders, over 600 participants were interviewed up to four times over a period of 5 years as part of the study. The sample was selected to reflect the diversity of people living with HIV in Ontario both in terms of region and sociodemographic factors.

ENGAGING COMMUNITIES IN RESEARCH

As a community-based study, every step of Positive Spaces Healthy Places was guided by the needs of people living with HIV, who actively led and shaped the process. As part of the study's commitment to the greater and meaningful involvement of people living with HIV or AIDS (GIPA/MIPA) principle,[3,4] people living with HIV were leaders of the study. In addition, peer research associates (people living with HIV) were hired, trained, and engaged in every stage of the research process. Using peer research associates made it easier to engage and retain hard-to-reach and underrepresented participants, ensured more complete data collection, and established strong connections between people living with HIV and the research.

Using collaborative and respectful research methods was as important to the Positive Spaces Healthy Places research team as answering the study's research questions. Researchers placed high value on the interconnection between evidence-based practice and practice-based evidence ("a range of treatment approaches and supports that are derived from, and supportive of, the positive cultural attributes of the local society and traditions"[5] [p. 16]), research as a culture, not just an activity, and solving problems together, through partnership and collaboration. Positive Spaces Healthy Places succeeded because of the values shared by the team and the strong relationships among academic, community, and policy partners.

Each group provided unique skills and knowledge that strengthened the study as a whole, allowing it to achieve what no one partner could have accomplished alone. Community partners ensured the meaningful engagement and involvement of the community, enhanced community morale, and showed leadership in moving research into action. Academic partners, who published findings in peer-reviewed journals, helped build a rigorous evidence-based case for investing in housing as a health service. The study's policy partners connected with key stakeholders and provided strategic advice to influence programs and services. Through the research process, peer research associates developed research skills, secured gainful employment, saw improvements in their quality of life, and helped shape the research directly affecting them and their community.

FINDINGS

Positive Spaces Healthy Places demonstrated that housing instability, including inappropriate and unsafe housing, is significantly associated with poorer mental and physical health among people living with HIV. Participants in the study who were unstably housed were more likely to have substance use issues, experience depression and higher levels of stress, have lower CD4 counts, have higher viral loads, and have higher rates of mortality. These same individuals were less likely to access medical and social services and adhere to antiretroviral medications.

Data from Positive Spaces Healthy Places were also used to form a picture of what healthy housing looks like, emphasizing safety, housing and economic security, a sense of belonging and community, and social inclusion as facilitators to well-being.

VALUE ADDED

Positive Spaces Healthy Places provided quantifiable data about housing issues for people living with HIV in Ontario. Findings from Positive Spaces Healthy

Places have led to increased funding, collaboration, awareness, policy changes, and more research.

Data have been used by local, national, and international organizations to secure additional funding and support for housing—including over $20 million for supportive housing in Ontario for people living with HIV. On the policy level, study findings were cited in an Ontario Human Rights Commission report and leveraged to ensure people living with HIV in Ontario who have substance use issues are now eligible for new supportive housing for people with addictions.

As a result of the study, researchers have built relationships with partners worldwide. At a recent International AIDS housing meeting, more than 150 Canadian, US, and European delegates endorsed a declaration asking policy makers to "recognize housing as a human right and address the lack of adequate housing as a barrier to effective HIV prevention, treatment, and care." The Positive Spaces Healthy Places study model is now being replicated across Canada, adding to the body of research.

Salud es Cultura (Southwest US-Mexico Border Region)

THE COMMUNITY NEED

The US-Mexico border represents one of the highest risk communities for a myriad of health disparities, including HIV. While Latinos represented approximately 16% of the US population, in 2010[6] they accounted for 21% of those newly diagnosed with HIV and 19% of people living with HIV in the same year.[7-9] Underserved Latino populations on both sides of the border are more vulnerable to acquiring HIV largely due to the social determinants of health that contribute to this disparity. Thousands of individuals, whether for work or home, engage in daily border crossings.[10]

Recent immigration policy enforcement, in combination with anti-immigrant legislation in states such as Arizona, has increased fear associated with accessing health and human services, and exacerbated the stigma associated with speaking Spanish and immigrant status within the United States.[11,12] Given these contextual factors, formidable barriers exist when attempting to manage HIV vulnerability. Thus, innovative methods are required to reach Latinos in a culturally and linguistically relevant manner, particularly in places within close proximity to the US-Mexico border.

ENGAGING COMMUNITIES IN RESEARCH

Salud es Cultura, a Latino-focused HIV prevention intervention, resulted from a series of collaborative activities with three community-based organizations, two of which are Federally Qualified Health Centers (FQHCs). FQHCs serve a vulnerable and underserved area or population, offer a sliding fee scale, provide comprehensive services, and have quality assurance oversight. These collaborative activities included involvement in a national needs assessment that included individual, in-depth interviews, and focus groups with Latinos living with or at-risk of HIV to determine HIV risks and contexts that increase vulnerabilities for their communities. In addition, the principal investigator's close collaboration with organizational leaders in HIV and AIDS advocacy both regionally and nationally, and her work with the organizations as they established peer health educator programs, facilitated community engagement. These collaborative efforts spanned nearly a decade.

The intervention also developed as the result of lived disparities and trust gained through interactions over time that facilitated both dialogue and a collective search for solutions. Early in the national needs assessment[13] and largely due to the needs assessment's qualitative nature, a new, Latino-specific definition of HIV risk emerged that did not completely conform to the risk categories associated with being gay or bisexual, having multiple sex partners, and engaging in unsafe injection drug use practices. Data from 121 interviews and 18 focus groups (n = 201) revealed that Latinos often experienced vulnerability due to (1) marriage-related sexual experiences, perceived sexual obligation ("*sexo es un deber*"—sex as a duty that is often associated with women's economic dependence on male partners; not engaged in because of desire); (2) men's lack of condom use with their "good women" or wives; (3) Latinas' inability to assert condom use within a relationship wherein they had little social and economic power; (4) Mexican women's inability to find employment on the Mexican side of the border after becoming mothers, which resulted in survival sex work during the day on the US side of the border; (5) women's inability to evade both physical and psychological abuse from their husbands for a myriad of reasons; (6) homophobia and the inability of gay or bisexual men to live openly, which often resulted in marriage followed by "down-low" sexual relations; (7) resistance on the part of both men and women to use condoms regularly; (8) lack of both knowledge of, and access to, culturally and linguistically relevant healthcare and HIV testing; (9) lack of HIV and AIDS-related knowledge; and, (10) low socioeconomic status and history of racism, both external and internalized, and discrimination.

Given the multifaceted nature of stigma associated with HIV combined with the risk-exacerbating factors listed above, extensive dialogue was warranted to clearly discuss stigma and its relationship to HIV risk. These processes were facilitated through CBPR techniques. In-depth discussions with HIV positive community health workers in San Ysidro revealed that the word "stigma" in and of itself was highly problematic, due to its relation to the word "*stigmata*" in Spanish, or "marks of God." The predominant fear was that stigma itself would be interpreted as marks of God, therefore potentially demarcating those with HIV. For this reason, stigma was only discussed in the intervention sessions after it had been fully and clearly defined.

The team's collective task was to find a way to mitigate the adverse effects of stigma by facilitating an understanding of how it impacts health access and issues surrounding HIV status. Given the fear associated with being Latino, participants extensively discussed ways in which to confront hardships through cultural values and narratives. From these dialogues, the project team developed the title *Salud es Cultura* to demonstrate the inextricable link between health and culture.

These multiple focus groups and dialogues resulted in the development of a 45-minute intervention and materials including an educational *rotafolio* or flip chart that could be easily transported to diverse settings, a facilitator's guide, and an evaluation plan. San Ysidro–based community health workers (people living with or affected by HIV) led the development of all project elements. Throughout the study, project staff met with community health worker teams in Los Angeles and El Paso to help ensure utility and effectiveness, given the diverse geographic regions involved. This process occurred until each site reached agreement regarding the anticipated usefulness of the intervention materials for the local community. Community health workers from each site then engaged in a one-day training in which communications methodology, an undergirding of the importance of culturally relevant communication techniques, and extensive role-playing were taught to ensure that each community health worker demonstrated competence in delivering the health *charla* (or "conversation"), the descriptive word used instead of the term "intervention." Community health workers were also trained in institutional review board procedures and were tested to ensure that they clearly understood problems associated with coercion as well as the importance of informed consent.

FINDINGS

Salud es Cultura was led by community health workers (*promotores de salud*) and engaged underserved Latinos in three southwestern US communities. All 579 participants were Latino adults from either El Paso, Texas ($n = 204$); San Ysidro, California ($n = 175$); or Los Angeles, California ($n = 200$). The purpose of the intervention was to decrease HIV-related stigma and increase HIV knowledge and perception of potential infection. *Promotores* delivered interactive group-based *charlas* to groups of Latinos in Spanish and English. To decrease stigma and motivate behavioral and attitudinal change, *charlas* emphasized positive Latino cultural values.

HIV stigma scores decreased significantly ($p < .001$) pre- to post-intervention, with participants demonstrating significant increases in HIV knowledge ($p < .001$), willingness to discuss HIV with one's sexual partner ($p < .001$), and perceptions of vulnerability or risk of exposure to HIV ($p = .006$). While these findings are positive, the length and resources associated with the project did not allow for development and testing of the potential effects of multiple *charlas*. Whether due to having to rely on a sole *charla* or other limitations associated with the project length and resources, willingness to test for HIV 3 months post intervention was not significantly associated with increased testing. Female participants demonstrated a greater reduction in HIV-related stigma scores compared to their male counterparts, which may have been related to a greater increase in HIV knowledge scores ($p = .016$ and $p = .007$, respectively). This may also be explained by the emphasis placed on familism/*familismo* and the importance of open dialogue about sexual risk behaviors and reduction measures so as to protect all family members from HIV.

VALUE ADDED

The effectiveness of this program and its resonance with community-based organizations working to reduce HIV vulnerability led to its further dissemination through four regional training sessions. Over 90 *promotores* were trained in Portland, Oregon; New York City; Washington, DC; and Oakland, California. The program's popularity led to further dissemination and training sessions in Mayaguez and Ponce, Puerto Rico, and Ft. Lauderdale, Florida.

Furthermore, the deidentified data and results garnered from each site were shared electronically and in the form of site-specific reports with each community-based organization. All partners reported using these data and elements from the report to further their respective agencies' grant and programmatic efforts.

Promotores-led interventions appear to reduce stigma overall, as well as stigma associated with sexual and reproductive health within underserved communities. These interventions also help build trust and facilitate CBPR engagement as well as collaborative efforts to mitigate health inequities among diverse contexts and communities. Additionally, because *promotores* programs are based within their respective communities, the skills and knowledge associated with their delivery resides within the community.

Building a Safe House on Firm Ground (International, Led by Salamander Trust)

THE COMMUNITY NEED AND VISION

In 2013, the World Health Organization's (WHO) Department of Reproductive Health and Research started the process of updating its 2006 guidelines on the sexual and reproductive health and human rights of women living with HIV, in light of rapidly changing treatment policies. In the 2006 guidelines, only one of the women acknowledged in the document was known to be living openly with HIV. For this update, the WHO decided to start the review process with a values and preferences survey of women living with HIV. Salamander Trust was selected to lead this process, and partnered with the ATHENA Network, the International Community of Women living with HIV (ICW Global), the Global Network of People living with HIV (GNP+), the Transgender Law Center, *Red de Jóvenes de Latinoamérica y el Caribe*, ICW Asia-Pacific, and ICW Zimbabwe.

The core study team included two women living with HIV, both of whom were former chairs of the International Community of Women living with HIV/AIDS (ICW), who had established a certain level of trust among this community. One had a background in participatory approaches to development and social anthropology; the other was a translator and linguist and community mobiliser. Other core team members included an expert in community involvement, with a long track record of monitoring and evaluation in relation to gender justice; a human rights lawyer with a public health background; and a doctor with expertise in complex obstetrics and ethics. All had long track records in gender justice and commitment to community involvement. This was the first online participatory international community-based survey of women living with HIV.

ENGAGING COMMUNITIES IN RESEARCH

To ensure the meaningful involvement of people living with HIV throughout the survey, the core team invited 14 women living with HIV with diverse backgrounds, ages, and experiences from around the world to form the "Global Reference Group" (GRG). The role of this group was to support the core team in shaping and validating the research process. This was done through Skype-based calls, sharing of articles to inform GRG members about the guidelines update process, and e-mail discussions.

The researchers sought to take a holistic approach to sexual and reproductive health and human rights. They designed a short holistic "quality of life and well-being" exercise which GRG members were asked to complete, in consultation with peers if preferred. This exercise invited them to reflect on the physical, sexual, psychological, material, and spiritual causes and consequences of their sexual and reproductive health and human rights. This presurvey process enabled GRG and core team members to develop a general understanding of the breadth and depth of causes and consequences of sexual and reproductive health and human rights experienced by women living with HIV, beyond a more conventional biomedical framework.

Another key part of the process from the outset was to adopt an appreciative inquiry approach to the process since, as one GRG member aptly stated, "often research on us asks us questions such as how we acquired our HIV which immediately throws us back into the trauma of what has happened to us. This can often reignite that trauma and can feel very disempowering." By contrast this approach sought to focus on well-being ("what has worked well for you?") and on suggested future priorities ("how can your health-care provider best help you to. . .?").

After discussion with the WHO Reproductive Health and Research Department and members of Guidelines Review Committee, institutional review board approval for the survey was not sought, as this study was a consultative element of the guidelines development process. Ethical considerations were undertaken in line with the WHO 2001 Ethical and Safety Recommendations for Research on Domestic Violence against Women and the ICW 2004 ethical guidelines on involving women with HIV in research.[14,15]

The results of the presurvey exercise enabled the core team to shape questions, which covered all the issues raised by GRG members through the holistic exercise. These questions, designed to elicit a mixture of quantitative and qualitative responses, were piloted and pretested by GRG members before finalizing them. The resulting online survey included one mandatory section and eight optional sections based on priorities defined by the GRG. Survey questions were available in English as well as seven other languages (Spanish, Russian, French, Portuguese, Arabic, Bahasi-Indonesian, and Chinese). In order to extend access to the survey to women living with HIV who had no Internet access, and to act as a cross-check for online survey responses, focus group discussions (FGDs) were also conducted in seven countries. Six of the facilitators of these FGDs were also women living openly with HIV and these and other facilitators were already well known and trusted by respondents.

RESULTS

A total of 832 women living with HIV from 94 countries responded to the survey. Further, 113 women from 7 countries took part in 11 FGDs. The results produced a wide range of recommendations which, to reflect the holistic approach, were presented in the form of different sections of a house (Figure 15.2). Once again, the results were reviewed and validated by GRG members before finalization. The FGD responses echoed those of the online survey responses.

DISSEMINATION

In order to ensure that all English-speaking respondents could access the results of the survey and make use of the findings in their own work, the resulting report was disseminated widely through e-mail, Internet, and social media. It was also translated into Spanish. To continue to ensure community involvement throughout the process, four peer-reviewed articles were coauthored by all core group members and some of the GRG members. Thus, each article had a majority of coauthors who are women living with HIV. These articles, highlighting the high levels of gender-based violence (GBV) and mental health issues (MH) experienced by women living with HIV, and explaining the participatory methodology, have all been published in open access peer-reviewed journals.[16-20] The GBV and MH articles, which highlight the critical lack of attention to these issues in global HIV

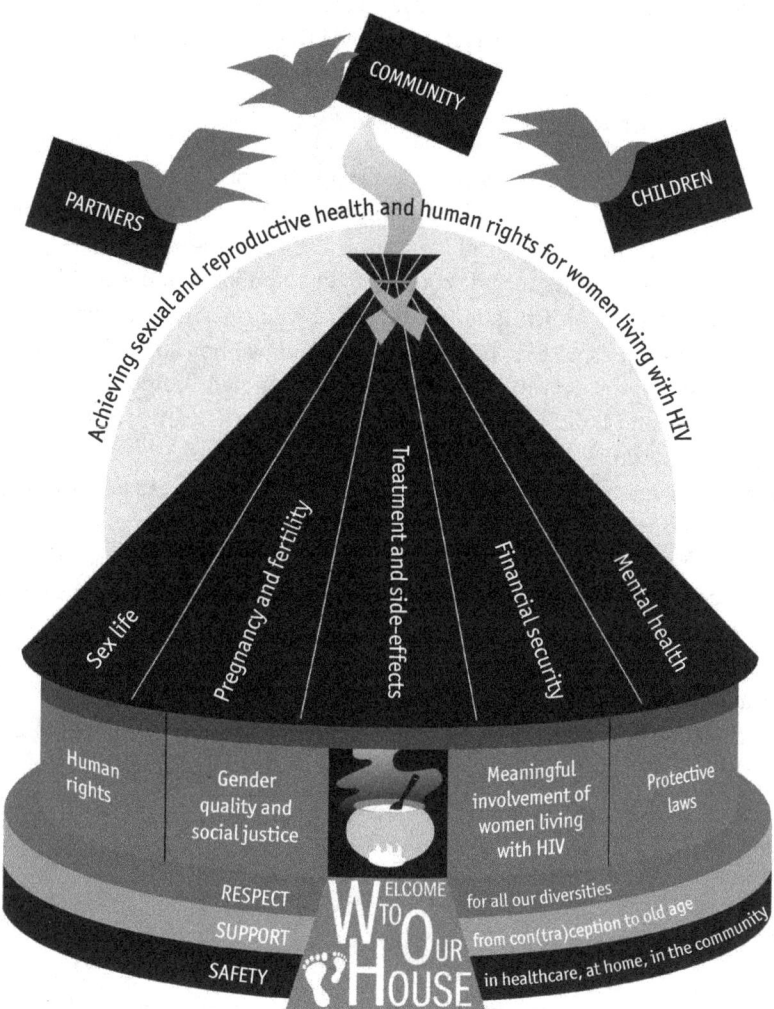

Figure 15.2 Recommendations for how to achieve sexual and reproductive health and human rights for women living with HIV.

policy guidelines for women with HIV, have also been translated into Spanish. Further dissemination has included a Spanish-language webinar for Latin Americans; an abstract regarding UK-based findings has been accepted as a poster for the British HIV Association; another abstract regarding reported treatment side effects has been submitted to the Durban International AIDS Conference; and specific analysis of the Russian language findings was presented at the Eastern Europe and Central Asia AIDS Conference in March 2016. The original survey in Russian is also in use in a national-level research process among women living with HIV in the Ukraine. The survey questions and responses are also available for other women living with HIV to use via the Salamander Trust website.[21]

CROSS-CASE ANALYSIS

This presentation of three case studies using CBPR principles in HIV research demonstrates the power of CBPR to improve overall health and well-being for people living with HIV while contributing to the HIV research knowledge base. Similarities across studies include commitment to building and sustaining trust among communities, which is inherent in CBPR, inclusion of priorities of the affected communities within the research agenda (e.g., housing, addressing contexts of risks appropriate to their lives, recognizing and promoting sexual and health rights), and building capacity among those participating in the research process so that knowledge and resources remain with them.

Differences among the case studies examined here illustrate that CBPR does not require uniform methodologies. All three case studies used mixed-methods approaches that coupled qualitative and quantitative formal and participatory measurement tools. Community participation in the development of the research design and measurement tools also enhanced the quality and rigor of the data. Additionally, approaches can build on varied theoretical frameworks, as shown by those used in the case studies.

All three case studies meaningfully engaged people living with HIV in the research process. The outcomes also benefited society by providing evidence for policies to enhance quality of life for people living with HIV and increase self-efficacy for HIV prevention.

Discussion

While this chapter focuses on the added value of community involvement in research through the use of CBPR principles, the authors also recognize that there are challenges to adhering to these principles for many academic researchers. While this chapter focuses on the intersections of CBPR and HIV, the effectiveness of participatory methodologies has also been discussed in relation to other health issues and social determinants of health, including violence against women and girls[22] and in rural and international development. Intimate partner violence against women is discussed by Steven Coughlin in chapter 14 in this volume.

Ultimately, if social justice efforts in HIV prevention and CBPR take hold, health workforce development will involve ensuring that individuals from underserved communities become a substantial part of the research and prevention workforce, as they are well placed to analyse what happened to them and advise others on how they might learn from their own experiences. These efforts may serve not just to eliminate disparities in HIV but also for other conditions associated with morbidity and mortality. Some of the most meaningful results of the CBPR process are not the research findings themselves, but rather the facilitation of empowerment that occurs within the communities and residents involved.

Acknowledgments

Positive Spaces Healthy Places: The researchers thank all participants who contributed their personal information in the hopes of establishing the link between the social determinants of health, housing, and personal well-being. Without them, there would have been no opportunity to move this field of study forward. Their contributions are helping others affected by HIV across Canada. The authors also acknowledge the valuable contributions of the study's community partners and peer research associates. Funding for Positive Spaces Healthy Places was provided by the Ontario HIV Treatment Network; AIDS Bureau, Ontario Ministry of Health and Long-Term Care; Canadian Institutes of Health Research (CIHR); Ontario AIDS Network; and The Wellesley Institute.

Salud es Cultura: The researchers thank the participants, the more than 90 *promotores de salud* who shared in both the development and implementation of the intervention, and project staff Liany Arroyo, Ana Carricchi, Cristina Delgado, and Gabriela Diaz. We also offer our gratitude to the staff and the leadership in the three communities—Richard Zaldivar, CEO, of The Wall/*Las Memorias* in Los Angeles; Ana Danzinger of *La Clinica de Salud Familiar la Fe* in El Paso; and Brenda Huerta and Rosana Escolari of the San Ysidro Health Center—for sharing our vision to facilitate health equity and honor the cultural capital and resilience of three underserved, yet thriving, communities.

Building a Safe House on Firm Ground: The researchers would like to thank all of the participants who contributed their personal information to the survey. We acknowledge core team members and report authors: Luisa Orza MA (lead author); Alice Welbourn PhD; Susan Bewley MA, MD, FRCOG; E. Tyler Crone JD, MPH; and MariJo Vazquez as well as our global reference group: Nukshinaro Ao, Coordinator, ICW Asia-Pacific; Cecilia Chung, Senior Strategist, Transgender Law Center; Sophie Dilmitis; Calorine Kenkem, Chair, Cameroonian Community of Women Living with HIV (CCAF+); Svetlana Moroz, Eurasian Women's Network on AIDS; Suzette Moses-Burton, Executive Director of the Global Network of People Living with HIV (GNP+); Hajjarah Nagadya; Angelina Namiba; L'Orangelis Thomas Negrón; Gracia Violeta Ross; Sophie Strachan, advisory member for GNP+ and UNAIDS Dialogue Platform member; Martha Tholanah, ICW Zimbabwe; Patricia Ukoli, Pan African Women Coalition and ICW West Africa; and Rita Wahab, Vivre Positif and MENA-Rosa. We also acknowledge the contributions of our translators—Zhen Li and Yuan Wenli (Chinese); Svetlana Moroz (Russian); Isabel Nunez (Portuguese); Sindi Putri (Indonesian), MariJo Vazquez (Spanish); Marion Zibelli (French)—and focus group discussion facilitators—Nukshinaro Ao and Yathip Lakkanasirorat, Asia-Pacific Network of People Living with HIV (ANP+); Yadanar Aung, Young Women's Christian Association (YWCA) Yangon; Abdelkader Bacha and Amandine Bollinger, UNICEF; Olive Edwards, Jamaica Community of Women Living with HIV (JCW+); Hereni Melesse, ATHENA Network; Gelila Sherifaw, Millennium Raey Women's Association; Chan Aye San, Myanmar Positive Women's Network Initiative; Debo Sow, KARLENE; Liz Tremlett, Salamander Trust; Aida Zerbo, Handicap International. Finally, we thank Dr. Manjulaa Narasimhan of the WHO Reproductive Health and Research Department, who suggested the survey, provided funding, and is leading the guidelines-updating process.

References

1. Brizay, U., Golob, L., Globerman, J., et al. "Community-Academic Partnerships in HIV-Related Research: A Systematic Literature Review of Theory and Practice." *Journal of the International AIDS Society* 18.1 (2015): 19354.
2. Israel, B.A., Schulz, A.J., and Parker, E.A. "Review of Community-Based Research: Assessing Partnership Approaches to Improve Public Health." *Annual Review of Public Health* 19 (1998): 173–202. <https://depts.washington.edu/ccph/pdf_files/annurev.publhealth.19.1.pdf>
3. UNAIDS Policy Brief. "The Greater Involvement of People Living with HIV (GIPA)." 2007. <http://www.unaids.org/en/resources/documents/2007/20070410_jc1299-policybrief-gipa_en.pdf>
4. SAfAIDS. "Mainstreaming the Meaningful Involvement of People Living with or Affected by AIDS/HIV (MIPA) into AIDS Programming." n.d. <http://www.safaids.net/content/mainstreaming-principle-mipa-hiv-and-aids-programming-brochure-safaids>
5. Isaacs, M.R., Huang, L.N., Hernandez, M., Echo-Hawk, H. The road to evidence: The intersection of evidence-based practices and cultural competence in children's mental health. Alliance of Multi-ethnic Behavioral Health Associations; (2005).
6. US Census Bureau. *Population Estimates, 2010.*
7. Centers for Disease and Control. "HIV Surveillance Supplemental Report." 17.4, December 2012. <http://www.cdc.gov/hiv/pdf/statistics_hssr_vol_17_no_4.pdf>
8. Centers for Disease and Control. "Fact Sheet: HIV in the United States." 2013. <http://www.cdc.gov/hiv/pdf/statistics_basics_factsheet.pdf>
9. Centers for Disease and Control. "HIV Surveillance Supplemental Report." 18.5, October 2013. <http://www.cdc.gov/hiv/pdf/2011_Monitoring_HIV_Indicators_HSSR_FINAL.pdf>
10. US Department of Transportation. "Research and Innovative Technology Administration, Bureau of Transportation Statistics, Based on Data from the Department of Homeland Security, U.S. Customs and Border Protection, Office of Field Operations." n.d. <http://transborder.bts.gov/programs/international/transborder/TBDR_BC/TBDR_BCQ.html>
11. Steinberg, E.M., Valenzuela-Araujo, D., Zickafoose, J.S., Kieffer, E., and DeCamp, L.R. "The 'Battle' of Managing Language Barriers in Health Care." *Clinical Pediatrics* (2016): 1–10.
12. Martinez, O., Wu, E., Sandfort, T., et al. "Evaluating the Impact of Immigration Policies on Health Status Among Undocumented Immigrants: A Systematic Review." *Journal of Immigrant and Minority Health* 17.3 (2015): 947–70.
13. Rios-Ellis, B. and Gutierrez, J.A. "Latinas and Deadly Sex: The Politics of HIV/AIDS Reporting." *Journal of Latino-Latin American Studies* 2.3 (2007): 120–37.
14. World Health Organization. "WHO Putting Women First: Ethical and Safety Recommendations for Research on Domestic Violence Against Women." 2015. <http://www.who.int/gender/violence/womenfirtseng.pdf>

15. International Community of Women Living with HIV/AIDS. "Guidelines on Ethical Participatory Research with HIV Positive Women." 2015. <http://www.icw.org/files/EthicalGuidelinesICW-07-04.pdf>

16. Narasimhan, M., Orza, L., Welbourn, A., Bewley, S., Cronee, T. and Vazquez, M. "Sexual and Reproductive Health and Human Rights of Women Living with HIV: A Global Community Survey." *Bulletin of the World Health Organization* (2016): 14.150912.

17. Namiba, A., Orza, L., Bewley, S., Crone, E.T., Vazquez, M. and Welbourn, A. "Ethical, Strategic and Meaningful Involvement of Women Living with HIV Starts at the Beginning." *Journal of Virus Eradication* 2 (2016): e8–9.

18. Orza, L., Bewley, S., Chung, C., Tyler Crone, E., Nagadya, H., Vazquez, M. and Welbourn, A. "Violence. Enough already": findings from a global participatory survey among women living with HIV. *Journal of the International AIDS Society* 18(6(Suppl 5) (2015). Available at: <http://www.jiasociety.org/index.php/jias/article/view/20285/pdf_1> [Accessed 1 Dec. 2015].

19. Orza, L., Bewley, S., Logie, C., Crone, E., Moroz, S., Strachan, S., Vazquez, M. and Welbourn, A. How does living with HIV impact on women's mental health? Voices from a global survey. *Journal of the International AIDS Society*, [online] 18(Suppl 5) (2015). Available at: <http://www.jiasociety.org/index.php/jias/article/view/20289> [Accessed 1 Dec. 2015].

20. Orza, L., Welbourn, A., Bewley, S., Crone, E. and Vazquez, M. *Construir una casa segura en terreno firme Hallazgos clave de la encuesta global sobre valores y preferencias en relación a la salud sexual y reproductiva y los derechos humanos de las mujeres viviendo con VIH.* [online] (2015). Salamander Trust. Available at: <http://salamandertrust.net/resources/SalT_Building_safe_house_report_ES_web.pdf> [Accessed 17 May 2016].

21. Salamander Trust. "Building a Safe House on Firm Ground: Key Findings from a Global Values and Preferences Survey Regarding the Sexual and Reproductive Health and Human Rights of Women Living with HIV." 2014. <http://www.athenanetwork.org/assets/files/General%20-%20publications/BuildingASafeHouseOnFirmGroundFINALreport190115.pdf>

22. Raab, M. and Stuppert, W. "Review of Evaluation Approaches and Methods for Interventions Related to Violence Against Women and Girls (VAWG)." (2014). <https://assets.publishing.service.gov.uk/media/57a089b440f0b652dd00037e/61259-Raab_Stuppert_Report_VAWG_Evaluations_Review_DFID_20140626.pdf>

16

Engaging Communities in Translational Research

STEVEN S. COUGHLIN, PHD

AND CAROLYN M. JENKINS, DRPH, MSN, RN, RD, LD, FAAN

Speaking broadly, translational research refers to the application of research findings, from basic science to practice-based and community research, to improve public health. Several authors have proposed more specific definitions to distinguish between the various phases of translation. This chapter provides an overview of the National Institutes of Health (NIH) Clinical and Translational Science Awards (CTSA) program, including CTSA community-engagement programs; frameworks and models for community engagement; community advisory boards (CABs) and their role in CTSA community engagement; academic–community partnerships evaluation; CTSA pilot study grant programs; and CTSA training programs in community-based participatory research (CBPR). Suggestions for future directions in community engagement in translational research are also discussed. In addition to increased efficiency and impact of biomedical research, the promise of the CTSA program is paradigm-shifting community-engaged, translational research aimed at improving health and alleviating suffering in diverse communities.

Community engagement involves scientific research conducted in communities in collaboration or partnership with researchers. As noted by the National Institute of Environmental Health Sciences,[1] "The process of scientific inquiry is such that community members, persons affected by the health condition, disability, or issue under study, or other key stakeholders in the community's health have the opportunity to be full participants in each phase of the work." This includes translational research aimed at turning observations in the laboratory, clinic, and community into interventions that improve the health of individuals and the public.[2] Translational science is the field of investigation focused on understanding the scientific and operational principles underlying each step of the translational process.[2] The translational science spectrum extends across several stages including basic and applied scientific research (preclinical and animal studies, T0), translation to humans (proof of concept Phase I clinical trials, T1), translation to patients (Phase 2 and Phase 3 clinical trials, T2), translation to practice (Phase 4 clinical trials and clinical outcomes research, T3), and translation to community (population-level outcome research, T4). Stages T3 and T4 involve translation of new data into the clinic, community, and health decision-making for populations.

The Clinical and Translational Science Awards Program

As discussed throughout this book, academic institutions must collaborate with community organizations to identify and address public health needs. Since it was established in 2006, the CTSA program at the NIH has supported a broad range of activities that engage communities in health studies and clinical research.[3] The CTSA program was designed to develop innovative solutions that will improve the efficiency, quality, and impact of the process for turning observations in the laboratory, clinic, and community into interventions that improve the health of individuals and the public. The CTSA program does not directly fund or conduct large-scale clinical and translational research. However, some individual CTSAs do support pilot studies, and some CTSAs are joining efforts to initiate collaborative pilot studies to improve health in communities.[4] The CTSA program supports the development and application of shared resources, infrastructure, and innovative technologies for clinical and translational research.[4] In 2011, the CTSA program became a part of the newly formed National Center for Advancing Translational Sciences. With an annual budget of approximately a billion dollars per year, it is the largest program at the NIH.[5] Currently about 62 medical research institutions in 31 US states and the District of Columbia are active member institutions. Some CTSA-funded institutions such as the University of Massachusetts Medical School in Worcester, collaborate with community-based groups, healthcare providers, researchers, and public health professionals to develop methods of effective community dialogue and research, ensure that up-to-date health information is widely available, and provide information about studies and access to clinical trials.[3] To address community needs, CTSA-supported investigators conduct research and outreach efforts through neighborhood service and community centers. Community members provide input on health programs and clinical studies by serving on advisory boards to CTSA institutions.[3]

To integrate translational science across its multiple phases and disciplines within diverse populations and across the individual lifespan, the CTSA Integration Across the Lifespan Domain Task Force focuses on (1) integrating translational science across the entire life span to attain improvements in health for all, (2) launching efforts to study special population differences in the progress and treatment of disease, and (3) developing an integrated approach to translational science across all phases of research.

Part of the CTSA mission is the education and training of translational researchers to ensure that investigators have the skills needed to effectively accelerate health discoveries.[6] All CTSA institutions offer research training to scholars who already have an MD, PhD, or equivalent doctoral degree. Many also include programs that provide predoctoral trainees with an introduction to clinical and translational research.[6] The CTSA Working Groups and Key Function Committee have developed core competency documents including core competencies in clinical and translational research.[7]

In 2013, the Institute of Medicine (IOM) released a report, *The CTSA Program at NIH: Opportunities for Advancing Clinical and Translational Research.*[4] The IOM concluded that the CTSA Awards program has been successful in establishing CTSAs as academic focus points for clinical and translational research and has begun to build a national network that will need to be fully integrated and collaborative to catalyze further progress. The IOM also concluded that the CTSA Awards program is contributing significantly to the advancement of clinical and translational research and is a worthwhile investment that would benefit from a variety of revisions to make it more efficient and effective. Key opportunities noted by the IOM include engaging in additional substantive and productive collaborations and building on initial successes in community engagement.[4] To build on the strengths of individual CTSAs, the IOM recommended that CTSAs build partnerships with industry, other research networks, community groups, and other stakeholders. The IOM recommended that (1) CTSAs should ensure that patients, family members, health care providers, clinical researchers, and other community stakeholders are involved across the continuum of clinical and translational research; (2) community engagement be defined broadly; (3) active and substantive community participation in priority setting and decision-making be ensured across all phases of clinical and translational research and in the leadership and governance of the CTSA program; (4) best practices in community engagement be disseminated; and (5) opportunities and incentives be explored to engage a more diverse community.[4]

Holzer and Kass[8] conducted a qualitative document analysis of the community engagement section of 12 original and 10 renewal grant applications of the 12 institutions awarded CTSA funding in 2006 and renewed in 2010. Institutions employed capacity-building and research engagement strategies. Research engagement strategies ranged from those that involved little input from communities (e.g., announcements) to those that allowed for a large amount of input from communities (e.g., community–researcher teams).[8] Capacity-building included a community liaison and consultation services for researchers and practitioners to evaluate ongoing studies and to assess the impact of studies on the community. In-depth interviews were also conducted with CTSA Community Engagement Core leaders and staff from the 2006 cohort of CTSAs.[9] All of the respondents

(n = 17) reported that the CTSA principal investigator was supportive of community engagement. Six themes related to challenges were identified: need for capacity-building, lack of positive relationships with communities, lack of leadership, funding constraints, time and staff constraints, and unsustainable models.[9]

To examine the roles of community representatives in CTSA activities and evaluate the extent of integration into the organizational and governance structures, Wilkins et al.[10] conducted an online survey of 60 CTSAs. Forty-seven (78%) completed the survey. The mean number of community representatives at each CTSA was 21.4.[10] Most CTSAs (89%) had CABs, and 94% included community representatives in community engagement cores.[10]

Frameworks and Models for Community Engagement

Several models or frameworks have been proposed for community engagement.[11,12] Community-engaged research includes outreach, consultation, and collaboration with community partners such as members of patient advocacy organizations, community-based organizations, and other stakeholders. As discussed by Coughlin and Yoo in chapter 2 in this volume, community-engaged research occurs across a continuum of increasing involvement of community members. At one end of the continuum, community members share leadership of studies with academic researchers. Communities and representative partners are empowered by having control over factors and decisions that affect their health and lives. When community members are true partners, there is equity for all involved, with shared goals and values, shared decision-making, shared resources, and colearning. In community-placed studies that are not truly participatory, researchers may still obtain ideas and strategies from community members, as in focus groups or in-depth interviews of key informants.

Community Advisory Boards and Their Role in CTSA Community Engagement

To incorporate engagement with communities in regions served by CTSA awards, CABs or community advisory committees often provide a systems-level infrastructure for academic–community partnerships and promote institutionalization and sustainability of the partnerships and their products.[13] Many of the local CTSAs mention CABs or committees as contributors to their research activities; however, membership and recruitment of membership are not discussed. Two frameworks[14,15] identified potential organizations or systems that could contribute to research networks. Concannon et al.[14] report that no common taxonomy exists to guide researchers and stakeholders in stakeholder-engaged research. Thus, the researchers proposed the 7Ps Framework to Identify Stakeholders and recommend that this framework be used as a guide, but not a strict formula.[14] The 7Ps include (1) the public and patients; (2) providers such as nurses, physicians, mental health counselors, pharmacists, and other providers of care such as EMS agencies, nursing homes, and so forth, that provide care to patients and populations; (3) purchasers such as employers or others underwriting costs of healthcare; (4) payers such as insurers; (5) policy makers; (6) product makers such as drug and device manufacturers; and (7) principal investigators and other researchers. The Stroke Investigative Research and Education Network (SIREN) uses a Community Systems Wheel, which places the community of individuals at the center of the wheel and as spokes includes systems that can contribute to the research process, including health and social services, politics and government, safety and transportation, education, physical environment, faith-based organizations, recreation, economics, and communication. The Community Systems Wheel also provides a guiding framework for CABs, and selection of members is based on each research community.

Best practices for CABs were identified by Newman et al.[13] based on previously published articles and analyses by the authors. These are summarized in Table 16.1.

Evaluating Academic–Community Partnerships

Several resources are available for evaluating academic–community partnerships and for planning community-engaged research. Researchers at the South Carolina Clinical and Translational Research (SCTR) Institute at the Medical University of South Carolina created a toolkit for academic–community partnerships that are preparing for CBPR.[16,17] The toolkit defines CBPR partnership readiness "the degree to which academic/community partners fit and have the capacity and operations necessary to plan, implement, evaluate, and disseminate CBPR projects that were informed by a partnership readiness model that will facilitate mutual growth of the partnership and positively influence targeted social and health needs in the community."[16] In addition to using a trained facilitator to guide the process, the authors offered several suggestions for using the toolkit (Box 16.1).

The National Institute of Environmental Health Sciences published the *Partnerships for Environmental Public Health Evaluation Metrics Manual*, which provides examples of metrics that Partnerships for Environmental Public Health grantees and program staff can use for program planning, implementation, and evaluation.[18] Evaluation tools are included for grantees and program staff to measure the effectiveness of partnerships and the impact of research on public health

Table 16.1 **Best Practices for Community Advisory Boards (CABs)**[13]

Formation of CAB	
Clarifying purpose, functions, and roles	Potential purpose, function, and roles may include: 1. community perceptions, preferences, and priorities in the development of a research agenda and research processes 2. advising on study protocol design and implementation, facilitating community consent, evaluating and communicating the risks and benefits of research, helping provide resources, evaluating education materials, disseminating information, and using research findings to advocate for policy change 3. partner or advisor; clarification of role is essential
Determining membership composition and recruitment strategies	To select appropriate board members: 1. specific inclusion criteria should be established that reflect the goals of the research and the intended functions and purpose of the CAB 2. assess community and capacity to guide identification of potential partners 3. create a "potential member matrix" that includes the types of organizations to be considered; their reputation, activities, and achievements in the community; their capability to contribute resources; their self-interests; and their potential conflicts 4. screen through telephone and personal interviews 5. invite through personal invitations and follow-up with letter to organization 6. review the potential member's intended role and clarify expectations, including and defining mechanisms of communication to help ensure a shared understanding of the requirements of the board member position 7. signed letter of commitment provides documentation of the agreement and helps to minimize potential misunderstandings

Operations	
Establish operating procedures and principles	Operating procedures guide how the team works together to complete tasks and include: 1. setting the agenda and documenting minutes 2. considering group dynamics and accepted social norms, listening to all, letting members agree to disagree 3. having all members participate in board meetings and activities, which start and end on time. Members periodically reassess and revise the procedures, on the basis of process evaluations, to maintain an equitable balance of power Defining community values or principles that guide research is another initial task of a CAB, and this provides the opportunity to integrate the local context, develop trust, and build relationships among board members

Table 16.1 **Continued**

Operations	
Establishing leadership, balancing power, and making decisions	Fair and appropriate distribution of power and leadership may be addressed with community and academic cochairs
	Effective leadership and balancing of power supports members' satisfaction, participation, and overall effectiveness by using democratic and consensus-based decision-making
	Establish process for decision-making and consensus decisions but increase group solidarity

Maintenance	
Evaluating partnership processes	A multimethod approach to collecting evaluation data increases the likelihood of well-rounded assessment of CAB structure and processes and may include:

1. key informant interviews, meeting observations, focus groups, documents such as activity logs, and member surveys to provide different perspectives of the partnership and enhance the comprehensiveness and credibility of evaluation
2. qualitative methods, such as key informant interviews, provide a platform for CAB partners to address frustrations and concerns
3. quantitative methods, such as surveys, provide a standardized measure of partnership processes that allows a baseline measure to be established and reevaluated over time to gauge continued effectiveness
4. measures of process evaluation incorporate items to assess group dynamics within a CAB partnership framework, including shared leadership, open communication, mechanisms for resolving conflicts, and trust and cohesion
5. evaluation of CAB leadership considers whether leaders provide praise and recognition, seek out members' opinions, and approach members for help with specific tasks
6. process evaluation also includes assessment of more pragmatic issues such as turnover rate of board members, success in recruiting members with specific skills or connections to influential leaders, members' perceptions of the benefits and costs of participation, and the degree to which members perceive the partnership to be effective and sustainable over time
7. evaluations that address partnership priorities increase the likelihood that partnership collaboration continues, thus promoting sustainability

(continued)

Table 16.1 **Continued**

Maintenance	
Sustainability	Develop plan for sustainability early in the life of the CAB
	Recognition of CAB members' contributions of time, resources, and expertise, through some type of compensation, promotes continued engagement in partnership
	Continuing relationships informally during gaps in funding or activities helps to maintain communication between partners and provides opportunity for brainstorming about next steps for partnership
	When sustainability is not possible, clear communication between researchers, CAB, and community members will leave door open for future collaborations

---

Box 16.1 **Recommendations for Using the "Are We Ready? Toolkit for Academic–Community Partnerships for Community-Based Participatory Research," South Carolina Clinical and Translational Research Institute**

1. Schedule a retreat in which all partners can participate (1–2 days): or
2. Plan five to six 2-hour sessions in which each section can be reviewed and discussed by all partners.
3. Each partner should have his/her own workbook.
4. Before the retreat or scheduled sessions, each partner should review and complete the reading materials for the planned session.
5. When the partners meet to discuss the assigned sections, individual responses are shared, discussed as a team, and tentative action plans are made. A trained facilitator will help guide this process. At the end of all of the sessions, the team will derive a final comprehensive action plan to guide next steps.
6. Prior to starting the first session, the partnership may want to decide on principles or ground rules to guide this process. For example, honest and transparent communications are vital for the team to make accurate assessments of the partnership readiness and growth opportunities to leverage the partnership for future success.[16]

at local, regional, and national levels.[18] The manual explains how to use a systematic, strategic analysis of program activities (actions that use available resources), outputs (direct products of activities), and impacts (benefits or changes resulting from activities and outputs) to identify meaningful metrics that can be used to document program achievements. For example, under "Output 3: Translation of scientific findings among partners," several potential metrics are listed in the manual (Box 16.2).

Szilagyi et al.[19] proposed a framework for evaluating the community engagement activities of academic medical centers. The framework includes broad goals and specific activities within each goal; goals and activities are evaluated using a health services research framework consisting of structure, process, and outcomes. In the framework, "structure represents the administrative arrangements and committees that are developed, the new organizations established to enhance community engagement goals, any new facilities or space, and financial as well as non-financial arrangements regarding community engagement."[19] Szilagyi et al.[19] recommended both qualitative and quantitative process assessments of activities (for example, What services were delivered? Were they appropriate and necessary? Were they delivered with fidelity and rigor, and in a timely, patient-centered, and culturally sensitive manner?).[19] The framework is likely to be helpful for evaluating the effectiveness and return on investment of academic medical center community engagement activities.

Box 16.2 **Example Metrics for Output 3: Translation of Scientific Findings Among Partners,** *Partnerships for Environmental Public Health Evaluation Metrics Manual*

- Number and description of materials that translate findings.
- Lists of coauthorship on materials that demonstrate a mix of partners.
- Description of subsequent funding for translation efforts.
- Description of support provided by target audience for translation efforts.
- Number of publications that report on translation activities.
- Description and counts of how partners are using findings in other settings.
- Number of requests for translated information by partners.
- Description of requests for materials by others.
- Anecdotal evidence indicating successful translation of scientific findings to new audiences.
- Number and description of materials or products produced by partners that include research finding.[18]

To lay the groundwork for evaluating community–academic contributions to research conducted by CTSAs, Eder et al.[12] proposed a typology consisting of three relationship types: engagement, collaboration, and shared leadership. The authors defined engagement as "an intention to exchange information and possibly resources (including money) through an individual event or a short-term series of events (including clinical trials)."[12] They defined collaboration as "an intention for members of a partnership to cooperate over time for the purpose of achieving specified goals," which may or may not be shared.[12] In addition, they defined shared leadership as "an intention for the partnership to achieve shared goals."[12] Rather than focusing on specific community–academic activities, the typology encourages CTSAs to measure the strength of relationships using synergy and trust as core metrics.[12]

Models that have been proposed for evaluating translational research,[5,20–23] may also be useful for evaluating community-engaged research. After considering prominent models of translational research and identifying their commonalities, Trochim et al.[23] proposed a process marker model for evaluating translational research. The model identifies key operational and measureable markers along a generalized process pathway from research to practice.[23] According to the model, translational research is a continuous process that moves from basic biomedical research through clinical and practice-based research, and ultimately to health policies, outcomes, and impacts.[23] The model assumes that this process may be bidirectional, variable, and complex and that there are many potential markers along this process.[23] The process marker model proposed by Trochim et al.,[23] which is grounded in process modeling research,[19,24] provides a useful framework for evaluating interventions aimed at improving translational research (for example, interventions designed to reduce the relatively long time from discovery to routine use and health impact).

CTSA Pilot Study Grant Programs

An increasing number of CTSAs have offered funding for pilot studies through small grant programs. For example, the Colorado Clinical and Translational Sciences Institute (CCTSI) initiated a Community Engagement Pilot Grants program that accepts proposals from either community or academic applicants. The program requires that at least half of requested grant funds go to a community partner.[25] One funding track (up to $10,000) is for developing new community–academic partnerships and the other (up to $30,000) is to strengthen existing partnerships through community translational research projects.[25] The initial investment of $272,742 led to over $2.8 million dollars in additional grant funding, and strengthened the capacity of community–academic partnerships and the rigor and relevance of their research.[25] The Harvard CTSA provided seed funding to community partners through a CBPR initiative.[26] The purpose of the initiative was to stimulate community–academic relationships necessary for improved translational research.[26] The goals were to (1) engage communities and empower them to select a research problem for study; (2) facilitate community understanding of the value of evidence and how to incorporate it into programs; and (3) facilitate partnership with an academic researcher or gather preliminary evidence.[26] The CAB for the Harvard CTSA Community Engagement program provided guidance for the funding program. The initiative facilitated relevant and innovative research. Some of the challenges that were encountered included variable community research readiness, insufficient project time, and difficulties identifying investigators for new partnerships.[26] Thompson et al. used a community grants program to directly fund community-based organizations to plan, implement, and evaluate pilot studies.[27] A request for applications (RFA) was developed and circulated widely throughout the Yakima Valley, in Washington State. The RFA sought proposals to address health disparities in cancer education, prevention, and treatment among Hispanics living in the Valley.[27] Funds available were $2,500.00–$3,500.00 for a 1-year project. To help evaluate the progress of the RFA community projects according to the perspectives of the CAB, an open-ended, semistructured interview was developed and administered by a former staff member to CAB members. In 4 years, 10 small grants proposed by community members were funded. The total funds allocated were about $25,000.[27] Interviews with CAB members indicated that the RFA program was perceived positively, but there were concerns about sustainability. The community grants program resulted in the implementation of several cancer prevention programs conducted by community organizations.[27] Rodgers et al.[28] proposed a model for building collaborative research capacity that focuses on the distribution of RFAs for pilot studies, awarding grants to community-based organizations of $15,000, and matching community-based organizations to university faculty. The model was developed by the Community Engagement Research Program of the Atlanta Clinical and Translational Science Institute (ACTSI), which is part of NIH's CTSA program.[28] The RFA resulted in 29 applications, and four community-based organizations in Atlanta and southwest Georgia were selected for funding. Technical assistance and training were provided to community-based organization staff on community assessment, program planning, evaluation, and grant writing.[28]

CTSA Training Programs in Community-Based Participatory Research

In addition to the training offered to community-based organization staff in Atlanta and southwest Georgia on community assessment, program planning, evaluation, and grant writing as part of the ACTSI model for building collaborative research capacity,[28] several additional training programs have been offered in the United States to enhance community–academic research. For example, the Center for Clinical and Translational Science and Training (CCTST) at the Cincinnati Children's Hospital Medical Center and University of Cincinnati College of Medicine in Ohio holds a 6-week leadership development training program designed to enhance academic–community research, integrate the interests of community leaders and academic health center researchers, and build research capacity and competencies within the community.[29] The curriculum was based on literature reviews, input from the Community Partner Council, and recommendations from academic health center members and those experienced with CBPR.[29] Participants attend nine, 3-hour interactive sessions designed to build skills and confidence and address challenges. Each session consists of didactic instruction, exercises, group discussion, skills development, and networking. An evaluation of outcome data for the first 2 years of the training program indicated that the Community Leaders Institute is achieving its goals of engaging faculty as trainer-scholars and promoting academic–community partnerships that are consistent with community and academic health center priorities.[29] Community Leaders Institute graduates are serving on academic health center committees (e.g., steering, research ethics).[29]

The South Carolina Clinical and Translational Research Institute holds the Community Engaged Scholars Program.[30] The program offers simultaneous training to CBPR teams, with each team consisting of at least one community partner and one academic partner.[30] The program includes 12 interactive group sessions, mentorship, and apprenticeship opportunities over 12 months.[30] After completing the Community Engaged Scholars Program, participants are expected to meet the competencies shown in Box 16.3. Among the challenges encountered are group instructions with varying levels of readiness among the CBPR partners, navigating the institutional review board process with community coinvestigators, and

---

Box 16.3 **Expected Competencies of Participants in the Community Engaged Scholars Program, South Carolina Clinical and Translational Research Institute**

- Understand the concepts and components of CBPR.
- Assess and leverage domains and key indicators of CBPR readiness for the partnership and potential research project.
- Integrate CBPR principles in grant proposals and research implementation.
- Communicate with audiences in both academic and community settings about CBPR principles and components.
- Implement a pilot CBPR initiative, and
- Build foundations for sustainability of the partnership and CBPR products.[30]

identifying appropriate academic investigators to match community research interests.[30]

   The University of New Mexico Health Sciences (NMHS) Center for Participatory Research holds a Summer Institute, Community Based Participatory Research Institute for Health: Indigenous and Critical Methodologies.[31] The annual summer institute is intended for graduate students, postdoctoral fellows, faculty, community partners, academic–community teams, and others. The institute explores how CBPR intersects with indigenous and critical methodologies, including the challenges for academic researchers and community members to discover knowledge for improved community health.[31]

Discussion

Speaking broadly, translational research has referred to the application of research findings, from basic science to practice-based and community research, to improve public health.[32] Several authors have proposed more specific definitions to distinguish between the various phases of translation.[5,20–22] The goal of community engagement is to involve those traditionally left out of the research process.[32] Although community engagement in research has a long history, the CTSA program has greatly increased its profile in biomedical research.[9]

   Recent studies have identified barriers to community-engaged translational research as well as substantial opportunities for further successes and innovations in academic-community partnerships. One potential barrier to community-engaged translational research is a lack of positive relationships between academic medical centers and potential community partners, which may stem from historical or more recent events (e.g., research viewed as harmful or insensitive to a community).[9] Yarborough et al.[33] noted that good relationships between research institutions and communities are an essential (but sometimes neglected) part of translational research. To build positive relationships, they recommended recruiting community advisors to each research team, which is consistent with the practice of forming CABs. Yarborough et al.[33] also called for a more equitable sharing of the economic benefits of research. To better understand how clinical and translational research is defined and perceived by community service providers, Martinez et al.[32] conducted focus groups in three neighborhoods in Tufts University's catchment area. Participants were asked about their experience with and perceptions of clinical and translational research. Exploitation and a lack of mutual respect emerged as key themes.[32] Participants reported that at times, community members have felt like "guinea pigs" in research or felt talked down to by researchers. Participants were interested in a long-term investment, and relationships with academic researchers that took into account mutual interest and had direct benefit to their community.[32] Effective communication in collaborative efforts was seen as key. The findings indicated that mistrust and cultural disconnects exist between research and community partners, which are potential barriers to community research partnerships.[32]

This chapter has identified several advances and innovations in CTSA community-engagement programs including new frameworks and models for community engagement; toolkits and new approaches for evaluating academic–community partnerships; CTSA pilot study grant programs; and CTSA training programs in CBPR. To facilitate academic–community partnerships, innovative community-engagement consulting services and a community-engagement "studio" have also been implemented.[34,35] Potential future directions include developing best practices for engaging the community in the dissemination, implementation, and improvement of health research,[36] and an increased emphasis on community engagement in research on health disparities through translational, transformational, and transdisciplinary approaches.[37] As noted by Dankwa-Mullan et al.,[37] "History teaches us that pioneering research achievements have been the result of a systemized integrative effort." In addition to increased efficiency and impact of biomedical research, the promise of the CTSA program is paradigm-shifting community-engaged, translational research aimed at improving health and alleviating suffering in diverse communities.

References

1. National Institute of Environmental Health Sciences. "Community-Based Participatory Research." <www.niehs.nih.gov/translat/cbpr/cbpr.htm>
2. National Center on Advancing Translational Science. "2014 Report." <https://ncats.nih.gov/files/NCATS_2014_report.pdf>
3. National Center for Advancing Translational Sciences. "Communities & Research." <http://ncats.nih.gov/ctsa/community>
4. Institute of Medicine. *The CTSA Program at NIH: Opportunities for Advancing Clinical and Translational Research.* Washington, DC: National Academy Press, 2013.
5. Sung, N.S., Crowley, W.F.J., Genel, M., et al. "Central Challenges Facing the National Clinical Research Enterprise." *Journal of the American Medical Association* 289 (2003): 1278–87.
6. Clinical and Translational Science Awards. "Integration Across the Lifespan Domain Task Force." <https://ctsacentral.org/consortium/education-and-training/>
7. Clinical and Translational Science Awards. "Core Competencies for Clinical and Translational Research." <https://ctsacentral.org/consortium/best-practices/335-2/>
8. Holzer, J. and Kass, N. "Community Engagement Strategies in the Original and Renewal Applications for CTSA Grant Funding." *Clinical Translation Science* 7 (2014): 38–43.
9. Holzer, J. and Kass, N. "Understanding the Supports of and Challenges to Community Engagement in the CTSAs." *Clinical Translation Science* 8 (2015): 116–22.
10. Wilkins, C.H., Spofford, M., Williams, N., et al. "Community Representatives Involvement in Clinical and Translational Science Awardee Activities." *Clinical Translational Science* 6 (2013): 292–6.
11. Clinical and Translational Science Awards Consortium Community Engagement Key Function Committee Task Force on the Principles of Community Engagement. *Principles of Community Engagement* (2nd ed.). NIH Publication No. 11-7782. Printed June 2011. <http://www.stsdr.cdc.gov/communityengagement/pdf/PCE_Report_508_FINAL.pdf>

12. Eder, M.M., Carter-Edwards, L., Hurd, T.C., Rumala, B.B. and Wallerstein, N. "A Logic Model for Community Engagement Within the CTSA Consortium: Can We Measure What We Model?" *Academic Medicine* 88 (2013): 1430–6.

13. Newman, S., Andrews, J., Magwood, G., Jenkins, C., Cox, M. and Williamson, D. "Community Advisory Boards in Community-Based Participatory Research: A Synthesis of Best Practices." *Preventing Chronic Disease* 8 (2001). <http://www.cdc.gov/pcd/issues/2011/may/10_0045.htm>

14. Concannon, T.W., Meissner, P., Grunbaum, J.A., et al. "A New Taxonomy for Stakeholder Engagement in Patient-Centered Outcomes Research." *Journal of General Internal Medicine* 27 (2012): 985–91.

15. Jenkins, C., Arulogun, O.S., Singh, A. et al. "Stroke Investigative Research and Education Network: Community Engagement and Outreach Within Phenomics Core." *Health Education and Behavior* 43 Suppl 1 (2016): 82S–92S.

16. Andres, J.O., Neman, S.D., Cox, J.M. and Meadows, O. *Are We Ready? Toolkit for Academic-Community Partnerships for Community-Based Participatory Research.* Charleston: South Carolina Clinical & Translational Research Institute, Medical University of South Carolina. <http://academicdepartments.musc.edu/sctr/programs/community_engagement/Documents/SCTR%20CCHP%20Are%20We%20Ready%20Toolkit.pdf>

17. Andrews, J.O., Cox, M.J., Newman, S.D. and Meadows, O. "Development and Evaluation of a Toolkit to Assess Partnership Readiness for Community-Based Participatory Research." *Progress in Community Health Partnerships* 5 (2011): 183–8.

18. National Institute of Environmental Health Sciences. *Partnerships for Environmental Public Health Evaluation Metrics Manual.* NIH Publication No. 12-7825. 2012. <http://www.niehs.nih.gov/research/supported/assets/docs/a_c/complete_peph_evaluation_metrics_manual_508.pdf>

19. Szilagyi, P.G., Shone, L.P., Dozier, A.M., Newton, G.L., Green, T. and Bennett, N.M. "Evaluating Community Engagement in an Academic Medical Center." *Academic Medicine* 89 (2014): 585–95.

20. Westfall, J.M., Mold, J. and Fagnan, L. "Practice-Based Research—'Blue Highways' on the NIH Roadmap." *Journal of the American Medical Association* 297 (2007): 403–6.

21. Dougherty, D. and Conway, P.H. "The 3T's Road Map to Transform US Health Care." *Journal of the American Medical Association* 299 (2008): 231921.

22. Khoury, M.J., Gwinn, M., Yoon, P.W., Dowling, N., Moore, C.A. and Bradley, L. "The Continuum of Translation Research in Genomic Medicine: How Can We Accelerate the Appropriate Integration of Human Genome Discoveries into Health Care and Disease Prevention? *Genetics in Medicine* 9 (2007): 665–74.

23. Trochim, W., Kane, C., Graham, M. and Pincus, H.A. "Evaluating Translational Research: A Process Marker Model." *Clinical and Translational Science* 4 (2011): 153–62.

24. Dilts, D.M., Sandler, A.B., Cheng, S.K., et al. "Steps and Time to Process Clinical Trials at the Cancer Therapy Evaluation Program." *Journal of Clinical Oncology* 27 (2009): 1761–6.

25. Main, D.S., Felzien, M.C., Magid, D.J., et al. "A Community Translational Research Pilot Grants Program to Facilitate Community-Academic Partnerships: Lessons from Colorado's Clinical Translational Science Awards." *Progress in Community Health Partnerships* 6 (2012): 381–7.

26. Tendulkar, S.A., Chu, J., Opp, J., et al. "A Funding Initiative for Community-Based Participatory Research: Lessons from the Harvard Catalyst Seed Grants." *Progress in Community Health Partnerships* 5 (2011): 35–44.

27. Thompson, B., Ondelacy, S., Godina, R. and Coronado, G.D. "A Small Grants Program to Involve Communities in Research." *Journal of Community Health* 25 (2010): 294–301.

28. Rodgers, K.C., Akintobi, T., Thompson, W.W., Evans, D., Escoffery, C. and Kegler, M.C. "A Model for Strengthening Collaborative Research Capacity: Illustrations from the Atlanta Clinical Translational Science Institute." *Health Education and Behavior* 41 (2014): 267–74.

29. Crosby, L.E., Par, W., Smith, T. and Mitchell, M.J. "The Community Leaders Institute: An Innovative Program to Train Community Leaders in Health Research." *Academic Medicine* 88 (2013): 335–42.

30. Andrews, J.O., Cox, M.J., Newman, S.D., et al. "Training Partnership Dyads for Community-Based Participatory Research: Strategies and Lessons Learned from the Community Engaged Scholars Program." *Health Promotion Practice* 14 (2013): 524–33.

31. University of New Mexico Center for Participatory Research. "Summer Institute: Community Based Participatory Research Institute for Health: Indigenous and Critical Methodologies." <http://cpr.unm.edu/curricula-classes/index.html>

32. Martinez, L.S., Russell, B., Rubin, C.L., Leslie, L.K. and Brugge, D. "Clinical and Translational Research and Community Engagement: Implications for Researcher Capacity Building." *Clinical Translation Science* 5 (2012): 329–32.

33. Yarborough, M., Edwards, K., Espinoza, P., et al. "Relationships Hold the Key to Trustworthy and Productive Translational Science: Recommendations for Expanding Community Engagement in Biomedical Research." *Clinical Translational Science* 6 (2013): 310–3.

34. Carter-Edwards, L., Cook, J.L., McDonald, M.A., Weaver, S.M., Chukwuka, K. and Eder, M. "Report on CTSA Consortium Use of the Community Engagement Consulting Service." *Clinical Translation Science* 6 (2013): 34–39.

35. Joosten, Y.A., Israel, T.L., Williams, N.A., et al. "Community Engagement Studios: A Structured Approach to Obtaining Meaningful Input from Stakeholders to Inform Research." *Academic Medicine* 90 (2015): 1646–50.

36. Bodison, S.C., Sankare, I., Anaya, H., et al., and the Community Engagement Workgroup. "Engaging the Community in the Dissemination, Implementation, and Improvement of Health-Related Research." *Clinical Translation Science* 8 (2015): 814–9.

37. Dankwa-Mullan, I., Rhee, K.B., Stoff, D.M., et al. "Moving Toward Paradigm-Shifting Research in Health Disparities Through Translational, Transformational, and Transdisciplinary Approaches." *American Journal of Public Health* 100 Suppl 1 (2010): S19–24.

17

Summary and Conclusions

STEVEN S. COUGHLIN, PHD

This concluding chapter provides a summary of recent trends and remaining issues and draws several major conclusions. Future directions in community-based participatory research (CBPR) are also discussed. Trends evident from the chapters in this book include the extension of CBPR into new communities and population subgroups, continued innovation and creativity in CBPR, the incorporation of CBPR approaches into dissemination and implementation research, and the adaptation of accepted principles of CBPR principles to specific cultural groups and into language that is understandable to a wide range of people. Evaluative research is needed to examine the relative costs, benefits, and effectiveness of CBPR and other types of public health research. There is a need for additional CBPR studies involving adolescents and elders who are in the oldest decades of life. When academic researchers and community partners work together, CBPR is an effective way to promote greater equity in healthcare access and alleviate health disparities in diverse communities across the life span. Continued efforts are needed to ensure that CBPR studies and evaluation projects are sustainable over time and that adequate resources are available. The incorporation of CBPR approaches into the translational sciences is a paradigm-shifting event that is likely to result in major advances in our understanding of the causes of and solutions to complex health challenges in diverse communities.

The chapters in this volume illustrate the many strengths and advantages of CBPR. Community-based participatory research explores the knowledge and perceptions of members of the local community, aligns the goals of research with community priorities, allows for the adaptation of existing resources in innovative ways, and brings together research partners who have varied skills, knowledge, and expertise to address complex health problems.[1-3] The collaborative nature of CBPR provides a forum that can bridge cultural differences among the academic and community partners and help to address the lack of trust that community members may have about academic researchers or institutions.[1,3]

Recent Trends in Community-Based Participatory Research

One trend evident from this book is the extension of CBPR into new communities and population subgroups. For example, although many early community-engaged studies of HIV/AIDS focused on gay and bisexual men in major urban centers such as Los Angeles, San Francisco, and New York, a growing number of CBPR studies have addressed HIV prevention and referral for treatment among African Americans and Hispanic men and women, and other important population subgroups.[4] As an additional example, CBPR and participatory action research on infant mortality have primarily been conducted in the United States and in Asian countries such as Nepal and India.[5-12] More recent studies are addressing infant mortality in countries in sub-Saharan Africa and other parts of the world.[13-15] As a further example, faith-based CBPR studies (which have sometimes been referred to as church-based studies) are no longer limited to those that engage members of church congregations; an increasing number of CBPR studies involve members of mosques, temples, and synagogues.[16-19]

Another trend has been continued innovation and creativity in CBPR. Creative approaches for engaging and empowering community members are hallmarks of CBPR.[20] As discussed in chapter 1, "photovoice" methods, a means of telling personal stories and community stories through photographs, have been used in CBPR as an approach for health needs assessment.[20-24] Community arts events have also been incorporated into CBPR projects.[25] For example, as part of a CBPR project involving African American youth in two urban neighborhoods, Yonas et al.[26] used the creative arts (writing, drawing, and painting activities) to obtain information about the participants' perspectives about community safety and violence. Recent studies have used CBPR approaches to develop smartphone applications for promoting pregnancy and interconception health among African American women at risk for adverse birth outcomes[27] and for enhancing dietary intake and physical activity among African American breast cancer survivors.[28]

As detailed by Oyana in chapter 4, Geographic Information System/Global Positioning System (GIS/GPS) technologies are being used to collect and analyze environmental (geospatial) datasets, which offer new scientific knowledge and insights into health problems. Robust and unbiased geospatial data and knowledge about communities is being used to deepen our understanding of public health problems, target interventions to reduce health disparities, and achieve health equity. Participatory GIS methods and analytical techniques are enhancing community-engaged health research. As discussed by Kim and Haynes in chapter 13, CBPR studies are being enhanced using novel technology for environmental and biological sampling. These new technologies are combining GPS with air monitoring and health outcome data. Community residents are being equipped with new tools to engage with researchers and collect their own data (i.e., citizen's science).

Another trend has been the incorporation of CBPR approaches into dissemination and implementation research as discussed by Coughlin and Yoo in chapter 2 and by Smith et al. in chapter 11. This is an important development as the dissemination, implementation, and adaptation of well-packaged CBPR interventions into new communities greatly extend their reach and potential benefits. Dissemination refers to the active promotion or support of a health program to encourage its widespread adoption.[29] This includes the adaptation, evaluation, implementation, and maintenance of an intervention that has been shown to be effective. The dissemination and translation of CBPR findings to address public health problems helps to ensure that the research has pragmatic results that lead to the greatest possible benefits. In addition to dissemination and implementation research, CBPR approaches have been integrated into informatics health research[30] and the clinical and translational sciences.[31]

A further trend has been the adaptation of accepted principles of CBPR principles[32,33] to specific cultural groups and into language that is understandable to a wide range of people. For example, as part of a community-engaged study of intimate partner violence, Burke et al.[34] conducted a workshop in which 18 participants were introduced to CBPR and accepted principles of CBPR were discussed.[32,33] The participants were critical of the language used to illustrate the principles and felt strongly that CBPR principles should be revised using more common words so that there would be less ambiguity about how the research would proceed. Smith et al.[35] noted that several sets of principles have been developed to guide the conduct of CBPR. They tend to be written in language that is most appropriate for academics and other research professionals and may not help lay people from the community understand CBPR. As part of a large-scale dissemination and implementation research (the Educational Program to Increase Colorectal Cancer Screening Study), Smith et al.[35] engaged community members of the National Black Leadership Initiative on Cancer in developing culturally specific principles for conducting academic–community collaborative research. A set of CBPR principles was developed that was intended to resonate with African American community members.[35]

Future Directions

Evaluative research is needed to examine the relative costs, benefits, and effectiveness of CBPR and other types of public health research. For example, relative to nonparticipatory research studies that do not involve partnerships with community residents or organizations, to what extent are findings from CBPR studies more likely to be disseminated to diverse audiences and to be translated into useful outcomes such as improvements in policy?[36] The evaluation of CBPR approaches to address public health concerns would be facilitated by enhancing ongoing systematic literature reviews such as the Guide to Community Preventive Services (www.thecommunityguide.org) so that community-engaged studies— and CBPR studies in particular—are distinguished from those that are not community engaged.

Another future direction is the need for additional CBPR studies involving adolescents and elders who are in the oldest decades of life. For a variety of health topics, the vast majority of published CBPR studies have involved adults or recently retired persons. However, studies indicate that CBPR approaches can successfully address the health concerns of teenagers[7,8,26,37–47] and people who are in the oldest decades of life.[48,49] Community-based participatory research is an effective approach for addressing disparities in both adolescent health and gerontology.

Future directions should include additional CPBR studies of adult-onset chronic illnesses such as diabetes, cardiovascular disease, and obesity involving communities in middle-income countries such as India, China, and Brazil, where the prevalence of overweight and obesity is rising rapidly.[50] In addition, CBPR projects that have been conducted to address malaria in low-income countries in sub-Saharan Africa should be translated to address other arthropod-borne diseases such as Chikungunya virus infection and Zika virus infection.[51,52]

Major Conclusions

When academic researchers and community partners work together, CBPR is an effective way to promote greater equity in healthcare access and alleviate health disparities. Community-based participatory research approaches are useful for addressing health disparities in communities that have been marginalized, oppressed, discriminated against, and stigmatized, or have otherwise experienced historical or contemporary injustices. Several chapters included in this volume highlight the important role of CBPR in addressing health disparities in diverse communities. As discussed by Coughlin et al. in chapter 1, pronounced health disparities exist in the United States and many other countries across population groups defined by race, ethnicity, sexual orientation, sexual identity, socioeconomic status, geographic locality, and other factors.[53] Many immigrant populations also experience health disparities, a topic dealt with by Vaughn and Jacquez in chapter 8. Racial minorities in the United States are more likely than their White counterparts to die from many common diseases including breast cancer, cardiovascular disease, diabetes, HIV/AIDS, and infant mortality.[53] Racial and ethnic minority populations are also more likely to be exposed to environmental toxicants, as discussed by Kim and Haynes in chapter 13. Despite the complexity and intractability of many public health problems (for example, interpersonal violence, substance abuse, and mental illness), evidence-based solutions do exist. Innovative CBPR studies, such as the one discussed by Akintobi et al. in chapter 9, are addressing multiple priority health concerns. The integrative approach employed by Akintobi et al. is examining mental and behavioral health practices in at-risk African American neighborhoods in Atlanta, Georgia, specifically as those practices relate to eating habits and access to nutritional foods; physical activity and environmental impact; and access to and use of primary care services for mental and behavioral health needs.

Continued efforts are needed to ensure that CBPR studies and evaluation projects are sustainable over time, and that adequate resources are available. To an increasing extent, major funding agencies such as the Centers for Disease Control, the National Institutes of Health (NIH), and the Patient-Centered Outcomes Research Institute require grant applicants to provide a plan for sustainability of the health intervention. Israel et al.[32] suggested that the endpoint of action research should be the establishment of sustainability mechanisms for the project such as searching for additional sources of funding and training community partners on how to secure additional funding. As noted by Kitzman-Ulrich and Holt in chapter 6, the sustainability of evidence-based health promotion in faith-based organizations depends on the extent to which it is institutionalized into the routine operations of the organizations.

Health needs assessments and pilot studies that are completed to lay the ground work for larger-scale CBPR studies of important public health problems often do not achieve their longer-term goals due to a lack of funding or other resources. Several factors can contribute to this problem, including the highly competitive nature of funding from agencies such as the National Institutes of Health, conflicting institutional priorities, turnover in academic researchers, and the challenges that many CBPR researchers have in obtaining tenure or promotion after devoting years to studies that require patience and substantial time spent engaging community partners.

Progress in science includes the gradual accumulation of knowledge within disciplines (e.g., the acquisition of evidence from community-engaged studies about effective interventions for promoting healthy behaviors in diverse populations) and nonlinear progress resulting from scientific breakthroughs or new scientific methods, resources, or strategies.[54] One example of this is the NIH Clinical and Translational Science Award program, which is increasing the efficiency and impact of biomedical research and furthering community-engaged, translational research aimed at improving health and well-being in communities.[31,55] The incorporation of CBPR approaches into the translational sciences is a paradigm-shifting event that is likely to result in major advances in our understanding of the causes of and solutions to complex health challenges in diverse communities.

References

1. Holkup, P.A., Tripp-Reimer, T., Salois, E.M. and Weinert, C. "Community-Based Participatory Research: An Approach to Intervention Research with a Native American Community." *ANS Advances in Nursing Science* 27 (2004): 162–75.

2. Stevens, P.E. and Hall, J.M. "Participatory Action Research for Sustaining Individual and Community Change: A Model of HIV Prevention Education." *AIDS Education and Prevention* 10 (1998): 387–402.

3. Israel, B.A., Shulz, A.J., Parker, E.A. and Becker, A.B. "Community-Based Participatory Research: Policy Recommendations for Promoting a Partnership Approach in Health Research." *Education for Health* 14 (2001): 182–97.

4. Coughlin, S.S. "Community-Based Participatory Research Studies on HIV/AIDS Prevention, 2005–2014." *Jacobs Journal of Community Medicine* 2 (2016): 19.

5. Chao, S.M., Donatoni, G., Bemis, C., et al. "Integrated Approaches to Improve Birth Outcomes: Perinatal Periods of Risk, Infant Mortality Review, and the Los Angeles Mommy and Baby Project." *Maternal and Child Health Journal* 14 (2010): 827–37.

6. Salihu, H.M., August, E.M., Alio, A.P., et al. "Community-Academic Partnerships to Reduce Black-White Disparities in Infant Mortality in Florida." *Progress in Community Health Partnerships* 5 (2011): 53–66.

7. Richards, J. and Mousseau, A. "Community-Based Participatory Research to Improve Preconception Health Among North Plains American Indian Adolescent Women." *American Indian Alaska and Native Mental Health Research* 19 (2012): 154–85.

8. Barlow, A., Mullany, B., Neault, N., et al. "Paraprofessional-Delivered Home-Visiting Intervention for American Indian Teen Mothers and Children: 3-Year Outcomes from a Randomized Controlled Trial." *American Journal of Psychiatry* 172 (2015): 154–62.

9. Manandhar, D.S., Osrin, D., Shrestha, B.P., et al. "Effect of a Participatory Intervention with Women's Groups on Birth Outcomes in Nepal: Cluster-Randomised Controlled Trial. *Lancet* 364 (2004): 970–9.

10. Azad, K., Barnett, S., Banerjee, B., et al. "Effect of Scaling Up Women's Groups on Birth Outcomes in Three Rural Districts in Bangladesh: A Cluster-Randomised Controlled Trial." *Lancet* 375 (2010): 1193–1202.

11. Tripathy, P., Nair, N., Barnett, S., et al. "Effect of a Participatory Intervention with Women's Groups on Birth Outcomes and Maternal Depression in Jharkhand and Orissa, India: A Cluster-Randomised Controlled Trial." *Lancet* 375 (2010): 1182–92.

12. More, N.S., Bapat, U., Das, S., et al. "Community Mobilization in Mumbai Slums to Improve Perinatal Care and Outcomes: A Cluster Randomized Controlled Trial." *PLoS Medicine* 9 (2012): e1001257.

13. Lewycka, S., Mwansambo, C., Rosato, M., et al. "Effect of Women's Groups and Volunteer Peer Counselling on Rates of Mortality, Morbidity, and Health Behaviours in Mothers and Children in Rural Malawi (MaiMwana): A Factorial, Cluster-Randomised Controlled Trial." *Lancet* 381 (2013): 1721–35.

14. Findley, S.E., Uwemedimo, O.T., Doctor, H.V., et al. "Early Results of an Integrated Maternal, Newborn, and Child Health Program, Northern Nigeria, 2009 to 2011." *BMC Public Health* 13 (2013): 1034 <http://www.biomedcentral.com/1471-2458/13/1034>

15. Colbourn, T., Nambiar, B., Bondo, A., et al. "Effects of Quality Improvement in Health Facilities and Community Mobilization Through Women's Groups on Maternal, Neonatal and Perinatal Mortality in Three Districts of Malawi: MaiKhanda, a Cluster Randomized Controlled Effectiveness Trial." *International Health* 5 (2013): 180–95.

16. McCabe, O.L., Marum, F., Mosley, A., et al. "Community Capacity-Building in Disaster Mental Health Resilience: A Pilot Study of an Academic/Faith Partnership Model." *International Journal of Emergency Mental Health* 14 (2012): 112–22.

17. Shirazi, M., Shirazi, A. and Bloom, J. "Developing a Culturally Competent Faith-Based Framework to Promote Breast Cancer Screening Among Afghan Immigrant Women." *Journal of Religion and Health* 54 (2015): 153–9.

18. Murray, K.E., Mohamed, A.S., Dawson, D.B., Syme, M., Abdi, S. and Barnack-Taviaris, J. "Somali Perspectives on Physical Activity: PhotoVoice to Address Barriers and Resources in San Diego." *Progress in Community Health Partnerships* 9 (2015): 83–90.

19. Killawi, A., Heisler, M., Hamid, H. and Padela, A.I. "Using CBPR for Health Research in American Muslim Mosque Communities." *Progress in Community Health Partnerships* 9 (2015): 65–74.

20. Wallerstein, N. and Duran, B. "The Conceptual, Historical, and Practice Roots of Community-Based Participatory Research and Related Participatory Traditions." In *Community-Based Participatory Research for Health*, ed. M. Minkler and N. Wallerstein. San Francisco, CA: Jossey-Bass, 2003; pp. 27–52.

21. Wang, C., Yuan, Y.L. and Feng, M.L. "Photovoice as a Tool for Participatory Evaluation: The Community's View of Process and Impact." *Journal of Contemporary Health* 4 (1996): 47–9.

22. Wang, C. and Pies, C. "Family, Maternal, and Child Health Through Photovoice." *Maternal and Child Health Journal* 8 (2004): 95–102.

23. Moffitt, P. and Vollman, A. "Photovoice: Picturing the Health of Aboriginal Women in a Remote Northern Community." *Canadian Journal of Nursing Research* 36 (2004): 189–201.

24. Castleden, H., Garvin, T. and Huu-ay-aht First Nation. "Modifying Photovoice for Community-Based Participatory Indigenous Research." *Social Sciences and Medicine* 66 (2008): 1393–405.

25. Chung, B., Jones, L., Jones, A., et al. "Using Community Arts Events to Enhance Collective Efficacy and Community Engagement to Address Depression in an African American Community." *American Journal of Public Health* 99 (2009): 237–44.

26. Yonas, M.A., Burke, J.G., Rak, K., Kelly, A.B.V. and Gielen, A.C. "A Picture's Worth a Thousand Words: Engaging Youth in CBPR Using the Creative Arts." *Progress in Community Health Partnerships* 3 (2009): 349–58.

27. Foster, J., Miller, L., Isbell, S., Shields, T., Worthy, N. and Dunlop, A.L. "mHealth to Promote Pregnancy and Interconception Health Among African-American Women at Risk for Adverse Birth Outcomes: A Pilot Study." *mHealth* 1 (2015). <http://dx.doi.org/10.3978/j.issn.2306-9740.2015.12.01>

28. Smith, S.A., Whitehead, M., Sheats, J.Q., Mastromonico, J., Yoo, W. and Coughlin, S.S. "A Community-Engaged Approach for Developing a Mobile Cancer Prevention App: The mCPA Study Protocol." *JMIR Research Protocols* 5 (2016): e34.

29. Glasgow, R.E., Marcus, A.C., Bull, S.S. and Wilson, K.M. "Disseminating Effective Cancer Screening Interventions." *Cancer* 101 Suppl 5 (2004): 1239–50.

30. Unertl, K.M., Schaefbauer, C.L., Campbell, T.R., et al. "Integrating Community-Based Participatory Research and Informatics Approaches to Improve the Engagement and Health of Underserved Populations." *Journal of the American Medical Informatics Association* 23 (2016): 60–73.

31. National Center for Advancing Translational Sciences. "Communities and Research." <http://ncats.nih.gov/ctsa/community>

32. Israel, B.A., Schultz, A.J., Parker, E.A., Becker, A.B., Allen, A.J., III, and Guzman, J.R. "Critical Issues in Developing and Following Community-Based Participatory Research Principles. In M. Minkler and N. Wallerstein, ed. *Community-Based Participatory Research for Health*. San Francisco: Jossey-Bass, 2003; pp. 53–76.

33. Viswanathan, M., Eng, E., Ammerman, A., et al. *Community-Based Participatory Research: Assessing the Evidence*. Evidence Report/Technology Assessment no. 99. Rockville, MD: Agency for Healthcare Research and Quality, 2004.

34. Burke, J.G., Hess, S., Hoffmann, K., et al. "Translating Community-Based Participatory Research (CBPR) Principles into Practice: Building a Research Agenda to Reduce Intimate Partner Violence." *Progress in Community Health Partnerships* 7 (2013): 115–22.

35. Smith, S.A., Whitehead, M.S., Sheats, J.Q., Ansa, B.E., Coughlin, S.S. and Blumenthal, D.S. "Community-Based Participatory Research Principles for the African American Community." *Journal of the Georgia Public Health Association* 5 (2015): 52–6.

36. Balazs, C.L. and Morello-Frosch, R. "The Three R's: How Community Based Participatory Research Strengthens the Rigor, Relevance and Reach of Science." *Environmental Justice* 6 (2013). doi:10.1089/env.2012.0017.

37. Kulbok, P.A., Meszaros, P.S., Bond, D.C., et al. "Youths as Partners in a Community Participatory Project for Substance Use Prevention." *Family and Community Health* 38 (2015): 3–11.

38. Bardwell, G., Morton, C., Chester, A., et al. "Feasibility of Adolescents to Conduct Community-Based Participatory Research on Obesity and Diabetes in Rural Appalachia." *Clinical and Translational Science* 2 (2009): 340–9.

39. Ferrera, M.J., Sacks, T.K., Perez, M., Nixon, J.P., Asis, D. and Coleman, W.L. "Empowering Immigrant Youth in Chicago: Utilizing CBPR to Document the Impact of a Youth Health Service Corps Program." *Family and Community Health* 38 (2015): 12–21.

40. Coughlin, S.S. and Smith, S.A. "Community-Based Participatory Research to Promote Healthy Diet and Nutrition and Prevent and Control Obesity Among African-Americans: A Literature Review." *Journal of Racial and Ethnic Health Disparities* 3 (2016): [Epub ahead of print].

41. Lightfoot, A.F., Taggart, T., Woods-Jaeger, B.A., Riggins, L., Jackson, M.R. and Eng, E. "Where Is the Faith? Using a CBPR Approach to Propose Adaptations to an Evidence-Based HIV Prevention Intervention for Adolescents in African American Faith Settings." *Journal of Religion and Health* 53 (2014): 1223–35.

42. Jacquez, F., Vaughn, L.M. and Wagner, E. "Youth as Partners, Participants or Passive Recipients: A Review of Children and Adolescents in Community-Based Participatory Research (CBPR)." *American Journal of Community Psychology* 51 (2013): 176–89.

43. Ford, T., Rasmus, S. and Allen, J. "Being Useful: Achieving Indigenous Youth Involvement in a Community-Based Participatory Research Project in Alaska." *International Journal of Circumpolar Health* 71 (2012): 1–7.

44. Brown, B.D., Harris, K.J., Harris, J.L., Parker, M., Ricci, C. and Noonan, C. "Translating the Diabetes Prevention Program for Northern Plains Indian Youth Through Community-Based Participatory Research Methods." *Diabetes Education* 36 (2010): 924–35.

45. Peterson, T.H., Dolan, T. and Hanft, S. "Partnering with Youth Organizers to Prevent Violence: An Analysis of Relationships, Power, and Change." *Progress in Community Health Partnerships* 4 (2010): 235–42.

46. Mathews, J.R., Mathews, T.L. and Mwaja, E. "Girls Take Charge: A Community-Based Participatory Research Program for Adolescent Girls." *Progress in Community Health Partnerships* 4 (2010): 17–24.

47. Coker-Appiah, D.S., Akers, A.Y., Banks, B., et al. "In Their Own Voices: Rural African American Youth Speak Out About Community-Based HIV Prevention Interventions." *Progress in Community Health Partnerships* 3 (2009): 301–12.

48. Dong, X. "Addressing Health and Well-Being of U.S. Chinese Older Adults Through Community-Based Participatory Research: Introduction to the PINE Study." *Journals of Gerontology Series A* 69 Suppl 2 (2014): S1–6.

49. Lucero, R., Sheehan, B., Yen, P., Velez, O., Nobile-Hernandez, D. and Tiase, V. "Identifying Consumer's Needs of Health Information Technology Through an Innovative Participatory Design Approach Among English- and Spanish-Speaking Urban Older Adults." *Applied Clinical Informatics* 5 (2014): 943–57.

50. Swinburn, B.A., Sacks, G., Hall, K.D., et al. "The Global Obesity Pandemic: Shaped by Global Drivers and Local Environments." *Lancet* 378 (2011): 804–14.

51. Opiyo, P., Mukabana, W.R., Kiche, I., Mathenge, E., Killeen, G.F. and Fillinger, U. "An Exploratory Study of Community Factors Relevant for Participatory Malaria Control on Rusinga Island, Western Kenya." *Malaria Journal* 6 (2007): 48.

52. Okeibunor, J.C., Orji, B.C., Brieger, W., et al. "Preventing Malaria in Pregnancy Through Community-Directed Interventions: Evidence from Akwa Ibom State, Nigeria." *Malaria Journal* 10 (2011): 227.

53. Adler, N.E. and Rehkopf, D.H. "U.S. Disparities in Health: Descriptions, Causes, and Mechanisms." *Annual Review of Public Health* 29 (2009): 235–52.

54. Hebert, J.R., Brandt, H.M., Armstead, C.A., Adams, S.A. and Steck S.E. "Interdisciplinary, Translational, and Community-Based Participatory Research: Finding a Common Language to Improve Cancer Research." *Cancer Epidemiology Biomarkers and Prevention* 18 (2009): 1213–7.

55. Institute of Medicine. *The CTSA Program at NIH: Opportunities for Advancing Clinical and Translational Research.* Washington, DC: National Academy Press, 2013.

Index

academia, advancement and promotion for
researchers in, 27–29
academic-community partnerships, 236, 236f. *See
also under* HIV
evaluating, 255, 258b, 259–60
reasons for failure of, 34
action research (AR), 235
Adderley-Kelly, B., 91
African American churches, 75–76
example of CBPR in, 95–96
African American groups, CBPR among, 91–92
reaching people where they are, 92–94
African Americans (and health disparities), 173
cancer and, 171, 171t, 172f, 173, 181, 186
cardiovascular disease (CVD) morbidity and
mortality rates, 134f, 134–35, 139, 141, 141t
AIDS. *See* HIV
Airhihenbuwa, C.O., 83
American Indians and Alaskan Natives (AIAN),
CBPR with, 100–102
advantages of using, 102–3
steps for conducting, 102
American Public Health Association (APHA), 136
AMIGAS: Ayundando a las Mujeres con
Informacion, Guia, y Amor para su Salud
(helping women with information,
guidance, and love for their health), 197t
analysis of variance (ANOVA), 15
Asian Americans
barriers to utilization of healthcare, 97–99
CBPR among, 96–97
barriers to research participation, 97–99
examples of successful, 99–100
health risks and behaviors, 97
asset mapping and tracking, 52
Atlanta, Georgia. *See* Morehouse School of
Medicine Prevention Research Center

Bangladeshi health promoters in New York, 119–20
Bartholomew Eldredge, L. Kay, 84–85
Behavioral Risk Factor Surveillance System
(BRFSS), 173

Bennet, J. M., 83
Blacks. *See* African Americans
Blumenthal, Daniel S., 62
breast cancer
disparities in the United States, 186
in diverse communities, role of CBPR in
addressing, 188–90, 200
prevention of
CBPR in action for, 188–90
primary, 186–87
the public health importance of, 185–86
breast cancer screening, 200–201
CBPR studies, and how CBPR influenced the
study activities, 190, 191–99t, 200–201
early detection through mammography, 187–88
Building a Safe House on Firm Ground, 242–48

cancer. *See also* breast cancer; cervical cancer;
colorectal cancer
racial/ethnic disparities, 171, 171t, 172f, 173,
181, 186
cardiovascular disease (CVD) and type II diabetes
mellitus (DMII), 131–33, 148–49. *See also*
Morehouse School of Medicine Prevention
Research Center
age-adjusted rates of, 141, 141t
correlates of, 133, 137
defined, 133
economic impacts, 133–34
framing the local context through CBPR, 138–42
intervention approaches for addressing, 138
limitations of existing community-clinical
linkages, 136
mental health and, 137
mortality rates for Blacks and Whites, 134f, 134–
35, 141, 141t
policy, systems, and environmental (PSE) change
approaches and, 136
racial/ethnic disparities, 134–35
risk factors for
behavioral, 135
structural, 135–36